Teen Health Series

Allergy Information For Teens, Second Edition

Health Tips About Allergic Reactions To Food, Pollen, Mold, And Other Substances

Including Facts About Diagnosing, Treating, And Preventing Allergic Responses And Complications

Edited by Karen Bellenir

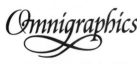

155 W. Congress, Suite 200
Detroit, MI 48226

Bibliographic Note

Because this page cannot legibly accommodate all the copyright notices, the Bibliographic Note portion of the Preface constitutes an extension of the copyright notice.

Edited by Karen Bellenir

Teen Health Series
Karen Bellenir, *Managing Editor*
David A. Cooke, M.D., *Medical Consultant*
Elizabeth Collins, *Research and Permissions Coordinator*
EdIndex, *Services for Publishers, Indexers*

* * *

Omnigraphics, Inc.
Matthew P. Barbour, *Senior Vice President*
Kevin M. Hayes, *Operations Manager*

* * *

Peter E. Ruffner, *Publisher*
Copyright © 2013 Omnigraphics, Inc.
ISBN 978-0-7808-1288-8
E-ISBN 978-0-7808-1289-5

Library of Congress Cataloging-in-Publication Data

Allergy information for teens : health tips about allergic reactions to food, pollen, mold, and other substances, including facts about diagnosing, treating, and preventing allergic responses and complications / edited by Karen Bellenir. -- Second edition.
    pages cm. -- (Teen health series)
  Audience: 9 to 12.
  Includes bibliographical references and index.
  Summary: "Provides basic consumer health information for teens about allergies, including facts about treating and preventing allergic reactions and complications, and tips for coping with allergies at home and school. Includes index and resource information"--Provided by publisher.
  ISBN 978-0-7808-1288-8 (hardcover : alk. paper) 1. Allergy. 2. Allergy in children. 3. Food allergy. 4. Insect allergy. I. Bellenir, Karen, editor.
  RC584.A45 2013
  618.9297'5--dc23

2012038514

Table of Contents

Preface

Part Three: Food Allergies And Intolerances

Part Four: Other Common Allergy Triggers

Part Five: Managing Allergies In Daily Life

Part Six: If You Need More Information

Preface

About This Book

According to the Centers for Disease Control and Prevention (CDC) four out of every 100 people under the age of 18 have a food allergy, and their numbers appear to be increasing. In the decade from 1997 to 2007, the prevalence of food allergy among people in this age group increased by 18%. Other types of allergies are also common. For example, one recent CDC survey found that 11.5% of respondents reported respiratory allergies and 12.6% reported skin allergies.

The consequences of allergic diseases vary considerably. For some people, the symptoms are merely a transient annoyance—occasional sniffles, sneezes, or mild itching. Others endure persistent, more severe symptoms that can disrupt education and relationships, hamper the adoption of healthy lifestyle choices, and hinder overall well-being. Chronic symptoms can lead to additional health concerns, such as the development of asthma. In some people with severe allergies, the consequences can even be deadly. The Asthma and Allergy Foundation of America reports that more than 500 people in the U.S. die every year as a result of serve allergic reactions to drugs, foods, insects, and latex.

Allergy Information For Teens, Second Edition provides updated information about a wide variety of allergic reactions, including common symptoms, diagnostic tools, and prevention strategies. It recounts what is currently known about the causes of allergies and the role the immune system plays in their development. It presents facts about rhinitis, sinusitis, dermatitis, urticaria (hives), anaphylaxis, and other types of symptoms produced by encounters with allergens. It also looks at the substances responsible for triggering these types of symptoms, including specific foods, animals, pollens, and chemicals. A special section on managing allergies in daily life outlines ways to avoid allergy triggers, handle medication at school, and cope with other challenges. The book concludes with resource directories for learning more about allergies and finding recipes to aid in the management of food allergies.

How To Use This Book

This book is divided into parts and chapters. Parts focus on broad areas of interest; chapters are devoted to single topics within a part.

Part One: Allergy Overview explains the biological processes that lead to the development of allergies and how allergy symptoms are detected and differentiated from symptoms due to other causes. It also provides facts about some of the most commonly used allergy treatments and the use of epinephrine injections for life-threatening allergic reactions.

Part Two: Allergy Symptoms And Complications provides details about the various ways allergic reactions can be identified and how they impact health. It discusses signs that may indicate breathing is being affected, and it explains how allergies can lead to the development of chronic respiratory illnesses. Other allergic symptoms, including those that affect the eyes and skin, are also discussed, and the part concludes with a chapter on anaphylaxis—a systemic allergic reaction that can result in death if not treated promptly.

Part Three: Food Allergies And Intolerances describes the differences between allergies and other adverse biological reactions to ingested substances. Individual chapters address the foods that are most commonly involved in allergic reactions, including nuts, grains, milk, eggs, and seafood. The most common intolerances and sensitivities—those to lactose, gluten, histamine, and sulfites—are also addressed.

Part Four: Other Common Allergy Triggers discusses some of the most frequently encountered substances in the indoor and outdoor environments that elicit allergic responses. These include allergies to pollens, pet dander, mold, and medications. Allergies to specific chemicals, including latex, nickle, and those that are frequently used in cosmetics, toiletries, clothing, and household products are also explained.

Part Five: Managing Allergies In Daily Life provides tips for people with allergies about minimizing the exacerbation of symptoms and maintaining an optimal quality of life. It discusses the rights of students to carry allergy-related medications in schools, offers suggestions for the safe use of cosmetics and skin care products, and provides additional suggestions for people with food allergies.

Part Six: If You Need More Information includes a directory of organizations able to provide further information about allergies and a list of online and print resources for allergen-free recipes.

Bibliographic Note

This volume contains documents and excerpts from publications issued by the following government agencies: Centers for Disease Control and Prevention (CDC); Environmental Protection Agency (EPA); National Cancer Institute; National Center for Complementary and Alternative Medicine; National Heart, Lung, and Blood Institute; National Institute of Allergy and Infectious Diseases; National Institute of Arthritis and Musculoskeletal and Skin Diseases; National Institute of Diabetes and Digestive and Kidney Diseases; National Institute of Environmental Health Sciences; National Library of Medicine; and the U.S. Food and Drug Administration (FDA).

In addition, this volume contains copyrighted documents and articles produced by the following individuals and organizations: A.D.A.M., Inc.; About.com; Allergy and Asthma Network Mothers of Asthmatics (AANMA); Allergy/Asthma Information Association; American Association for Clinical Chemistry; American College of Allergy, Asthma, and Immunology; American Rhinologic Society; American Society of Health-System Pharmacists; Asthma and Allergy Foundation of America; Asthma and Allergy Foundation of America, New England Chapter; Australasian Society of Clinical Immunology and Allergy; Food Allergy Initiative; Victoria Groce; Kids with Food Allergies; Daniel More; National Eczema Association; National Jewish Health; Nemours Foundation; New Zealand Dermatological Society; Regents of the University of California (Food and Drug Allergy Care Center at UCLA); Regents of the University of Michigan (Kellogg Eye Center); Frank J. Twarog; University of Florida (Institute of Food and Agriculture Sciences Extension); and Vickerstaff Health Services, Inc.

The photograph on the front cover is © LSO Photo/iStockphoto.

Full citation information is provided on the first page of each chapter. Every effort has been made to secure all necessary rights to reprint the copyrighted material. If any omissions have been made, please contact Omnigraphics to make corrections for future editions.

Acknowledgements

In addition to the organizations listed above, special thanks are due to Liz Collins, research and permissions coordinator; Zachary Klimecki, editorial assistant, Lisa Bakewell, verification assistant; and WhimsyInk, prepress services provider.

About The *Teen Health Series*

At the request of librarians serving today's young adults, the *Teen Health Series* was developed as a specially focused set of volumes within Omnigraphics' *Health Reference Series*. Each volume deals comprehensively with a topic selected according to the needs and interests of people in middle school and high school.

Teens seeking preventive guidance, information about disease warning signs, medical statistics, and risk factors for health problems will find answers to their questions in the *Teen Health Series*. The *Series*, however, is not intended to serve as a tool for diagnosing illness, in prescribing treatments, or as a substitute for the physician/patient relationship. All people concerned about medical symptoms or the possibility of disease are encouraged to seek professional care from an appropriate health care provider.

If there is a topic you would like to see addressed in a future volume of the *Teen Health Series*, please write to:

Editor
Teen Health Series
Omnigraphics, Inc.
155 W. Congress, Suite 200
Detroit, MI 48226

A Note About Spelling And Style

Teen Health Series editors use *Stedman's Medical Dictionary* as an authority for questions related to the spelling of medical terms and the *Chicago Manual of Style* for questions related to grammatical structures, punctuation, and other editorial concerns. Consistent adherence is not always possible, however, because the individual volumes within the *Series* include many documents from a wide variety of different producers and copyright holders, and the editor's primary goal is to present material from each source as accurately as is possible following the terms specified by each document's producer. This sometimes means that information in different chapters or sections may follow other guidelines and alternate spelling authorities. For example, occasionally a copyright holder may require that eponymous terms be shown in possessive forms (Crohn's disease *vs.* Crohn disease) or that British spelling norms be retained (leukaemia *vs.* leukemia).

Locating Information Within The *Teen Health Series*

The *Teen Health Series* contains a wealth of information about a wide variety of medical topics. As the *Series* continues to grow in size and scope, locating the precise information needed by a specific student may become more challenging. To address this concern, information about books within the *Teen Health Series* is included in *A Contents Guide to the Health Reference Series*. The *Contents Guide* presents an extensive list of more than 16,000 diseases, treatments, and other topics of general interest compiled from the Tables of Contents and major index headings from the books of the *Teen Health Series* and *Health Reference Series*. To access *A Contents Guide to the Health Reference Series*, visit www.healthreferenceseries.com.

Our Advisory Board

We would like to thank the following advisory board members for providing guidance to the development of this *Series*:

Dr. Lynda Baker, Associate Professor of Library and Information Science, Wayne State University, Detroit, MI

Nancy Bulgarelli, William Beaumont Hospital Library, Royal Oak, MI

Karen Imarisio, Bloomfield Township Public Library, Bloomfield Township, MI

Karen Morgan, Mardigian Library, University of Michigan-Dearborn, Dearborn, MI

Rosemary Orlando, St. Clair Shores Public Library, St. Clair Shores, MI

Medical Consultant

Medical consultation services are provided to the *Teen Health Series* editors by David A. Cooke, M.D. Dr. Cooke is a graduate of Brandeis University, and he received his M.D. degree from the University of Michigan. He completed residency training at the University of Wisconsin Hospital and Clinics. He is board-certified in internal medicine. Dr. Cooke currently works as part of the University of Michigan Health System and practices in Ann Arbor, MI. In his free time, he enjoys writing, science fiction, and spending time with his family.

Part One
Allergy Overview

Chapter 1

Allergies: The Basic Facts

Your eyes itch, your nose is running, you're sneezing, and you're covered in hives. It's allergy season again, and all you want to do is curl up into a ball of misery.

There has to be something you can do to feel better. After all, doctors seem to have a cure for everything, right? Not for allergies. But there are ways to relieve allergy symptoms or avoid getting the symptoms, even though you can't actually get rid of the allergies themselves.

What Are Allergies?

Allergies are abnormal immune system reactions to things that are typically harmless to most people. When you're allergic to something, your immune system mistakenly believes that this substance is harmful to your body. (Substances that cause allergic reactions, such as certain foods, dust, plant pollen, or medicines, are known as allergens.)

In an attempt to protect the body, the immune system produces IgE antibodies to that allergen. Those antibodies then cause certain cells in the body to release chemicals into the bloodstream, one of which is histamine (pronounced: his-tuh-meen).

The histamine then acts on the eyes, nose, throat, lungs, skin, or gastrointestinal tract and causes the symptoms of the allergic reaction. Future exposure to that same allergen will trigger this antibody response again. This means that every time you come into contact with that allergen, you'll have an allergic reaction.

About This Chapter: "Allergies," July 2009, reprinted with permission from www.kidshealth.org. This information was provided by KidsHealth®, one of the largest resources online for medically reviewed health information written for parents, kids, and teens. For more articles like this, visit www.KidsHealth.org, or www.TeensHealth .org. Copyright © 1995-2012 The Nemours Foundation. All rights reserved.

> ### How Fast Is A Sneeze?
>
> If your sneeze were a car, it would get a ticket for speeding. When you sneeze, particles fly out of your nose at 100 mph. A sneeze is the body's way of getting rid of something that's irritating the nose. Your nose feels a tickle and the sneeze center in your brain responds by coordinating muscles in your belly, chest, and diaphragm to sneeze out the irritant.

Allergic reactions can be mild, like a runny nose, or they can be severe, like difficulty breathing. An asthma attack, for example, is often an allergic reaction to something that is breathed into the lungs by a person who is susceptible.

Some types of allergies produce multiple symptoms, and in rare cases, an allergic reaction can become very severe—this severe reaction is called anaphylaxis (pronounced: an-uh-fuh-lak-sis). Signs of anaphylaxis include difficulty breathing, difficulty swallowing, swelling of the lips, tongue, and throat or other parts of the body, and dizziness or loss of consciousness.

Anaphylaxis usually occurs minutes after exposure to a triggering substance, such as a peanut, but some reactions might be delayed by as long as four hours. Luckily, anaphylactic reactions don't occur often and can be treated successfully if proper medical procedures are followed.

Why Do People Get Allergies?

The tendency to develop allergies is often hereditary, which means it can be passed down through your genes. (Thanks a lot, Mom and Dad.) However, just because a parent or sibling has allergies doesn't mean you will definitely get them, too. A person usually doesn't inherit a particular allergy, just the likelihood of having allergies.

What Things Are People Are Allergic To?

Some of the most common allergens are:

- **Foods:** Food allergies are most common in infants and often go away as people get older. Although some food allergies can be serious, many simply cause annoying symptoms like an itchy rash, a stuffy nose, and diarrhea. The foods that people are most commonly allergic to are milk and other dairy products, eggs, wheat, soy, peanuts and tree nuts, and seafood.

- **Insect Bites And Stings:** The venom (poison) in insect bites and stings can cause allergic reactions, and can be severe and even cause an anaphylactic reaction in some people.

- **Airborne Particles:** Often called environmental allergens, these are the most common allergens. Examples of airborne particles that can cause allergies are dust mites (tiny bugs that live in house dust); mold spores; animal dander (flakes of scaly, dried skin, and dried saliva from your pets); and pollen from grass, ragweed, and trees.

- **Medicines:** Antibiotics—medications used to treat infections—are the most common type of medicines that cause allergic reactions. Many other medicines, including over-the-counter medications (those you can buy without a prescription), also can cause allergic-type reactions.

- **Chemicals:** Some cosmetics or laundry detergents can make people break out in an itchy rash (hives). Usually, this is because someone has a reaction to the chemicals in these products. Dyes, household cleaners, and pesticides used on lawns or plants also can cause allergic reactions in some people.

How Do Doctors Diagnose And Treat Allergies?

If your family doctor suspects you might have an allergy, he or she might refer you to an allergist (a doctor who specializes in allergy treatment) for further testing. The allergist will ask you about your own allergy symptoms (such as how often they occur and when) and about whether any family members have allergies. The allergist also will perform tests to confirm an allergy—these will depend on the type of allergy someone has and may include a skin test or blood test.

The most complete way to avoid allergic reactions is to stay away from the substances that cause them (called avoidance). Doctors can also treat some allergies using medications and allergy shots.

Avoidance

In some cases, like food allergies, avoiding the allergen is a life-saving necessity. That's because, unlike allergies to airborne particles that can be treated with shots or medications, the only way to treat food allergies is to avoid the allergen entirely. For example, people who are allergic to peanuts should avoid not only peanuts, but also any food that might contain even tiny traces of them.

What's A Pollen Count?

Pollen counts measure how much pollen is in the air and can help people with allergies determine how bad their symptoms might be on any given day. Pollen counts are usually higher in the morning and on warm, dry, breezy days and lowest when it's chilly and wet. Although not always exact, the local weather report's pollen count can be helpful when planning outside activities.

Avoidance can help protect people against non-food or chemical allergens, too. In fact, for some people, eliminating exposure to an allergen is enough to prevent allergy symptoms and they don't need to take medicines or go through other allergy treatments.

Here are some things that can help you avoid airborne allergens:

- Keep family pets out of certain rooms, like your bedroom, and bathe them if necessary.

- Remove carpets or rugs from your room (hard floor surfaces don't collect dust as much as carpets do).

- Don't hang heavy drapes and get rid of other items that allow dust to accumulate.

- Clean frequently (if your allergy is severe, you may be able to get someone else to do your dirty work)

- Use special covers to seal pillows and mattresses if you're allergic to dust mites.

- If you're allergic to pollen, keep windows closed when pollen season's at its peak, change your clothing after being outdoors—and don't mow lawns.

- If you're allergic to mold, avoid damp areas, such as basements, and keep bathrooms and other mold-prone areas clean and dry.

Medications

Medications such as pills or nasal sprays are often used to treat allergies. Although medications can control the allergy symptoms (such as sneezing, headaches, or a stuffy nose), they are not a cure and can't make the tendency to have allergic reactions go away. Many effective medications are available to treat common allergies, and your doctor can help you to identify those that work for you.

Another type of medication that some severely allergic people will need to have on hand is a shot of epinephrine (pronounced: eh-puh-neh-frin), a fast-acting medicine that can help offset an anaphylactic reaction. This medicine comes in an easy-to-carry container that looks like a pen. Epinephrine is available by prescription only. If you have a severe allergy and your doctor thinks you should carry it, he or she will give you instructions on how to use it.

Shots

Allergy shots are also referred to as allergen immunotherapy. By receiving injections of small amounts of an allergen, your body can gradually develop antibodies and undergo other immune system changes that help reduce the reaction to that allergen.

Immunotherapy is only recommended for specific allergies, such as allergies to things you might breathe in (like pollen, pet dander, or dust mites) or insect allergies. Immunotherapy doesn't help with some allergies, like food allergies.

Although many people find the thought of allergy shots unsettling, shots can be highly effective—and it doesn't take long to get used to them. Often, the longer someone receives allergy shots, the more they help the body build up antibodies that fight the allergies. Although the shots don't cure allergies, they do tend to raise a person's tolerance when exposed to the allergen, which means fewer or less severe symptoms.

If you're severely allergic to bites and stings, talk to a doctor about getting venom immunotherapy (shots) from an allergist.

Is It A Cold Or Allergies?

If the spring and summer seasons leave you sneezing and wheezing, you might have allergies. Colds, on the other hand, are more likely to occur at any time (though they're more common in the colder months).

Colds and allergies produce similar symptoms, but colds usually last only a week or so. And although both may cause your nose and eyes to itch, colds and other viral infections can also cause a fever, aches and pains, and colored mucus. Cold symptoms often worsen as the days go on and then gradually improve, but allergies begin immediately after exposure to the offending allergen and last as long as that exposure continues.

If you're not sure whether your symptoms are caused by allergies or a cold, talk with your doctor.

Dealing With Allergies

So once you know you have allergies, how do you deal with them? First and foremost, try to avoid things you're allergic to.

If you have a food allergy, that means avoiding foods that trigger symptoms and learning how to read food labels to make sure you're not consuming even tiny amounts of allergens. People with environmental allergies should keep their house clean of dust and pet dander and watch the weather for days when pollen is high. Switching to perfume-free and dye-free detergents, cosmetics, and beauty products (you may see non-allergenic ingredients listed as hypoallergenic on product labels) also can help.

If you're taking medication, follow the directions carefully and make sure your regular doctor is aware of anything an allergist gives you (like shots or prescriptions). If you have a severe allergy, consider wearing a medical emergency ID (such as a MedicAlert bracelet), which will explain your allergy and who to contact in case of an emergency.

If you've been diagnosed with allergies, you have a lot of company. The National Institutes of Health (NIH) report that more than 50 million Americans are affected by allergic diseases. The good news is that doctors and scientists are working to better understand allergies, to improve treatment methods, and to possibly prevent allergies altogether.

Chapter 2

What Causes Allergies?

Why Are Allergies Increasing?

The occurrence of allergic disease is skyrocketing, and some estimates are that as many as one-in-five Americans have an allergic condition. Allergies are specific and reproducible undesired and unpleasant immune responses that are triggered by naturally occurring substances such as foods, pollens, or other influences in our surroundings. Overwhelming evidence from various studies suggests that the "hygiene hypothesis" explains most of the allergy epidemic.

The Hygiene Hypothesis

The hygiene hypothesis states that excessive cleanliness interrupts the normal development of the immune system, and this change leads to an increase in allergies. In short, our "developed" lifestyles have eliminated the natural variation in the types and quantity of germs our immune systems needs for it to develop into a less allergic, better regulated state of being. These concepts are illustrated in Figure 2.1.

Figure 2.2 simplifies the immune system into two separate tendencies: T_H1 and T_H2 responses. On the left, we see that exposures to germs, "dirt," and certain types of infection are part of the natural development of our immune response from a "default" T_H2-based system

About This Chapter: This chapter includes "Why Are Allergies Increasing?" by Melinda Braskett, M.D., Medical Director, Food and Drug Allergy Care Center at the University of California Los Angeles. © 2012 Regents of the University of California. All rights reserved. Reprinted with permission. For additional information from the Food and Drug Allergy Care Center at UCLA, visit http://fooddrugallergy.ucla.edu.

at birth to a "mature" T_H1-based system. On the right, we see how some cultural choices can interrupt the course of the immune system, and allow the T_H2 response to continue to dominate and promote allergic conditions. Therefore, many of the advances of modernization, such as good sanitation and eradicating parasitic (helminth) infections, may actually be fueling this epidemic of allergies.

What Causes Allergies?

The substances that cause allergic disease in people are known as allergens. *Antigens*, or protein particles like pollen, food, or dander, enter our bodies through a variety of ways. If the antigen causes an allergic reaction, that particle is considered an *allergen*—an antigen that triggers an allergic reaction. These allergens can get into our body in several ways:

- **Inhaled Into The Nose And The Lungs:** Examples are airborne pollens of certain trees, grasses, and weeds; house dust that includes dust mite particles, mold spores, cat and dog dander, and latex dust.

- **Ingested By Mouth:** Frequent culprits include shrimp, peanuts, and other nuts.

- **Injected:** Such as medications delivered by needle, like penicillin or other injectable drugs, and venom from insect stings and bites.

- **Absorbed Through The Skin:** Plants such as poison ivy, sumac, and oak, and latex are examples.

Source: Excerpted from "What Causes Allergies?" reprinted with permission from the Asthma and Allergy Foundation of America (www.aafa.org), © 2011.

Why Are Food Allergies Increasing?

Food allergies are increasing as part of the overall trend of increasing allergies due to the hygiene hypothesis. However, there are some specific reasons that food allergies are increasing.

Delayed Introduction Of Foods

The recent practice of delaying the introduction of some foods, such as peanut, with high potential for allergy may be associated with higher rates of food allergy. Evidence for this theory comes from the fact that cultures that introduce peanut earlier have less food allergy while those that delay introduction of potentially allergic foods have seen an increase in food allergy. But this may be due to other factors. The LEAP study (www.leapstudy.co.uk)

Environment

Rural environments	"Modernized" environments
Low level of sanitation	High levels of sanitation
Large families or daycare	Small family size
Rare use of antibiotics	Frequent use of antibiotics
Variable intestinal bacteria	Stable intestinal bacteria
Parasitic infections	Elimination of parasites

"Less Allergic"   "More Allergic"

Genetic and Other Factors

Figure 2.1. Modernization and other environmental changes associated with a "developed" lifestyle promote allergies.

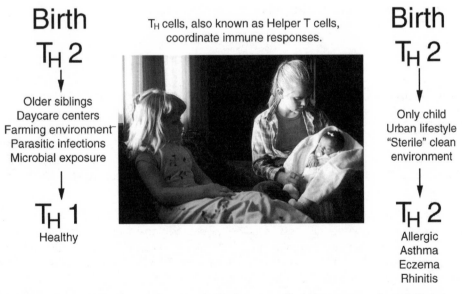

Birth

$T_H 2$

T_H cells, also known as Helper T cells, coordinate immune responses.

Birth

$T_H 2$

Older siblings
Daycare centers
Farming environment
Parasitic infections
Microbial exposure

Only child
Urban lifestyle
"Sterile" clean
environment

$T_H 1$
Healthy

$T_H 2$
Allergic
Asthma
Eczema
Rhinitis

Figure 2.2. In the absence of natural challenges, the immune system fails to mature. This situation can promote the development of allergic conditions (photograph courtesy National Cancer Institute, AV-8007-4356).

is a well-designed investigation that attempts to answer this question with respect to peanut allergy. Specifically, this large, on-going study seeks to determine which approach is associated with less peanut allergy: extended avoidance or the early introduction of peanut in high doses. Current guidelines from U.S.-based pediatric allergists recommend delaying solids until about four to six months. Beyond this age, there are no further recommendations to delay the introduction of at-risk foods for allergic reasons, but there are still restrictions about food for developmental and infectious reasons.

Form Of Food We Eat

Different forms of the same food appear to be more likely to provoke an allergic response, specifically roasting peanuts rather than boiling them makes them much more likely to cause an allergic reaction. Also, many people with milk or egg allergy can tolerate baked forms of these foods.

Increased Awareness And Reporting

Heightened awareness among doctors, parents, teachers and the general public about the symptoms and potential consequences of food allergies may contribute to the reason we are meeting more people with food allergy. Additionally, clinical research in food allergy is advancing rapidly, and earlier studies may have underestimated the rates of food allergy.

What Makes Some Pollen Cause Allergies, and Not Others?

Plant pollens that are carried by the wind cause most allergies of the nose, eyes, and lungs. These plants (including certain weeds, trees, and grasses) are natural pollutants produced at various times of the year when their small, inconspicuous flowers discharge literally billions of pollen particles.

Because the particles can be carried significant distances, it is important for you not only to understand local environmental conditions, but also conditions over the broader area of the state or region in which you live. Unlike the wind-pollinated plants, conspicuous wild flowers or flowers used in most residential gardens are pollinated by bees, wasps, and other insects and therefore are not widely capable of producing allergic disease.

Source: Excerpted from "What Causes Allergies?" reprinted with permission from the Asthma and Allergy Foundation of America (www.aafa.org), © 2011.

What Is The Role Of Heredity In Allergy?

Like baldness, height, and eye color, the capacity to become allergic is an inherited characteristic. Yet, although you may be born with the genetic capability to become allergic, you are not automatically allergic to specific allergens. Several factors must be present for allergic sensitivity to be developed:

- The specific genes acquired from parents.
- The exposure to one or more allergens to which you have a genetically programmed response.
- The degree and length of exposure.

A baby born with the tendency to become allergic to cow's milk, for example, may show allergic symptoms several months after birth. A genetic capability to become allergic to cat dander may take three to four years of cat exposure before the person shows symptoms. These people may also become allergic to other environmental substances with age.

On the other hand, poison ivy allergy (contact dermatitis) is an example of an allergy in which hereditary background does not play a part. The person with poison ivy allergy first has to be exposed to the oil from the plant. This usually occurs during youth, when a rash does not always appear. However, the first exposure may sensitize or cause the person to become allergic and, when subsequent exposure takes place, a contact dermatitis rash appears and can be quite severe. Many plants are capable of producing this type of rash. Substances other than plants, such as dyes, metals, and chemicals in deodorants and cosmetics, can also cause a similar dermatitis.

Source: Excerpted from "What Causes Allergies?" reprinted with permission from the Asthma and Allergy Foundation of America (www.aafa.org), © 2011.

Drug Allergies Are Also Due To The Immune System

Adverse Drug Reactions

Any unintended, undesired effect of a medication is called an adverse drug reaction. Allergic reactions are just one type of these reactions, caused by specific immune responses. It is important to know if an adverse reaction is actually an allergy due to an immune mechanism because these reactions can be unpredictable, and severe allergic reactions can be very dangerous. Also, allergic reactions generally respond to drug desensitization, but other adverse reactions do not.

Are Drug Allergies And Adverse Drug Reactions Increasing?

Only about 5–10 percent of adverse drug reactions are allergic reactions, and since we don't know the actual rate of drug allergy it is impossible to say if it is increasing. However, each new drug or supplement has possible unwanted and undesired side effects and the potential to cause allergic immune-mediated reactions. There is heighted awareness about the symptoms and potential consequences of drug allergies and adverse drug reactions by both doctors and patients. It is likely that both adverse drug reactions and drug allergies are increasing.

Does The Hygiene Hypothesis Affect Drug Allergies?

The hygiene hypothesis explains why there is an increase in allergies to foods, pollens, and other components of our environment. People with allergic conditions such as food allergy, eczema, asthma, and seasonal allergies or hay fever are not more likely to have drug allergies. However, people with underlying allergic conditions appear to be more likely to have severe and potentially dangerous allergic reactions to medications.

Chapter 3

The Immune System
And Its Role In Allergies

Introduction

The immune system is a network of cells, tissues, and organs that work together to defend the body against attacks by "foreign" invaders. These are primarily microbes—tiny organisms such as bacteria, parasites, and fungi that can cause infections. Viruses also cause infections, but are too primitive to be classified as living organisms. The human body provides an ideal environment for many microbes. It is the immune system's job to keep them out or, failing that, to seek out and destroy them.

When the immune system hits the wrong target, however, it can unleash a torrent of disorders, including allergic diseases, arthritis, and a form of diabetes. If the immune system is crippled, other kinds of diseases result.

The immune system is amazingly complex. It can recognize and remember millions of different enemies, and it can produce secretions (release of fluids) and cells to match up with and wipe out nearly all of them.

The secret to its success is an elaborate and dynamic communications network. Millions and millions of cells, organized into sets and subsets, gather like clouds of bees swarming around a hive and pass information back and forth in response to an infection. Once immune cells receive the alarm, they become activated and begin to produce powerful chemicals. These substances allow the cells to regulate their own growth and behavior, enlist other immune cells, and direct the new recruits to trouble spots.

About This Chapter: Excerpted from "Understanding the Immune System: How It Works," National Institute of Allergy and Infectious Diseases (www.niaid.nih.gov), 2007. Reviewed by David A. Cooke, MD, FACP, September 2012.

Self And Nonself

The key to a healthy immune system is its remarkable ability to distinguish between the body's own cells, recognized as *self*, and foreign cells, or *nonself*. The body's immune defenses normally coexist peacefully with cells that carry distinctive self marker molecules. But when immune defenders encounter foreign cells or organisms carrying markers that say nonself, they quickly launch an attack.

Anything that can trigger this immune response is called an antigen. An antigen can be a microbe such as a virus, or a part of a microbe such as a molecule. Tissues or cells from another person (except an identical twin) also carry nonself markers and act as foreign antigens. This explains why tissue transplants may be rejected.

In abnormal situations, the immune system can mistake self for nonself and launch an attack against the body's own cells or tissues. The result is called an autoimmune disease. Some forms of arthritis and diabetes are autoimmune diseases. In other cases, the immune system responds to a seemingly harmless foreign substance such as ragweed pollen. The result is allergy, and this kind of antigen is called an allergen.

The Structure Of The Immune System

The organs of the immune system are positioned throughout the body. They are called lymphoid organs because they are home to lymphocytes, small white blood cells that are the key players in the immune system. Bone marrow, the soft tissue in the hollow center of bones, is the ultimate source of all blood cells, including lymphocytes. The thymus is a lymphoid organ that lies behind the breastbone. Lymphocytes known as T lymphocytes or T cells ("T" stands for "thymus") mature in the thymus and then migrate to other tissues. B lymphocytes, also known as B cells, become activated and mature into plasma cells, which make and release antibodies.

Organs of the immune system are positioned throughout the body. They include tonsils, adenoids, lymph nodes and lymphatic vessels, appendix, thymus, spleen, Peyer's patches, and bone marrow.

Lymph nodes, which are located in many parts of the body, are lymphoid tissues that contain numerous specialized structures.

- T cells from the thymus concentrate in the paracortex.

- B cells develop in and around the germinal centers.

- Plasma cells occur in the medulla.

Lymphocytes can travel throughout the body using the blood vessels. The cells can also travel through a system of lymphatic vessels that closely parallels the body's veins and arteries.

Cells and fluids are exchanged between blood and lymphatic vessels, enabling the lymphatic system to monitor the body for invading microbes. The lymphatic vessels carry lymph, a clear fluid that bathes the body's tissues.

Small, bean-shaped lymph nodes are laced along the lymphatic vessels, with clusters in the neck, armpits, abdomen, and groin. Each lymph node contains specialized compartments where immune cells congregate, and where they can encounter antigens.

Immune cells, microbes, and foreign antigens enter the lymph nodes via incoming lymphatic vessels or the lymph nodes' tiny blood vessels. All lymphocytes exit lymph nodes through outgoing lymphatic vessels. Once in the bloodstream, lymphocytes are transported to tissues throughout the body. They patrol everywhere for foreign antigens, then gradually drift back into the lymphatic system to begin the cycle all over again.

The spleen is a flattened organ at the upper left of the abdomen. Like the lymph nodes, the spleen contains specialized compartments where immune cells gather and work. The spleen serves as a meeting ground where immune defenses confront antigens.

What Is *Lymph*?

Lymph: A transparent, slightly yellow fluid that carries lymphocytes, bathes the body tissues, and drains into the lymphatic vessels.

Lymph Node: A small bean-shaped organ of the immune system, distributed widely throughout the body and linked by lymphatic vessels. Lymph nodes are garrisons of B and T cells, dendritic cells, macrophages, and other kinds of immune cells.

Lymphatic Vessels: A body-wide network of channels, similar to the blood vessels, which transports lymph to the immune organs and into the bloodstream.

Lymphocyte: A small white blood cell produced in the lymphoid organs and essential to immune defenses. B cells, T cells, and NK T cells are lymphocytes.

Lymphoid Organ: An organ of the immune system where lymphocytes develop and congregate. These organs include the bone marrow, thymus, lymph nodes, spleen, and various other clusters of lymphoid tissue. Blood vessels and lymphatic vessels are also lymphoid organs.

Lymphokines: Powerful chemical substances secreted by lymphocytes. These molecules help direct and regulate the immune responses.

Other clumps of lymphoid tissue are found in many parts of the body, especially in the linings of the digestive tract, airways, and lungs—territories that serve as gateways to the body. These tissues include the tonsils, adenoids, and appendix.

Immune Cells And Their Products

The immune system stockpiles a huge arsenal of cells, not only lymphocytes but also cell-devouring phagocytes and their relatives. Some immune cells take on all intruders, whereas others are trained on highly specific targets. To work effectively, most immune cells need the cooperation of their comrades. Sometimes immune cells communicate by direct physical contact, and sometimes they communicate releasing chemical messengers.

The immune system stores just a few of each kind of the different cells needed to recognize millions of possible enemies. When an antigen first appears, the few immune cells that can respond to it multiply into a full-scale army of cells. After their job is done, the immune cells fade away, leaving sentries behind to watch for future attacks.

All immune cells begin as immature stem cells in the bone marrow. They respond to different cytokines and other chemical signals to grow into specific immune cell types, such as T cells, B cells, or phagocytes. Because stem cells have not yet committed to a particular future, their use presents an interesting possibility for treating some immune system disorders. Researchers currently are investigating if a person's own stem cells can be used to regenerate damaged immune responses in autoimmune diseases and in immune deficiency disorders, such as HIV infection.

B Cells

B cells and T cells are the main types of lymphocytes. B cells work chiefly by secreting substances called antibodies into the body's fluids. Antibodies ambush foreign antigens circulating in the bloodstream. They are powerless, however, to penetrate cells. The job of attacking target cells—either cells that have been infected by viruses or cells that have been distorted by cancer—is left to T cells or other immune cells (described below).

Each B cell is programmed to make one specific antibody. For example, one B cell will make an antibody that blocks a virus that causes the common cold, while another produces an antibody that attacks a bacterium that causes pneumonia. When a B cell encounters the kind of antigen that triggers it to become active, it gives rise to many large cells known as plasma cells, which produce antibodies.

- Immunoglobulin G, or IgG, is a kind of antibody that works efficiently to coat microbes, speeding their uptake by other cells in the immune system.

- IgM is very effective at killing bacteria.

- IgA concentrates in body fluids—tears, saliva, and the secretions of the respiratory and digestive tracts—guarding the entrances to the body.

- IgE, whose natural job probably is to protect against parasitic infections, is responsible for the symptoms of allergy.

- IgD remains attached to B cells and plays a key role in initiating early B cell responses.

T Cells

Unlike B cells, T cells do not recognize free-floating antigens. Rather, their surfaces contain specialized antibody-like receptors that see fragments of antigens on the surfaces of infected or cancerous cells. T cells contribute to immune defenses in two major ways: some direct and regulate immune responses, whereas others directly attack infected or cancerous cells.

Helper T cells, or T_H cells, coordinate immune responses by communicating with other cells. Some stimulate nearby B cells to produce antibodies, others call in microbe-gobbling cells called phagocytes, and still others activate other T cells.

Cytotoxic T lymphocytes (CTLs)—also called killer T cells—perform a different function. These cells directly attack other cells carrying certain foreign or abnormal molecules on their surfaces. CTLs are especially useful for attacking viruses because viruses often hide from other parts of the immune system while they grow inside infected cells. CTLs recognize small fragments of these viruses peeking out from the cell membrane and launch an attack to kill the infected cell.

In most cases, T cells only recognize an antigen if it is carried on the surface of a cell by one of the body's own major histocompatibility complex, or MHC, molecules. MHC molecules are proteins recognized by T cells when they distinguish between self and nonself. A self-MHC molecule provides a recognizable scaffolding to present a foreign antigen to the T cell. In humans, MHC antigens are called human leukocyte antigens, or HLA.

Although MHC molecules are required for T cell responses against foreign invaders, they also create problems during organ transplantations. Virtually every cell in the body is covered with MHC proteins, but each person has a different set of these proteins on his or her cells. If a T cell recognizes a nonself-MHC molecule on another cell, it will destroy the cell. Therefore, doctors must match organ recipients with donors who have the closest MHC makeup. Otherwise the recipient's T cells will likely attack the transplanted organ, leading to graft rejection.

Important Components Of An Immune Response

Antibody: A molecule (also called an immunoglobulin) produced by a mature B cell (plasma cell) in response to an antigen. When an antibody attaches to an antigen, it helps the body destroy or inactivate the antigen.

Antigen: A substance or molecule that is recognized by the immune system. The antigen can be from foreign material such as bacteria or viruses.

B Cell or B Lymphocyte: A small white blood cell crucial to the immune defenses. B cells come from bone marrow and develop into blood cells called plasma cells, which are the source of antibodies.

Basophil: A white blood cell that contributes to inflammatory reactions. Along with mast cells, basophils are responsible for the symptoms of allergy.

Complement Cascade: A precise sequence of events, usually triggered by antigen-antibody complexes, in which each component of the complement system is activated in turn.

Complement: A complex series of blood proteins whose action "complements" the work of antibodies. Complement destroys bacteria, produces inflammation, and regulates immune reactions.

Helper T Cells (T_H Cells): A subset of T cells that carry the CD4 surface marker and are essential for turning on antibody production, activating cytotoxic T cells, and initiating many other immune functions.

Human Leukocyte Antigen (HLA): A protein on the surfaces of human cells that identifies the cells as "self" and, like MHC antigens, performs essential roles in immune responses. HLAs are used in laboratory tests to determine whether one person's tissues are compatible with another person's, and could be used in a transplant. HLAs are the human equivalent of MHC antigens; they are coded for by MHC genes.

Natural killer (NK) cells are another kind of lethal white cell, or lymphocyte. Like CTLs, NK cells are armed with granules filled with potent chemicals. But CTLs look for antigen fragments bound to self-MHC molecules, whereas NK cells recognize cells lacking self-MHC molecules. Thus, NK cells have the potential to attack many types of foreign cells.

Both kinds of killer cells slay on contact. The deadly assassins bind to their targets, aim their weapons, and then deliver a lethal burst of chemicals.

Immune Response: Reaction of the immune system to foreign substances. Although normal immune responses are designed to protect the body from pathogens, immune dysregulation can damage normal cells and tissues, as in the case of autoimmune diseases.

Immunoglobulin: One of a family of large protein molecules, also known as antibodies, produced by mature B cells (plasma cells).

Inflammation: An immune system reaction to "foreign" invaders such as microbes or allergens. Signs include redness, swelling, pain, or heat.

Macrophage: A large and versatile immune cell that devours invading pathogens and other intruders. Macrophages stimulate other immune cells by presenting them with small pieces of the invaders.

Major Histocompatibility Complex (MHC): A group of genes that controls several aspects of the immune response. MHC genes code for "self" markers on all body cells.

Mast Cell: A granulocyte found in tissue. The contents of mast cells, along with those of basophils, are responsible for the symptoms of allergy.

Natural Killer (NK) Cell: A large granule-containing lymphocyte that recognizes and kills cells lacking self antigens. These cells' target recognition molecules are different from T cells.

NK T Cell: A T cell that has some characteristics of NK cells. It produces large amounts of cytokines when stimulated, and is activated by fatty substances (lipids) bound to non-MHC molecules called CD1d.

Spleen: A lymphoid organ in the abdominal cavity that is an important center for immune system activities.

T Cell or T Lymphocyte: A small white blood cell that recognizes antigen fragments bound to cell surfaces by specialized antibody-like receptors. "T" stands for the thymus gland, where T cells develop and acquire their receptors.

Tonsils and Adenoids: Prominent oval masses of lymphoid tissues on either side of the throat.

T cells aid the normal processes of the immune system. If NK T cells fail to function properly, asthma, certain autoimmune diseases—including type 1 diabetes—or the growth of cancers may result. NK T cells get their name because they are a kind of T lymphocyte that carries some of the surface proteins, called *markers*, typical of NK T cells. But these T cells differ from other kinds of T cells. They do not recognize pieces of antigen bound to self-MHC molecules. Instead, they recognize fatty substances (lipids and glycolipids) that are bound to a different class of molecules called CD1d. Scientists are trying to discover methods to control the timing and release of chemical factors by NK T cells, with the hope they can modify immune responses in ways that benefit patients.

Phagocytes And Their Relatives

Phagocytes are large white cells that can swallow and digest microbes and other foreign particles. Monocytes are phagocytes that circulate in the blood. When monocytes migrate into tissues, they develop into macrophages. Specialized types of macrophages can be found in many organs, including the lungs, kidneys, brain, and liver.

Macrophages play many roles. As scavengers, they rid the body of worn-out cells and other debris. They display bits of foreign antigen in a way that draws the attention of matching lymphocytes and, in that respect, resemble dendritic cells (described below). And they churn out an amazing variety of powerful chemical signals, known as monokines, which are vital to the immune response.

Granulocytes are another kind of immune cell. They contain granules filled with potent chemicals, which allow the granulocytes to destroy microorganisms. Some of these chemicals, such as histamine, also contribute to inflammation and allergy.

One type of granulocyte, the neutrophil, is also a phagocyte. Neutrophils use their prepackaged chemicals to break down the microbes they ingest. Eosinophils and basophils are granulocytes that *degranulate* by spraying their chemicals onto harmful cells or microbes nearby.

Mast cells function much like basophils, except they are not blood cells. Rather, they are found in the lungs, skin, tongue, and linings of the nose and intestinal tract, where they contribute to the symptoms of allergy.

Related structures, called blood platelets, are cell fragments. Platelets also contain granules. In addition to promoting blood clotting and wound repair, platelets activate some immune defenses.

Dendritic cells are found in the parts of lymphoid organs where T cells also exist. Like macrophages, dendritic cells in lymphoid tissues display antigens to T cells and help stimulate T cells during an immune response. They are called dendritic cells because they have branchlike extensions that can interlace to form a network.

T Cell Receptors

T cell receptors are complex protein molecules that peek through the surface membranes of T cells. The exterior part of a T cell receptor recognizes short pieces of foreign antigens that are bound to self-MHC molecules on other cells of the body. It is because of their T cell receptors that T cells can recognize disease-causing microorganisms and rally other immune cells to attack the invaders, or kill the invaders themselves.

Toll-like receptors (TLRs), which occur on cells throughout the immune system, are a family of proteins the body uses as a first line of defense against invading microbes. Like T cell receptors, some TLRs peek through the surface membranes of immune cells, allowing them to respond to microbes in the cells' environment.

Some TLRs are activated by molecules that make up viruses, whereas other TLRs respond to molecules that make up the cell walls of bacteria. Once activated, TLRs relay the alarm to other actors in the immune system. For example, some TLRs play important roles in the all-purpose first-responder arm of the immune system, also called the *innate immune system*. In short order, the innate immune system responds with a surge of chemical signals that together cause inflammation, fever, and other responses to infection or injury. Other TLRs help initiate responses from genetically identical groups of lymphocytes, called clones, that are already programmed to recognize specific antigens. Such responses are called adaptive immunity.

Overall, the cellular receptors important for the first-line responses of innate immunity are encoded by genes people inherit from their parents. In contrast, adaptive immune responses rely on antigen receptors that are pieced together in the genomes of lymphocytes during their development in various tissues of the body. In addition to TLRs, other kinds of innate immune receptors can stimulate phagocytosis by macrophages, trigger the inflammatory responses that help control local infections, and play a range of crucial roles in defending the body against invading microbes.

Cytokines

Cells of the immune system communicate with one another by releasing and responding to chemical messengers called cytokines. These proteins are secreted by immune cells and act on other cells to coordinate appropriate immune responses. Cytokines include a diverse assortment of interleukins, interferons, and growth factors.

Some cytokines are chemical switches that turn certain immune cell types on and off. One cytokine, interleukin 2 (IL-2), triggers the immune system to produce T cells. IL-2's immunity-boosting properties have traditionally made it a promising treatment for several illnesses. Clinical studies are underway to test its benefits in diseases such as cancer, hepatitis C, and HIV infection and AIDS. Scientists are studying other cytokines to see whether they can also be used to treat diseases.

One group of cytokines chemically attracts specific cell types. These so-called chemokines are released by cells at a site of injury or infection and call other immune cells to the region to help repair the damage or fight off the invader. Chemokines often play a key role in inflammation and are a promising target for new drugs to help regulate immune responses.

Complement

The complement system is made up of about 25 proteins that work together to assist, or *complement*, the action of antibodies in destroying bacteria. Complement also helps to rid the body of antibody-coated antigens (antigen-antibody complexes). Complement proteins, which cause blood vessels to become dilated and then leaky, contribute to the redness, warmth, swelling, pain, and loss of function that characterize an inflammatory response.

Complement proteins circulate in the blood in an inactive form. When the first protein in the complement series is activated—typically by an antibody that has locked onto an antigen—it sets in motion a domino effect. Each component takes its turn in a precise chain of steps known as the complement cascade. The end products are molecular cylinders that are inserted into—and that puncture holes in—the cell walls that surround the invading bacteria. With fluids and molecules flowing in and out, the bacterial cells swell, burst, and die. Other components of the complement system make bacteria more susceptible to phagocytosis or beckon other immune cells to the area.

Mounting An Immune Response

Infections are the most common cause of human disease. They range from the common cold to debilitating conditions like chronic hepatitis to life-threatening diseases such as AIDS (acquired immune deficiency syndrome). Disease-causing microbes (pathogens) attempting to get into the body must first move past the body's external armor, usually the skin or cells lining the body's internal passageways.

The skin provides an imposing barrier to invading microbes. It is generally penetrable only through cuts or tiny abrasions. The digestive and respiratory tracts—both portals of entry for a number of microbes—also have their own levels of protection. Microbes entering the nose often cause the nasal surfaces to secrete more protective mucus, and attempts to enter the nose or lungs can trigger a sneeze or cough reflex to force microbial invaders out of the respiratory passageways. The stomach contains a strong acid that destroys many pathogens that are swallowed with food.

If microbes survive the body's front-line defenses, they still have to find a way through the walls of the digestive, respiratory, or urogenital passageways to the underlying cells. These passageways are lined with tightly packed epithelial cells covered in a layer of mucus, effectively blocking the transport of many pathogens into deeper cell layers.

Mucosal surfaces also secrete a special class of antibody called IgA, which in many cases is the first type of antibody to encounter an invading microbe. Underneath the epithelial layer a variety of immune cells, including macrophages, B cells, and T cells, lie in wait for any microbe that might bypass the barriers at the surface.

Next, invaders must escape a series of general defenses of the innate immune system, which are ready to attack without regard for specific antigen markers. These include patrolling phagocytes, NK T cells, and complement.

Microbes cross the general barriers then confront specific weapons of the adaptive immune system tailored just for them. These specific weapons, which include both antibodies and T cells, are equipped with singular receptor structures that allow them to recognize and interact with their designated targets.

Bacteria, Viruses, And Parasites

The most common disease-causing microbes are bacteria, viruses, and parasites. Each uses a different tactic to infect a person, and, therefore, each is thwarted by different components of the immune system.

Most bacteria live in the spaces between cells and are readily attacked by antibodies. When antibodies attach to a bacterium, they send signals to complement proteins and phagocytic cells to destroy the bound microbes. Some bacteria are eaten directly by phagocytes, which signal to certain T cells to join the attack.

All viruses, plus a few types of bacteria and parasites, must enter cells of the body to survive, requiring a different kind of immune defense. Infected cells use their MHC molecules to put pieces of the invading microbes on their surfaces, flagging down CTLs to destroy the infected cells. Antibodies also can assist in the immune response by attaching to and clearing viruses before they have a chance to enter cells.

Parasites live either inside or outside cells. Intracellular parasites such as the organism that causes malaria can trigger T cell responses. Extracellular parasites are often much larger than

Immune System Dysfunction

Allergen: Any substance that causes an allergy.

Allergies: Diseases that occur when the immune system responds to a false alarm. A normally harmless material is mistaken for a threat and attacked.

Autoimmune Disease: Disease that results when the immune system mistakenly attacks the body's own tissues. Examples include multiple sclerosis, type 1 diabetes, rheumatoid arthritis, and systemic lupus erythematosus.

bacteria or viruses and require a much broader immune attack. Parasitic infections often trigger an inflammatory response in which eosinophils, basophils, and other specialized granule-containing cells rush to the scene and release their stores of toxic chemicals in an attempt to destroy the invaders. Antibodies also play a role in this attack, attracting the granule-filled cells to the site of infection.

Allergy Is A Disorder Of The Immune System

The most common types of allergic diseases occur when the immune system responds to a false alarm. In an allergic person, a normally harmless material such as grass pollen, food particles, mold, or house dust mites is mistaken for a threat and attacked.

Allergies such as pollen allergy are related to the antibody known as IgE. Like other antibodies, each IgE antibody is specific; one acts against oak pollen and another against ragweed, for example.

Chapter 4

The Respiratory System And How It Works

The Respiratory System

The respiratory system is a group of organs and tissues that help you breathe. The main parts of this system are the airways, the lungs and linked blood vessels, and the muscles that enable breathing.

Airways

The airways are pipes that carry oxygen-rich air to your lungs and carbon dioxide, a waste gas, out of your lungs. The airways include these components:

- Nose and linked air passages (called nasal cavities)
- Mouth
- Larynx, or voice box
- Trachea, or windpipe
- Tubes called bronchial tubes or bronchi, and their branches

Air first enters your body through your nose or mouth, which wets and warms the air. (Cold, dry air can irritate your lungs.) The air then travels through your voice box and down your windpipe. The windpipe splits into two bronchial tubes that enter your lungs.

A thin flap of tissue called the epiglottis covers your windpipe when you swallow. This prevents food or drink from entering the air passages that lead to your lungs.

About This Chapter: From "The Respiratory System?" National Heart Lung and Blood Institute (www.nhlbi.nih .gov), June 2010.

Except for the mouth and some parts of the nose, all of the airways have special hairs called cilia that are coated with sticky mucus. The cilia trap germs and other foreign particles that enter your airways when you breathe in air.

These fine hairs then sweep the particles up to the nose or mouth. From there, they're swallowed, coughed, or sneezed out of the body. Nose hairs and mouth saliva also trap particles and germs.

Lungs And Blood Vessels

Your lungs and linked blood vessels deliver oxygen to your body and remove carbon dioxide from your body. Your lungs lie on either side of your breastbone and fill the inside of your chest cavity. Your left lung is slightly smaller than your right lung to allow room for your heart.

Within the lungs, your bronchi branch into thousands of smaller, thinner tubes called bronchioles. These tubes end in bunches of tiny round air sacs called alveoli.

Each of these air sacs is covered in a mesh of tiny blood vessels called capillaries. The capillaries connect to a network of arteries and veins that move blood through your body.

The pulmonary artery and its branches deliver blood rich in carbon dioxide (and lacking in oxygen) to the capillaries that surround the air sacs. Inside the air sacs, carbon dioxide moves from the blood into the air. At the same time, oxygen moves from the air into the blood in the capillaries.

The oxygen-rich blood then travels to the heart through the pulmonary vein and its branches. The heart pumps the oxygen-rich blood out to the body.

The lungs are divided into five main sections called lobes. Some people need to have a diseased lung lobe removed. However, they can still breathe well using the rest of their lung lobes.

Muscles Used For Breathing

Muscles near the lungs help expand and contract (tighten) the lungs to allow breathing. These muscles include the diaphragm, intercostal muscles, abdominal muscles, and muscles in the neck and collarbone area.

The diaphragm is a dome-shaped muscle located below your lungs. It separates the chest cavity from the abdominal cavity. The diaphragm is the main muscle used for breathing.

The intercostal muscles are located between your ribs. They also play a major role in helping you breathe.

What Are the Lungs?

Your lungs are organs in your chest that allow your body to take in oxygen from the air. They also help remove carbon dioxide (a waste gas that can be toxic) from your body.

The lungs' intake of oxygen and removal of carbon dioxide is called gas exchange. Gas exchange is part of breathing. Breathing is a vital function of life; it helps your body work properly. Other organs and tissues also help make breathing possible.

Source: National Heart Lung and Blood Institute, 2010.

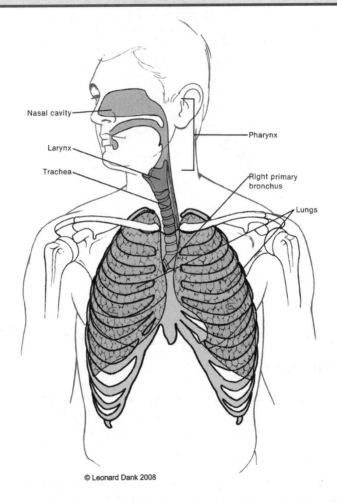

© Leonard Dank 2008

Figure 4.1. Organs of the Respiratory System (Source: The Inner Man DVD, © Leonard Dank; reprinted with permission).

Beneath your diaphragm are abdominal muscles. They help you breathe out when you're breathing fast (for example, during physical activity).

Muscles in your neck and collarbone area help you breathe in when other muscles involved in breathing don't work well, or when lung disease impairs your breathing.

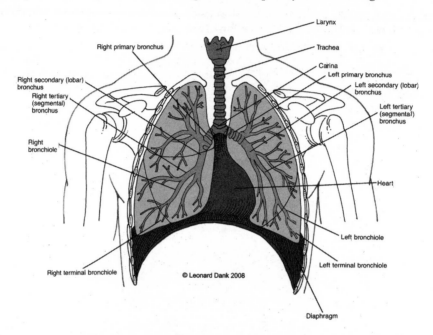

Figure 4.2. Bronchial Tree. (Source: The Inner Man DVD, © Leonard Dank; reprinted with permission.)

What Happens When You Breathe?

Breathing In (Inhalation)

When you breathe in, or inhale, your diaphragm contracts (tightens) and moves downward. This increases the space in your chest cavity, into which your lungs expand. The intercostal muscles between your ribs also help enlarge the chest cavity. They contract to pull your rib cage both upward and outward when you inhale.

As your lungs expand, air is sucked in through your nose or mouth. The air travels down your windpipe and into your lungs. After passing through your bronchial tubes, the air finally reaches and enters the alveoli (air sacs).

Through the very thin walls of the alveoli, oxygen from the air passes to the surrounding capillaries (blood vessels). A red blood cell protein called hemoglobin helps move oxygen from the air sacs to the blood.

At the same time, carbon dioxide moves from the capillaries into the air sacs. The gas has traveled in the bloodstream from the right side of the heart through the pulmonary artery.

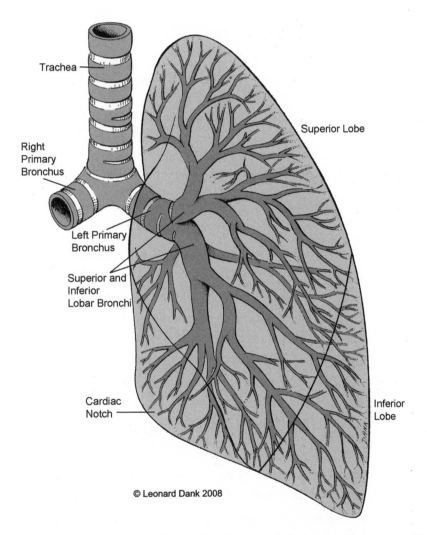

© Leonard Dank 2008

Figure 4.3. Lungs: Bronchopulmonary Segments(Source: The Inner Man DVD, © Leonard Dank; reprinted with permission.)

Oxygen-rich blood from the lungs is carried through a network of capillaries to the pulmonary vein. This vein delivers the oxygen-rich blood to the left side of the heart. The left side of the heart pumps the blood to the rest of the body. There, the oxygen in the blood moves from blood vessels into surrounding tissues.

Breathing Out (Exhalation)

When you breathe out, or exhale, your diaphragm relaxes and moves upward into the chest cavity. The intercostal muscles between the ribs also relax to reduce the space in the chest cavity.

As the space in the chest cavity gets smaller, air rich in carbon dioxide is forced out of your lungs and windpipe, and then out of your nose or mouth.

Breathing out requires no effort from your body unless you have a lung disease or are doing physical activity. When you're physically active, your abdominal muscles contract and push your diaphragm against your lungs even more than usual. This rapidly pushes out the air in your lungs.

What Controls Your Breathing?

A respiratory control center at the base of your brain controls your breathing. This center sends ongoing signals down your spine and to the nerves of the muscles involved in breathing.

These signals ensure your breathing muscles contract (tighten) and relax regularly. This allows your breathing to happen automatically, without you being aware of it.

To a limited degree, you can change your breathing rate, such as by breathing faster or holding your breath. Your emotions also can change your breathing. For example, being scared or angry can affect your breathing pattern.

Your breathing will change depending on how active you are and the condition of the air around you. For example, you need to breathe more often when you do physical activity. In contrast, your body needs to restrict how much air you breathe if the air contains irritants or toxins.

To adjust your breathing to changing needs, your body has many sensors in your brain, blood vessels, muscles, and lungs.

Sensors in the brain and in two major blood vessels (the carotid artery and the aorta) detect carbon dioxide or oxygen levels in your blood and change your breathing rate as needed.

Sensors in the airways detect lung irritants. The sensors can trigger sneezing or coughing. In people who have asthma, the sensors may cause the muscles around the airways in the lungs to contract. This makes the airways smaller.

Sensors in the alveoli (air sacs) detect a buildup of fluid in the lung tissues. These sensors are thought to trigger rapid, shallow breathing.

Sensors in your joints and muscles detect movement of your arms or legs. These sensors may play a role in increasing your breathing rate when you're physically active.

Is It A Cold Or An Allergy?

Symptoms	Cold	Airborne Allergy
Cough	Common	Sometimes
General Aches, Pains	Slight	Never
Fatigue, Weakness	Sometimes	Sometimes
Itchy Eyes	Rare or Never	Common
Sneezing	Usual	Usual
Sore Throat	Common	Sometimes
Runny Nose	Common	Common
Stuffy Nose	Common	Common
Fever	Rare	Never
Duration	3 to 14 days	Weeks (for example, 6 weeks for ragweed or grass pollen seasons)
Treatment	Antihistamines Decongestants Nonsteroidal anti-inflammatory medicines	Antihistamines Nasal steroids Decongestants
Prevention	Wash your hands often with soap and water Avoid close contact with anyone with a cold	Avoid those things that you are allergic to such as pollen, house dust mites, mold, pet dander, cockroaches
Complications	Sinus infection Middle ear infection Asthma	Sinus infection Asthma

Source: "Is it a Cold or an Allergy?" National Institute of Allergy and Infectious Diseases (www.niad.nih.gov), November 2008.

Lung Diseases And Conditions

Many steps are involved in breathing. If injury, disease, or other factors affect any of the steps, you may have trouble breathing.

For example, the fine hairs (cilia) that line your upper airways may not trap all of the germs you breathe in. These germs can cause an infection in your bronchial tubes (bronchitis) or deep in your lungs (pneumonia). These infections cause a buildup of mucus and/or fluid that narrows the airways and limits airflow in and out of your lungs.

If you have asthma, breathing in certain substances that you're sensitive to can trigger your airways to narrow. This makes it hard for air to flow in and out of your lungs.

Over a long period, breathing in cigarette smoke or air pollutants can damage the airways and the air sacs. This can lead to a condition called COPD (chronic obstructive pulmonary disease). COPD prevents proper airflow in and out of your lungs and can hinder gas exchange in the air sacs.

An important step to breathing is the movement of your diaphragm and other muscles in your chest, neck, and abdomen. This movement lets you inhale and exhale. Nerves that run from your brain to these muscles control their movement. Damage to these nerves in your upper spinal cord can cause breathing to stop, unless a machine is used to help you breathe. (This machine is called a ventilator or a respirator.)

A steady flow of blood in the small blood vessels that surround your air sacs is vital for gas exchange. Long periods of inactivity or surgery can cause a blood clot called a pulmonary embolism (PE) to block a lung artery. A PE can reduce or block the flow of blood in the small blood vessels and hinder gas exchange.

Chapter 5

Lung Function Tests For Breathing Problems

What Are Lung Function Tests?

Lung function tests, also called pulmonary function tests, measure how well your lungs work. These tests are used to look for the cause of breathing problems, such as shortness of breath.

Lung function tests measure several different elements involved in breathing:

- How much air you can take into your lungs. This amount is compared to that of other people your age, height, and sex. This allows your doctor to see whether you're in the normal range.

- How much air you can blow out of your lungs and how fast you can do it.

- How well your lungs deliver oxygen to your blood.

- The strength of your breathing muscles.

Doctors use lung function tests to help diagnose conditions such as asthma, pulmonary fibrosis (scarring of the lung tissue), and COPD (chronic obstructive pulmonary disease).

Lung function tests also are used to check the extent of damage caused by conditions such as pulmonary fibrosis and sarcoidosis. Also, these tests may be used to check how well treatments, such as asthma medicines, are working.

About This Chapter: From "Explore Lung Function Tests?" National Heart Lung and Blood Institute (www.nhlbi .nih.gov), August 2010.

Overview

Lung function tests include breathing tests and tests that measure the oxygen level in your blood. These are the breathing tests most often used:

- **Spirometry:** This test measures how much air you can breathe in and out. It also measures how fast you can blow air out.

- **Lung Volume Measurement:** This test, in addition to spirometry, measures how much air remains in your lungs after you breathe out fully.

- **Lung Diffusion Capacity:** This test measures how well oxygen passes from your lungs to your bloodstream.

These tests may not show what's causing breathing problems. So, you may have other tests as well, such as a cardiopulmonary exercise test. This test measures how well your lungs and heart work while you exercise on a treadmill or bicycle.

Two tests that measure the oxygen level in your blood are pulse oximetry and arterial blood gas tests. These tests also are called blood oxygen tests.

Pulse oximetry measures the blood oxygen level using a special light. For an arterial blood gas test, your doctor inserts a needle into an artery, usually in your wrist, and takes a sample of blood. The oxygen level of the blood sample is measured.

Outlook

Lung function tests usually are painless and rarely cause side effects. You may feel some discomfort during an arterial blood gas test when the needle is inserted into the artery.

Types Of Lung Function Tests

Breathing Tests

Spirometry

Spirometry measures how much air you breathe in and out and how fast you blow it out. This is measured two ways: peak expiratory flow rate (PEFR) and forced expiratory volume in one second (FEV1).

PEFR refers to the amount of air you can blow out as quickly as possible. FEV1 refers to the amount of air you can blow out in one second.

During the test, a technician will ask you to take a deep breath in. Then, you'll blow as hard as you can into a tube connected to a small machine. The machine is called a spirometer.

Your doctor may have you inhale a medicine that helps open your airways. He or she will want to see whether the medicine changes or improves the test results.

Spirometry helps check for conditions that affect how much air you can breathe in, such as pulmonary fibrosis (scarring of the lung tissue). The test also helps detect diseases that affect how fast you can breathe air out, like asthma and COPD (chronic obstructive pulmonary disease).

Lung Volume Measurement

This test measures the size of your lungs and how much air you can breathe in and out. During the test, you sit inside a glass booth and breathe into a tube that's hooked to a computer.

Sometimes you breathe in nitrogen or helium gas and then blow it out. The gas you breathe out is measured to test how much air your lungs can hold.

Lung volume measurement can help diagnose pulmonary fibrosis or a stiff and/or weak chest wall.

Lung Diffusion Capacity

This test measures how well oxygen passes from your lungs to your bloodstream. During this test, you breathe in a type of gas through a tube. You hold your breath for a brief moment and then blow out the gas.

Abnormal test results may suggest loss of lung tissue, emphysema (a type of COPD), very bad scarring of the lung tissue, or problems with blood flow through the body's arteries.

Tests To Measure Oxygen Level

Pulse oximetry and arterial blood gas tests show how much oxygen is in your blood. During pulse oximetry, a small sensor is attached to your finger or ear. The sensor uses light to estimate how much oxygen is in your blood. This test is painless and no needles are used.

For an arterial blood gas test, a blood sample is taken from an artery, usually in your wrist. The sample is sent to a laboratory, where its oxygen level is measured.

Testing In Infants And Young Children

Spirometry and other measures of lung function usually can be done in children older than six years, if they can follow directions well. Spirometry may be tried in children as young as five years. However, technicians who have special training with young children may need to do the testing.

Instead of spirometry, a growing number of medical centers measure respiratory system resistance. This is another way to test lung function in young children.

The child wears nose clips and has his or her cheeks supported with an adult's hands. The child breathes in and out quietly on a mouthpiece, while the technician measures changes in pressure at the mouth. During these lung function tests, parents can help comfort their children and encourage them to cooperate.

Very young children (younger than two years) may need an infant lung function test. This requires special equipment and medical staff. This type of test is available only at a few medical centers. The doctor gives the child medicine to help him or her sleep through the test. A technician places a mask over the child's nose and mouth and a vest around the child's chest.

The mask and vest are attached to a lung function machine. The machine gently pushes air into the child's lungs through the mask. As the child exhales, the vest slightly squeezes his or her chest. This helps push more air out of the lungs. The exhaled air is then measured.

In children younger than five years, doctors likely will use signs and symptoms, medical history, and a physical exam to diagnose lung problems.

Pulse oximetry and arterial blood gas tests can be used for children of all ages.

Diagnosing Lung Conditions

Your doctor will diagnose a lung condition based on your medical and family histories, a physical exam, and test results.

Medical And Family Histories

Your doctor will ask you questions, such as these:

- Do you ever feel like you can't get enough air?
- Does your chest feel tight sometimes?
- Do you have periods of coughing or wheezing (a whistling sound when you breathe)?
- Do you ever have chest pain?
- Can you walk or run as fast as other people your age?

Your doctor also will ask whether you or anyone in your family has ever had these experiences:

- Had asthma and/or allergies
- Had heart disease

- Smoked

- Traveled to places where they may have been exposed to tuberculosis

- Had a job that exposed them to dust, fumes, or particles (like asbestos)

Physical Exam

Your doctor will check your heart rate, breathing rate, and blood pressure. He or she also will listen to your heart and lungs with a stethoscope and feel your abdomen and limbs.

Your doctor will look for signs of heart or lung disease, or another disease that may be causing your symptoms.

Lung And Heart Tests

Based on your medical history and physical exam, your doctor will recommend tests. A chest x-ray usually is the first test done to find the cause of a breathing problem. This test takes pictures of the organs and structures inside your chest.

Your doctor may do lung function tests to find out even more about how well your lungs work.

Your doctor also may do tests to check your heart, such as an EKG (electrocardiogram) or a stress test. An EKG detects and records your heart's electrical activity. A stress test shows how well your heart works during physical activity.

What To Expect Before Lung Function Tests

If you take breathing medicines, your doctor may ask you to stop them for a short time before spirometry, lung volume measurement, or lung diffusion capacity tests.

No special preparation is needed before pulse oximetry and arterial blood gas tests. If you're getting oxygen therapy, your doctor may ask you to stop using it for a short time before the tests. This allows your doctor to check your blood oxygen level without the added oxygen.

Other Names For Lung Function Tests

- Lung diffusion testing; also called diffusing capacity and diffusing capacity of the lung for carbon monoxide, or DLCO
- Pulmonary function tests, or PFTs
- Arterial blood gas tests also are called blood gas analyses or ABGs.

What To Expect During Lung Function Tests

Breathing Tests

Spirometry may be done in your doctor's office or in a special lung function laboratory (lab). Lung volume measurement and lung diffusion capacity tests are done in a special lab or clinic. For these tests, you sit in a chair next to a machine that measures your breathing. For spirometry, you sit or stand next to the machine.

Before the tests, a technician places soft clips on your nose. This allows you to breathe only through a tube that's attached to the testing machine. The technician will tell you how to breathe into the tube. For example, you may be asked to breathe normally, slowly, or rapidly.

The deep breathing done in some of the tests may make you feel short of breath, dizzy, or light-headed, or it may make you cough.

Spirometry

For this test, you take a deep breath and then exhale as fast and as hard as you can into the tube. With spirometry, your doctor may give you a medicine that helps open your airways. Your doctor will want to see whether the medicine changes or improves the test results.

Lung Volume Measurement

For this test, you sit in a clear glass booth and breathe through the tube attached to the testing machine. The changes in pressure inside the booth are measured to show how much air you can breathe into your lungs.

Sometimes you breathe in nitrogen or helium gas and then exhale. The gas that you breathe out is measured.

Lung Diffusion Capacity

During this test, you breathe in gas through the tube, hold your breath for 10 seconds, and then rapidly blow it out. The gas contains a small amount of carbon monoxide, which won't harm you.

Tests To Measure Oxygen Level

Pulse oximetry is done in a doctor's office or hospital. An arterial blood gas test is done in a lab or hospital.

Pulse Oximetry

For this test, a small sensor is attached to your finger or ear using a clip or flexible tape. The sensor is then attached to a cable that leads to a small machine called an oximeter. The oximeter shows the amount of oxygen in your blood. This test is painless and no needles are used.

Arterial Blood Gas

During this test, your doctor or technician inserts a needle into an artery, usually in your wrist, and takes a sample of blood. You may feel some discomfort when the needle is inserted. The sample is then sent to a lab where its oxygen level is measured.

After the needle is removed, you may feel mild pressure or throbbing at the needle site. Applying pressure to the area for 5–10 minutes should stop the bleeding. You'll be given a small bandage to place on the area.

What To Expect After Lung Function Tests

You can return to your normal activities and restart your medicines after lung function tests. Talk with your doctor about when you'll get the test results.

What Do Lung Function Tests Show?

Breathing Tests

Spirometry

Spirometry can show whether you have these conditions:

- A blockage (obstruction) in your airways. This may be a sign of asthma, COPD (chronic obstructive pulmonary disease), or another obstructive lung disorder.

- Smaller than normal lungs (restriction). This may be a sign of heart failure, pulmonary fibrosis (scarring of the lung tissue), or another restrictive lung disorder.

Lung Volume Measurement

This test shows the size of your lungs. Abnormal test results may show that you have pulmonary fibrosis or a stiff and/or weak chest wall.

Lung Diffusion Capacity

This test can show a problem with oxygen moving from your lungs into your bloodstream. This may be a sign of loss of lung tissue, emphysema (a type of COPD), or problems with blood flow through the body's arteries.

Tests To Measure Oxygen Level

Pulse oximetry and arterial blood gas tests measure the oxygen level in your blood. These tests show how well your lungs are taking in oxygen and moving it into the bloodstream. A low level of oxygen in the blood may be a sign of a lung or heart disorder.

What Are The Risks Of Lung Function Tests?

Spirometry, lung volume measurement, and lung diffusion capacity tests usually are safe. These tests rarely cause problems.

Pulse oximetry has no risks. Side effects from arterial blood gas tests are rare.

Chapter 6

Patch Tests For Allergies

Patch Tests (Contact Allergy Testing)

Dermatologists apply patch tests in patients with dermatitis, to find out whether their skin condition may be caused or aggravated by a contact allergy. Patch tests are not the same as skin prick tests, which are used to diagnose hay fever allergy (house dust mite, grass pollens, and cat dander). Skin prick tests have very limited value for patients with skin rashes.

The patch testing described here is as it is undertaken in Hamilton, New Zealand. There may be slight differences in methods used at other centers—if you are having patch tests done, ask your dermatologist to explain.

A range of substances can be used for patch testing. The European Standard Series of allergens (or similar) is applied to nearly every patient, together with specific tests appropriate to the individual. Each substance (known as an allergen) has been tested to find the best concentration to demonstrate an allergic reaction without causing irritation to those who are not allergic to the material.

Sometimes the results can be inconclusive or misleading. Instead of one or two positive reactions, sometimes nearly all test areas become red and itchy. This is known as "angry back" and is most likely to occur in those with very active dermatitis (false positive result). At other times, there may be little or no apparent reaction to a substance that regularly causes dermatitis in that person (false negative result).

Further testing may be necessary. Patch tests do not always explain the cause of dermatitis.

The Appointments

The first appointment will take about half an hour. Tiny quantities of 25 to 150 materials in individual square plastic or round aluminium chambers are applied to the upper back. They are kept in place with special hypoallergenic adhesive tape. The patches stay in place undisturbed for 48 hours.

At the second appointment, usually two days later, the patches will be removed. Sometimes further patches are applied. The back is marked with an indelible black felt tip pen or other suitable marker to identify the test sites.

These marks must still be visible at the third appointment, usually two days later (four days after application). The back should be checked and if necessary remarked on several occasions between the second and third appointments.

The Results

The dermatologist will complete a record form at the second and third appointments (usually 48 and 96 hour readings). The result for each test site is recorded. The system we use is as follows:

- Negative (-)
- Irritant reaction (IR)
- Equivocal/uncertain (+/-)
- Weak positive (+)
- Strong positive (++)
- Extreme reaction (+++)

Irritant reactions include sweat rash, follicular pustules, and burn-like reactions. Uncertain reactions refer to a pink area under the test chamber. Weak positives are slightly elevated pink or red plaques. Strong positives are "papulovesicles," and extreme reactions are blisters or ulcers. The relevance depends on the site and type of dermatitis and the specific allergen. The interpretation of the results requires considerable experience and training.

Notes

- Do not expose your back to the sun for four weeks before your patch tests.
- Wear old clothing; felt tip pen marks can stain clothes.

- Do not swim, rub, or exercise, as the patches may come off.

- Keep the back dry, so no baths, showers, or unnecessary sweating.

- Arrange for someone to remark the test sites with indelible felt tip marker.

Bring Your Own Materials For Testing

Discuss the particular substances with which you come into contact with your dermatologist; you may be asked to bring materials from home or work.

- Provide your dermatologist with data sheets of industrial items with which you are in contact.

- Bring or send all chemical items for testing at least a week before the first appointment so that they can be prepared for testing if necessary.

- Only small quantities are required, for example, a few drops or grains.

- Label items carefully with their common and chemical names—provide data sheets if available.

- Identified food items and plants (if relevant) should be brought fresh to the first appointment; ice block trays are useful to separate items.

- Bring a selection of cosmetics to be tested (up to ten items) including nail varnish, moisturizer, sunscreen, perfume, shampoo. Soap is not usually tested (it always causes a reaction if left on the skin for two days).

- Bring all prescribed and non-prescribed ointments, creams, and lotions that you have used.

- Relevant clothing including rubber gloves and footwear can be tested; about one centimeter of material is needed, taken from seams or other unimportant areas in contact with the affected skin.

Photopatch Tests

Some patients have photopatch tests because their dermatitis develops on skin exposed to the sun (photosensitivity). Two sets of perfumes, antiseptics, plant materials, and sunscreens may be applied. After removal, one set is exposed to a small dose of ultraviolet radiation (UVA). This is not enough to cause a photosensitivity reaction on its own.

45

Adverse Reactions To Patch Tests

Positive patch test results are small areas of active eczema/dermatitis. They will be itchy and may require treatment with topical steroid.

- Occasionally patch test reactions persist for several weeks.

- Patch tests may provoke other areas of dermatitis to recur or to appear for the first time.

- Although hypoallergenic tape is used, occasionally people react to all areas in contact with the tape.

- An "angry back" reaction may arise, particularly in a patient with active dermatitis at the time of testing, or in someone who has multiple positive reactions. "Angry back" refers to false positives to many or all of the tested allergens.

- Rarely, sensitization to a new allergen may occur as a result of the test—this is revealed as a reaction occurring around 10 days after the test was applied.

- Retesting may be required, sometimes one allergen at a time, to confirm or clarify a reaction.

Chapter 7

Allergy Blood Testing

At A Glance

Why Get Tested?

To screen for allergies; sometimes to monitor the effectiveness of immunotherapy (desensitization) treatment.

When To Get Tested?

When you have symptoms such as hives, dermatitis, nasal congestion, red itchy eyes, asthma, or abdominal pain that your doctor suspects may be caused by an allergy.

Sample Required?

A blood sample drawn from a vein in your arm.

Test Preparation Needed?

None.

The Test Sample

What is being tested?

This test measures the amount of allergen-specific immunoglobulin E (IgE) in the blood in order to detect an allergy to a particular substance. IgE is a protein associated with allergic

About This Chapter: "Allergy Blood Testing: At a Glance, Test Sample, Test, Common Questions," © 2012 American Association for Clinical Chemistry. Reprinted with permission. For additional information about clinical lab testing, visit the Lab Tests Online website at www.labtestsonline.org.

reactions; it is normally found in very small amounts in the blood. IgE is an antibody that functions as part of the body's immune system, its defense against "intruders." When someone with a predisposition to allergies is exposed to a potential allergen, such as food, grass, or animal dander, for the first time, they become sensitized. Their body perceives the potential allergen as a foreign substance and produces a specific IgE antibody that binds to specialized mast cells in the skin, respiratory system, and gastrointestinal tract, and to basophils in the blood stream. With the next exposure, these attached IgE antibodies recognize the allergen and cause the mast and basophil cells to release histamine and other chemicals, resulting in an allergic reaction that begins at the exposure site.

Each allergen-specific IgE antibody test performed is separate and very specific: honeybee versus bumblebee, egg white versus egg yolk, giant ragweed versus western ragweed. Groupings of these tests, such as food panels or regional weed, grass, and mold panels, can be done. Alternatively, the doctor may pick and choose selectively from a long list of individual allergens suspected of causing a person's allergies.

The allergen-specific IgE test can be done using a variety of methods. The traditional method that has been used is the RAST (radioallergosorbent test), but it has been largely replaced in most laboratories with the newer IgE-specific immunoassay method. Some doctors refer to all IgE allergy tests as RAST even though this is a specific methodology and may not be the exact assay that the testing lab is using.

Allergy Blood Testing Terms

Also Known As: RAST test; Radioallergosorbent test; Allergy screen

Formal Name: Allergen-specific IgE antibody test

Related Tests: Total IgE; Complete blood count (CBC); White blood cell differential count; Eosinophil count; Basophil count

---

How is the sample collected for testing?

A blood sample is obtained by inserting a needle into a vein in the arm.

NOTE: If undergoing medical tests makes you or someone you care for anxious, embarrassed, or even difficult to manage, you might consider reading one or more of the following articles [available from the American Association for Clinical Chemistry online at http://labtestsonline.org]: "Coping with Test Pain, Discomfort, and Anxiety," "Tips on Blood

Testing," "Tips to Help Children through Their Medical Tests," and "Tips to Help the Elderly through Their Medical Tests." Another article, "Follow That Sample," provides a glimpse at the collection and processing of a blood sample and throat culture.

Is any test preparation needed to ensure the quality of the sample?

No test preparation is needed.

The Test

How is it used?

The allergen-specific IgE antibody test is a blood test used to screen for an allergy to a specific substance or substances if a person presents with acute or chronic allergy-like symptoms. This is especially true if symptoms are recurrent and appear to be tied to triggers, such as exposures to particular foods or environments, and if other family members are known to have allergies.

A variety of different types of allergy tests may be performed by exposing a person to different substances under careful medical supervision (see "Common Questions," #1, below). The usefulness of these tests, however, can be affected by skin conditions, such as significant dermatitis or eczema, and by medications, such as histamines and some anti-depressants. With some tests there is also the potential for severe reactions, including a severe reaction that may be life-threatening. In these cases, the allergen-specific IgE antibody test may be ordered as an alternative, as it is performed on a blood sample and does not have an effect on the person being tested.

The allergen-specific IgE antibody test may also be done to monitor immunotherapy (desensitization) or to see if a child has outgrown an allergy. It can only be used in a general way, however, as the level of IgE present does not correlate to the severity of an allergic reaction, and someone who has outgrown an allergy may have a positive IgE for many years afterward.

When is it ordered?

One or more allergen-specific IgE antibody tests are usually ordered when a person has signs or symptoms that suggest an allergy to one or more substances. Signs and symptoms may include:

- Hives
- Dermatitis

- Eczema

- Red itchy eyes

- Coughing, nasal congestion, sneezing

- Asthma

- Itching and tingling in the mouth

- Abdominal pain, or vomiting and diarrhea

A test may also be ordered occasionally to help evaluate the effectiveness of immunotherapy or to determine whether a child has outgrown an allergy.

What does the test result mean?

Negative results indicate that a person probably does not have a "true allergy," an IgE-mediated response to that specific allergen, but the results of allergen-specific IgE antibody tests must always be interpreted and used with caution and the advice of the doctor. Even if an IgE test is negative, there is still a small chance that a person does have an allergy.

Elevated results usually indicate an allergy, but even if the specific IgE test is positive, a person may or may not ever have an actual physical allergic reaction when exposed to that substance. The amount of specific IgE present does not necessarily predict the potential severity of a reaction. A person's clinical history and additional medically supervised allergy tests may be necessary to confirm an allergy diagnosis.

Is there anything else I should know?

Sometimes your doctor will look at other blood tests for an indirect indication of an ongoing allergic process, including a total IgE level or a complete blood count (CBC) and white blood cell differential (specifically eosinophils and basophils). Increases in these test results may suggest an allergy, but they may also be elevated for other reasons.

Common Questions

1. What other tests are available for allergy testing?

Skin prick or scratch tests, patch tests, and oral food challenges are usually done by an allergist or dermatologist. Your doctor may also try eliminating foods from your diet and then reintroducing them to find out what you are allergic to. It is important that these tests be done under close medical supervision, as a life-threatening anaphylactic reaction is possible.

2. My allergy test was negative, but I am having symptoms. What else could it be?

You could have a genetic hypersensitivity problem, such as sensitivity to gluten with celiac disease or have an enzyme deficiency, such as a lactase deficiency causing lactose intolerance. It could also be an allergy-like condition that is not mediated by IgE for which there are no specific laboratory tests. Or it could be another disease that is causing allergy-like symptoms. It is important to investigate your individual situation with your doctor's assistance.

3. My allergy symptoms are generally mild. How serious is this really?

Allergic reactions are very individual. They can be mild or severe, vary from exposure to exposure, get worse over time (or may not), involve the whole body, and can sometimes be fatal.

4. Will my allergies ever go away?

Although children do outgrow some allergies, adults usually do not. Allergies that cause the worst reactions, such as anaphylaxis caused by peanuts, do not usually go away. Avoidance of the allergen and advance preparation for accidental exposure, in the form of medications such as antihistamines and portable epinephrine injections, is the safest course. Immunotherapy can help decrease symptoms for some unavoidable allergies, but they won't work for food and the treatment, which usually consists of years of regular injections, may need to be continued indefinitely.

5. Why am I told to avoid fresh fruit when my allergy is to tree pollen?

There are cross-reactions between some airborne allergens and fruit proteins. Your body thinks it is detecting tree pollen and creates an allergic reaction to the fruit. It is, however, a relatively rare occurrence.

Chapter 8

Allergy Shots (Immunotherapy)

Immunotherapy (commonly called allergy shots) is a form of treatment to reduce an allergic reaction to allergens. Immunotherapy consists of a series of injections (shots) with a solution containing the allergens that cause your symptoms. Treatment usually begins with a weak solution given once or twice a week. The strength of the solution is gradually increased with each dose. Once the strongest dosage is reached, the injections are often given once a month to control symptoms. At that point, sensitivity to the allergens has been decreased, and a person has reached a maintenance level.

Though not a cure, allergy shots can significantly reduce allergy symptoms in some people who are unable to avoid allergens and who do not respond well to other medications.

Allergy shots should always be given at your healthcare provider's office.

Research has shown that allergy shots can reduce symptoms of:

- Allergic rhinitis (hay fever)

- Grass, weed and tree pollen allergies

- Allergic asthma

- Dust mites allergy

- Animal dander allergy

- Insect sting allergy

About This Chapter: "Allergy Shots (Immunotherapy)," December 2011. Copyright © National Jewish Health (www.njhealth.org). All rights reserved. Used by permission.

Allergy shots are less effective against molds and are not a useful method for the treatment of food allergy.

When To Consider Immunotherapy

If you are thinking of allergy shots, ask your healthcare provider about a referral to a board certified allergist. A board certified allergist will follow a number of steps to evaluate if allergy shots are right for you.

The allergist will ask you questions about your history, environment, and symptoms. This will help determine if skin testing is needed. Prick skin testing may be done. This will help identify the specific allergens that are causing your symptoms. Skin testing should only be done under the supervision of a board certified allergist.

Once an allergy has been identified, the next step is to decrease or eliminate exposure to the allergen. This is called environmental control. Evidence shows that allergy and asthma symptoms may improve over time, if the recommended environmental control changes are made. For example, removing furry or feathered pets or following control measures for house dust mites and cockroaches may decrease symptoms. Preventing your contact with grasses, weeds, and tree pollen may be more difficult. Closing outside doors and windows and using air conditioning decreases exposure in the home.

Next, your healthcare provider may recommend medication. Antihistamines and nasal medications may be recommended. Allergy shots may be recommended for people with severe hay fever. They may also be recommended for people with allergic asthma when the allergen cannot be avoided. Allergy shots should be prescribed only by a board certified allergist.

Length Of Time

Six months to a year of allergy shots may be required before you notice any improvement in symptoms. If your symptoms do not improve after this time, ask you allergist to review your overall treatment program. If the treatment is effective, the shots often continue three to five years, until the person is symptom-free or until symptoms can be controlled with mild medications for one year. In general, allergy shots should be stopped if they are not effective within two to three years.

Alternatives

There are a number of alternative treatments that claim to "cure" allergies. These methods are not supported by scientific studies, and they are not approved by the American Academy of Allergy and Immunology. Unapproved alternative treatments include:

- high-dose vitamin and mineral therapy

- urine injections

- bacterial vaccines

- exotic diets

It can be easy to feel overwhelmed or confused by the many different methods of allergy testing and treatment. It is best to work with a board certified allergist to evaluate and determine what is appropriate for you.

"Rush Immunotherapy"

"Rush immunotherapy" is a series of allergy shots. They are given over two to three days in a row. This "rushes" the initial phase of the treatment. Increasing doses of allergen extract are given every 30 minutes to hourly instead of every few days or weeks. There is an increased risk of a reaction with this procedure. Therefore, rush immunotherapy should only be done in a hospital or high-risk procedure area under very close supervision.

Chapter 9

Medications Used To Treat Allergic Symptoms

Antihistamines

Histamine is one of the chemicals released when antibodies overreact to allergens. It is the cause of many symptoms of allergic rhinitis. Antihistamines can help relieve:

- Itching, sneezing, and runny nose (unless combined with a decongestant, antihistamines do not work well for relieving nasal congestion).

- Other allergy symptoms unrelated to rhinitis, including hives and some rashes

If possible, patients should take antihistamines before an anticipated allergy attack.

Many antihistamines are available. They include short-acting and long-acting forms, and come in oral pill and nasal spray forms.

Antihistamines are generally categorized as first- and second-generation. First-generation antihistamines, which include diphenhydramine (Benadryl, generic) and clemastine (Tavist, generic) cause more severe side effects (such as drowsiness) than most newer second-generation antihistamines. For this reason, second-generation antihistamines are generally preferred and recommended over first-generation antihistamines.

There are some notes of caution when taking any antihistamine:

- Antihistamines may thicken mucus secretions and can worsen bacterial rhinitis or sinusitis.

- Antihistamines can lose their effectiveness over time, and a different one may need to be tried.

About This Chapter: Excerpted from "Allergic Rhinitis," © 2012 A.D.A.M., Inc. Reprinted with permission.

Second-generation antihistamines are sometimes referred to collectively as nonsedating antihistamines. However, cetirizine (Zyrtec, generic) and the nasal spray antihistamines (Astelin, Patanase) can cause drowsiness when taken at recommended doses. Loratadine (Claritin, generic) and desloratadine (Clarinex) can cause drowsiness when taken at doses exceeding the recommended dose.

Brand Names

Second-generation antihistamines in pill form include:

- Loratadine (Claritin, generic): Loratadine is available over-the-counter and is approved for children ages two and older. Loraine-D (Claritin-D) combines the antihistamine with the decongestant pseudoephedrine. Desloratadine (Clarinex) is similar to Claritin but stronger and longer-lasting. It is available only by prescription.

- Cetirizine (Zyrtec, generic): Cetirizine is approved for both indoor and outdoor allergies. It is the only antihistamine to date approved for infants as young as six months. It is available over-the-counter. Cetirizine-D (Zyrtec-D) is a pill that combines the antihistamine with the decongestant pseudoephedrine.

- Fexofenadine (Allegra, generic) is also available over-the-counter.

- Levocetirizine (Xyzal) is a prescription medication approved to treat seasonal allergic rhinitis in patients age two years and older. It is available in both pill and liquid form.

- Acrivastine and pseudoephedrine (Semprex-D) is a pill that combines an antihistamine and decongestant.

Second-generation antihistamines in nasal form are as good as or better than the oral forms for treatment of seasonal allergic rhinitis. However, they can cause drowsiness, and are not as effective for allergic rhinitis as nasal corticosteroids. Nasal spray antihistamines are available by prescription and include:

- Azelastine (Astelin, Astepro)

- Olopatadine (Patanase)

Side Effects And Precautions.

- Common side effects include headache, dry mouth, and dry nose. (These are often only temporary and go away during treatment.)

- Drowsiness occurs in about 10% of adults and in 2–4% of children. The nasal spray forms of second-generation antihistamines cause more drowsiness than the pill forms.

- Extended-release forms of loratadine and cetirizine have other ingredients that can cause other symptoms, including nervousness, restlessness, and insomnia.

Nasal Corticosteroids

Corticosteroids help reduce the inflammatory response associated with allergic reactions. Nasal-spray corticosteroids (commonly called steroids) are considered the most effective drugs for controlling the symptoms of moderate-to-severe allergic rhinitis. They are often used either alone or in combination with second-generation oral antihistamines. The benefits of nasal spray steroids include:

- Reducing inflammation and mucus production

- Improving night sleep and daytime alertness in patients with chronic allergic rhinitis

- Treating polyps in the nasal passages

Nasal-Spray Brands

Corticosteroids available in nasal spray form include:

- Triamcinolone (Nasacort, generic). Approved for patients age two and older.

- Mometasone furoate (Nasonex). Approved of patients age three and older.

- Fluticasone (Flonase, generic). Approved for patients age two and older.

- Beclomethasone (Beconase, Vancenase, generic). Approved for patients age six and older.

- Flunisolide (Nasarel, generic). Approved for patients age six and older.

- Budesonide (Rhinocort, generic). Approved for patients age six and older.

- Ciclesonide (Alvesco, Omnaris). Approved for patients age 12 and older.

Side Effects

Corticosteroids are powerful anti-inflammatory drugs. Although oral steroids can have many side effects, the nasal-spray form affects only local areas and has less risk for widespread side effects unless the drug is used excessively. Side effects of nasal steroids may include:

- Dryness, burning, stinging in the nasal passage

- Sneezing

- Headaches and nosebleed (uncommon but should be reported to your doctor immediately)

Possible Long-Term Complications

All corticosteroids suppress stress hormones. This effect is known to produce some serious long-term complications in people who take oral steroids. Researchers have found far fewer concerns with nasal administration or inhaled forms, but there may be certain problems:

- **Effect On Growth:** The major concern for children is whether nasal steroids, like other forms of steroids, will adversely affect growth. Different steroids may be absorbed differently or may stay longer in the body. Growth impairment from nasal corticosteroid sprays taken at correct dosages has not been demonstrated. Most children who take only recommended dosages of nasal sprays, and do not also take inhaled corticosteroids for asthma, will not have any problems.

- **Effect On Eyes:** Glaucoma is a known side effect of oral steroids. Some ophthalmologists have observed higher pressure in the eye (a sign of glaucoma) in some patients taking nasal steroid sprays, particularly those taking higher dosages or those who also take inhaled corticosteroids for asthma. However, studies to date have not shown an increased risk for glaucoma. Periodic eye examinations are advised.

- **Use During Pregnancy:** Steroids are most likely safe during pregnancy, but pregnant women should talk to their doctors before taking them.

- **Nasal Passage Injury:** Steroid sprays may injure the nasal septum (the bony area that separates the nasal passage) if the spray is directed onto it. This complication is very rare.

- **Lower Resistance To Infection:** People with any infectious disease or injury in the nose should not take these drugs until the disease or wound has been treated and cured.

Cromolyn

Cromolyn serves as both an anti-inflammatory drug and a specific blocker for allergens. The standard cromolyn nasal spray (Nasalcrom, generic) is not as effective as steroid nasal sprays but does work well for many people with mild allergies. It is one of the preferred first-line therapies for pregnant women with mild allergic rhinitis. It may take up to three weeks to experience full benefit.

Side Effects

Cromolyn has no major side effects, but minor ones include nasal congestion, coughing, sneezing, wheezing, nausea, nosebleeds, and dry throat. The spray can cause burning or irritation.

Leukotriene Antagonists

Leukotriene antagonists are oral drugs that block leukotrienes, powerful immune system factors that cause airway constriction and mucus production in allergy-related asthma. They appear to work as well as antihistamines for treatment of allergic rhinitis, but are not as effective as nasal corticosteroids.

Leukotriene antagonists include zafirlukast (Accolate) and montelukast (Singulair). These drugs are mainly used to treat asthma. Montelukast is also approved to treat seasonal allergies and indoor allergies.

The U.S. Food and Drug Administration (FDA) warns that these drugs have been associated with behavior and mood changes, including agitation, aggression, anxiousness, dream abnormalities, hallucinations, depression, insomnia, irritability, restlessness, tremor, and suicidal thinking and behavior. Patients who take a leukotriene antagonist drug such as montelukast should be monitored for signs of behavioral and mood changes. Doctors should consider discontinuing the drug if patients exhibit any of these symptoms.

Decongestants

Decongestants work by shrinking blood vessels in the nose. Many over-the-counter decongestants are available, which can be either taken by mouth or applied to the nose.

Nasal Decongestants

Nasal-delivery decongestants are applied directly into the nasal passages with a spray, gel, drops, or vapors. Nasal decongestants come in long-acting or short-acting forms. The effects of short-acting decongestants last about four hours. Long-acting decongestants last 6–12 hours. The active ingredients in nasal decongestants include oxymetazoline, xylometazoline, and phenylephrine. Nasal forms work faster than oral decongestants and may not cause as much drowsiness. However, they can cause dependency and rebound.

The major problem with nasal-delivery decongestants, particularly long-acting forms, is a cycle of dependency and rebound effects. The 12-hour brands pose a particular risk for this effect.

- With prolonged use (more than 3–5 days), nasal decongestants lose effectiveness and can cause swelling in the nasal passages.

- The patient then increases the frequency of the dose. As the congestion worsens, the patient may respond with even more frequent doses.

- This causes dependency and increased nasal congestion.

The following precautions are important for people taking nasal decongestants:

- When using a nasal spray, spray each nostril once. Wait a minute to allow absorption into the mucosal tissues, and then spray again.

- Do not share droppers and inhalers with other people.

- Discard sprayers, inhalers, or other decongestant delivery devices when the medication is no longer needed. Over time, these devices can become reservoirs for bacteria.

- Discard the medicine if it becomes cloudy or unclear.

- DO NOT USE NASAL DECONGESTANTS FOR LONGER THAN THREE DAYS.

Oral Decongestants

Oral decongestants also come in many brands, which have similar ingredients. The most common active ingredients are pseudoephedrine (Sudafed, other brands, generic) and phenylephrine, sometimes in combination with an antihistamine. Oral decongestants can cause side effects such as insomnia, irritability, nervousness, and heart palpitations. Taking pseudoephedrine in the morning, as opposed to later in the day or before bedtime, can help patients avoid these side effects.

Individuals At Risk For Complications From Decongestants

People who may be at higher risk for complications are those with certain medical conditions, including disorders that make blood vessels highly susceptible to contraction. Such conditions include:

- Heart disease
- High blood pressure
- Thyroid disease
- Diabetes

- Prostate problems that cause urinary difficulties

- Migraines

- Raynaud phenomenon

- High sensitivity to cold

- Emphysema or chronic bronchitis. (People with these conditions should particularly avoid high-potency, short-acting nasal decongestant.)

Anyone with these conditions should not use oral or nasal decongestants without a doctor's guidance. Other people who should not use decongestants without first consulting a doctor include:

- Pregnant women

- Children. Children appear to metabolize decongestants differently than adults. Decongestants should not be used at all in infants and children under the age of four years, and some doctors recommend not giving them to children under the age of 14. Children are at particular risk for central nervous system side effects, including convulsions, rapid heart rates, loss of consciousness, and death.

Decongestants can cause dangerous interactions when combined with certain types of medications, such as the antidepressant MAO inhibitors. They can also serious problems when combined with methamphetamines or diet pills. Be sure to tell your doctor about any drug or herbal remedy you are taking. Caffeine can also increase the stimulant side effects of pseudoephedrine.

Nasal Ipratropium

Ipratropium bromide (Atrovent, generic) is a prescription nasal spray that can help relieve runny nose. It works best when given in combination with a nasal corticosteroid. Side effects include nasal dryness, nosebleeds, and sore throat. It should not be used by people who have glaucoma or men who have an enlarged prostate gland.

Chapter 10

Epinephrine Injections For Life-Threatening Allergic Reactions

Why is this medicine prescribed?

Epinephrine injection is used along with emergency medical treatment to treat life-threatening allergic reactions caused by insect bites or stings, foods, medications, latex, and other causes. Epinephrine is in a class of medications called alpha- and beta-adrenergic agonists (sympathomimetic agents). It works by relaxing the muscles in the airways and tightening the blood vessels.

How should this medicine be used?

Epinephrine injection comes as a pre-filled automatic injection device containing a solution (liquid) to inject under the skin or into the muscle in the outer side of the thigh. It is usually injected as needed at the first sign of a serious allergic reaction. Use epinephrine injection exactly as directed; do not inject it more often or inject more or less of it than prescribed by your doctor.

You should inject epinephrine injection as soon as you suspect that you may be experiencing a serious allergic reaction. Signs of a serious allergic reaction include closing of the airways, wheezing, sneezing, hoarseness, hives, itching, swelling, skin redness, fast heartbeat, weak pulse, anxiety, confusion, stomach pain, losing control of urine or bowel movements, faintness, or loss of consciousness. Talk to your doctor about these symptoms and be sure you understand how to tell when you are having a serious allergic reaction and should inject epinephrine.

About This Chapter: "Epinephrine Injection," © American Society of Health-System Pharmacists (ASHP), 2013. All rights reserved. Any duplication in any form must be authorized by ASHP.

Brand Names

- Adrenaclick, Adrenalin Chloride Solution, EpiPen Auto-Injector, EpiPen Jr. Auto-Injector, Twinject

Keep your automatic injection device with you or available at all times so that you will be able to inject epinephrine quickly when an allergic reaction begins. Be aware of the expiration date stamped on the device and replace the device when this date passes. Look at the solution in the device from time to time. If the solution is discolored or contains particles, call your doctor to get a new injection device.

Epinephrine injection helps to treat serious allergic reaction but does not take the place of medical treatment. Get emergency medical treatment immediately after you inject epinephrine. Rest quietly while you wait for emergency medical treatment.

Most automatic injection devices contain enough solution for one dose of epinephrine. One type of automatic injection device (Twinject) can be used according to the package directions to inject two doses of epinephrine if needed to treat an allergic reaction. If your doctor has prescribed this device for you, be sure that you know how to inject the second dose and how to tell whether you should inject a second dose.

Ask your doctor or pharmacist to show you or the person who will be injecting the medication how to inject it. Before you use epinephrine injection for the first time, read the patient information that comes with it. This information includes directions for how to use the pre-filled automatic injection device. Be sure to ask your pharmacist or doctor if you have any questions about how to inject this medication.

Epinephrine should be injected only in the middle of the outer side of the thigh, and can be injected through clothing if necessary in an emergency. Do not inject epinephrine into the buttocks or any other part of your body.

After you inject a dose of epinephrine injection, some solution will remain in the injection device. This is normal and does not mean that you did not receive the full dose. Do not use the extra liquid; dispose of the remaining liquid and device properly. Take the used device with you to the emergency room or ask your doctor, pharmacist, or health care provider how to throw away used injection devices safely.

Do not put your thumb, fingers, or hand over the needle area of the automatic injection device. If epinephrine is accidently injected into the fingers, hands, toes, or feet, get emergency medical treatment immediately.

Are there other uses for this medication?

This medication may be prescribed for other uses; ask your doctor or pharmacist for more information.

What special precautions should I follow?

Before using epinephrine injection,

- tell your doctor and pharmacist if you are allergic to epinephrine, any other medications, sulfites, or any of the other ingredients in epinephrine injection. Your doctor may tell you to use epinephrine injection even if you are allergic to one of the ingredients because it is a life-saving medication. The epinephrine automatic injection device does not contain latex and is safe to use if you have a latex allergy.

- tell your doctor and pharmacist what other prescription and nonprescription medications, vitamins, nutritional supplements, and herbal products you are taking or plan to take. Be sure to mention any of the following: certain antidepressants such as amitriptyline (Elavil), amoxapine, clomipramine (Anafranil), desipramine (Norpramin), doxepin (Silenor), imipramine (Tofranil), maprotiline, mirtazapine (Remeron), nortriptyline (Pamelor), protriptyline (Vivactil), and trimipramine (Surmontil); antihistamines such as chlorpheniramine (Chlor-Trimeton) and diphenhydramine (Benadryl); beta blockers such as propranolol (Inderal); digoxin (Digitek, Lanoxicaps, Lanoxin); diuretics ("water pills"); ergot medications such as dihydroergotamine (D.H.E. 45, Migranal), ergoloid mesylates (Hydergine,), ergonovine (Ergotrate), ergotamine (in Cafergot, in Migergot), methylergonovine (Methergine), and methysergide (Sansert); levothyroxine (Levothroid, Levoxyl, Synthroid, Unithroid); and medications for irregular heartbeat such as quinidine. Also tell your doctor if you are taking a monoamine oxidase inhibitor such as isocarboxazid (Marplan), phenelzine (Nardil), selegiline (Eldepryl, Emsam, Zelapar), and tranylcypromine (Parnate) or have stopped taking it within the past two weeks. Your doctor may need to monitor you carefully for side effects.

- tell your doctor if you have or have ever had chest pain, irregular heartbeat, high blood pressure, or other heart disease; diabetes; hyperthyroidism (an overactive thyroid); depression or other mental illness; or Parkinson disease. If you will be using the Twinject device, tell your doctor if you have arthritis or difficulty using your hands.

- tell your doctor if you are pregnant, plan to become pregnant, or are breast-feeding. Talk to your doctor about whether and when you should use epinephrine injection if you are pregnant.

What side effects can this medicine cause?

Epinephrine injection may cause side effects. When you get emergency medical treatment after you inject epinephrine, tell your doctor if you are experiencing any of these side effects:

- difficulty breathing
- pounding, fast, or irregular heartbeat
- nausea
- vomiting
- sweating
- dizziness
- nervousness, anxiety, or restlessness
- weakness
- pale skin
- headache
- uncontrollable shaking of a part of your body

What should I know about storage and disposal of this medication?

Keep this medication in the plastic carrying tube it came in, tightly closed, and out of reach of children. Keep it at room temperature and away from light, excess heat, and moisture (not in the bathroom). Do not refrigerate epinephrine injection or leave it in your car, especially in hot or cold weather. If the pre-filled automatic injection device is dropped, check to see if it is broken or leaking. Throw away any medication that is damaged, outdated or no longer needed and be sure to have a replacement available. Talk to your pharmacist about the proper disposal of your medication.

What should I do in case of overdose?

In case of overdose, call your local poison control center at 1-800-222-1222. If the victim has collapsed or is not breathing, call local emergency services at 911.

Symptoms of overdose may include:

- sudden weakness or numbness on one side of the body
- sudden difficulty speaking

- slow or fast heart rate

- shortness of breath

- fast breathing

- confusion

- tiredness or weakness

- cold, pale skin

- decreased urination

What other information should I know?

Keep all appointments with your doctor.

Do not let anyone else take your medication. If you use a pre-filled automatic injection device, be sure to get a replacement right away. Ask your pharmacist any questions you have about refilling your prescription.

It is important for you to keep a written list of all of the prescription and nonprescription (over-the-counter) medicines you are taking, as well as any products such as vitamins, minerals, or other dietary supplements. You should bring this list with you each time you visit a doctor or if you are admitted to a hospital. It is also important information to carry with you in case of emergencies.

Part Two
Allergy Symptoms And Complications

Chapter 11

Coughing And Sneezing

What Is Cough?

A cough is a natural reflex that protects your lungs. Coughing helps clear your airways of lung irritants, such as smoke and mucus (a slimy substance). This helps prevent infections. A cough also can be a symptom of a medical problem. Prolonged coughing can cause unpleasant side effects, such as chest pain, exhaustion, light-headedness, and loss of bladder control. Coughing also can interfere with sleep, socializing, and work.

Overview

Coughing occurs when the nerve endings in your airways become irritated. The airways are tubes that carry air into and out of your lungs. Certain substances (such as smoke and pollen), medical conditions, and medicines can irritate these nerve endings.

A cough can be acute, subacute, or chronic, depending on how long it lasts.

An acute cough lasts less than three weeks. Common causes of an acute cough are a common cold or other upper respiratory infections. Examples of other upper respiratory infections include the flu, pneumonia, and whooping cough.

A subacute cough lasts three to eight weeks. This type of cough remains even after a cold or other respiratory infection is over.

A chronic cough lasts more than eight weeks. Common causes of a chronic cough are upper airway cough syndrome (UACS), asthma, and gastroesophageal reflux disease (GERD).

About This Chapter: From "Cough," National Heart Lung and Blood Institute (www.nhlbi.nih.gov), October 2010.

UACS is a term used to describe conditions that inflame the upper airways and cause a cough. Examples include sinus infections and allergies. These conditions can cause mucus to run down your throat from the back of your nose. This is called postnasal drip.

Asthma is a long-term lung disease that inflames and narrows the airways. GERD occurs if acid from your stomach backs up into your throat.

Outlook

The best way to treat a cough is to treat its cause. For example, asthma is treated with medicines that open the airways.

Your doctor may recommend cough medicine if the cause of your cough is unknown and the cough causes a lot of discomfort. Cough medicines may harm children. If you have a cough, talk with your doctor about how to treat it.

What Causes Cough?

Coughing occurs when the nerve endings in your airways become irritated. Certain irritants and allergens, medical conditions, and medicines can irritate these nerve endings.

Irritants And Allergens

An irritant is something you're sensitive to. For example, smoking or inhaling secondhand smoke can irritate your lungs. Smoking also can lead to medical conditions that can cause a cough. Other irritants include air pollution, paint fumes, or scented products like perfumes or air fresheners.

An allergen is something you're allergic to, such as dust, animal dander, mold, or pollens from trees, grasses, and flowers.

Coughing helps clear your airways of irritants and allergens. This helps prevent infections.

Medical Conditions

Many medical conditions can cause acute, subacute, or chronic cough. Common causes of an acute cough are a common cold or other upper respiratory infections. Examples of other upper respiratory infections include the flu, pneumonia, and whooping cough. Common causes of a chronic cough are upper airway cough syndrome (UACS), asthma, and gastroesophageal reflux disease (GERD).

Other conditions that can cause a chronic cough include the following:

- **Respiratory Infections:** A cough from an upper respiratory infection can develop into a chronic cough.

- **Chronic Bronchitis:** This condition occurs if the lining of the airways is constantly irritated and inflamed. Smoking is the main cause of chronic bronchitis.

- **Bronchiectasis:** This is a condition in which damage to the airways causes them to widen and become flabby and scarred. This prevents the airways from properly moving mucus out of your lungs. An infection or other condition that injures the walls of the airways usually causes bronchiectasis.

- **Chronic Obstructive Pulmonary Disease:** COPD is a disease that prevents enough air from flowing in and out of the airways.

- **Lung Cancer:** In rare cases, a chronic cough is due to lung cancer. Most people who develop lung cancer smoke or used to smoke.

- **Heart Failure:** Heart failure is a condition in which the heart can't pump enough blood to meet the body's needs. Fluid can build up in the body and lead to many symptoms. If fluid builds up in the lungs, it can cause a chronic cough.

Medicines

Certain medicines can cause a chronic cough. Examples of these medicines are ACE inhibitors and beta blockers. ACE inhibitors are used to treat high blood pressure (HBP). Beta blockers are used to treat HBP, migraine headaches, and glaucoma.

Who Is At Risk For Cough?

People at risk for cough include those with these characteristics:

- Are exposed to things that irritate their airways (called irritants) or things that they're allergic to (called allergens). Examples of irritants are cigarette smoke, air pollution, paint fumes, and scented products. Examples of allergens are dust, animal dander, mold, and pollens from trees, grasses, and flowers.

- Have certain conditions that irritate the lungs, such as asthma, sinus infections, colds, or gastroesophageal reflux disease.

- Smoke. Smoking can irritate your lungs and cause coughing. Smoking and/or exposure to secondhand smoke also can lead to medical conditions that can cause a cough.

- Take certain medicines, such as ACE inhibitors and beta blockers. ACE inhibitors are used to treat high blood pressure (HBP). Beta blockers are used to treat HBP, migraine headaches, and glaucoma.

- Women are more likely than men to develop a chronic cough.

What Are The Signs And Symptoms Of Cough?

When you cough, mucus (a slimy substance) may come up. Coughing helps clear the mucus in your airways from a cold, bronchitis, or other condition. Rarely, people cough up blood. If this happens, you should call your doctor right away.

A cough may be a symptom of a medical condition. Thus, it may occur with other signs and symptoms of that condition. For example, if you have a cold, you may have a runny or stuffy nose. If you have gastroesophageal reflux disease, you may have a sour taste in your mouth.

What Makes Me Sneeze?

AHHH . . . CHOO!

If you just sneezed, something was probably irritating or tickling the inside of your nose. Sneezing, also called sternutation, is your body's way of removing an irritation from your nose.

When the inside of your nose gets a tickle, a message is sent to a special part of your brain called the sneeze center. The sneeze center then sends a message to all the muscles that have to work together to create the amazingly complicated process that we call the sneeze.

Some of the muscles involved are the abdominal (belly) muscles, the chest muscles, the diaphragm (the large muscle beneath your lungs that makes you breathe), the muscles that control your vocal cords, and muscles in the back of your throat. Don't forget the eyelid muscles! Did you know that you always close your eyes when you sneeze?

It is the job of the sneeze center to make all these muscles work together, in just the right order, to send that irritation flying out of your nose. And fly it does—sneezing can send tiny particles speeding out of your nose at up to 100 miles per hour!

Most anything that can irritate the inside of your nose can start a sneeze. Some common things include dust, cold air, or pepper. When you catch a cold in your nose, a virus has made a temporary home there and is causing lots of swelling and irritation. Some people have allergies, and they sneeze when they are exposed to certain things, such as animal dander

A chronic cough can make you feel tired because you use a lot of energy to cough. It also can prevent you from sleeping well and interfere with work and socializing. A chronic cough also can cause headaches, chest pain, loss of bladder control, sweating, and, rarely, fractured ribs.

How Is The Cause Of Cough Diagnosed?

Your doctor will diagnose the cause of your cough based on your medical history, a physical exam, and test results.

Medical History

Your doctor will likely ask questions about your cough. He or she may ask how long you've had it, whether you're coughing anything up (such as mucus), and how much you cough. Your doctor also may ask about other things:

- About your medical history, including whether you have allergies, asthma, or other medical conditions.

(which comes from the skin of many common pets) or pollen (which comes from some plants).

Do you know anyone who sneezes when they step outside into the sunshine? About one out of every three people sneezes when exposed to bright light. They are called photic sneezers (photic means light). If you are a photic sneezer, you got it from one of your parents because it is an inherited trait. You could say that it runs in your family. Most people have some sensitivity to light that can trigger a sneeze.

Have you ever had the feeling that you are about to sneeze, but it just gets stuck? Next time that happens, try looking toward a bright light briefly (but don't look right into the sun)—see if that doesn't unstick a stuck sneeze!

ACHOO

When some people are exposed to bright light, they sneeze. This condition is called photic sneezing, but the scientific name is autosomal dominant compelling helio-ophthalmic outburst syndrome (helio means sun and ophthalmic means eyes). To make it easier to say and remember, scientists and doctors shortened it to ACHOO syndrome.

- Whether you have heartburn or a sour taste in your mouth. These may be signs of gastroesophageal reflux disease (GERD).

- Whether you've recently had a cold or the flu.

- Whether you smoke or spend time around others who smoke.

- Whether you've been around air pollution, a lot of dust, or fumes.

Physical Exam

To check for signs of problems related to cough, your doctor will use a stethoscope to listen to your lungs. He or she will listen for wheezing (a whistling or squeaky sound when you breathe) or other abnormal sounds.

Diagnostic Tests

Your doctor may recommend tests based on the results of your medical history and physical exam. For example, if you have symptoms of GERD, your doctor may recommend a pH probe. This test measures the acid level of the fluid in your throat.

Other tests may include some of these:

- An exam of the mucus from your nose or throat. This test can show whether you have a bacterial infection.

- A chest x-ray. A chest x-ray takes a picture of your heart and lungs. This test can help diagnose conditions such as pneumonia and lung cancer.

- Lung function tests. These tests measure how much air you can breathe in and out, how fast you can breathe air out, and how well your lungs deliver oxygen to your blood. Lung function tests can help diagnose asthma and other conditions.

- An x-ray of the sinuses. This test can help diagnose a sinus infection.

How Is Cough Treated?

The best way to treat a cough is to treat its cause. However, sometimes the cause is unknown. Other treatments, such as medicines and a vaporizer, can help relieve the cough itself.

Treating The Cause Of A Cough

Acute And Subacute Cough: An acute cough lasts less than three weeks. Common causes of an acute cough are a common cold or other upper respiratory infections. Examples of other upper respiratory infections include the flu, pneumonia, and whooping cough. An acute cough usually goes away after the illness that caused it is over. A subacute cough lasts three to eight weeks. This type of cough remains even after a cold or other respiratory infection is over.

Studies show that antibiotics and cold medicines can't cure a cold. However, your doctor may prescribe medicines to treat another cause of an acute or subacute cough. For example, antibiotics may be given for pneumonia.

Chronic Cough: Common causes of a chronic cough are upper airway cough syndrome (UACS), asthma, and gastroesophageal reflux disease (GERD). If you have a sinus infection, your doctor may prescribe antibiotics. He or she also may suggest you use a medicine that you spray into your nose. If allergies are causing your cough, your doctor may advise you to avoid the substances that you're allergic to (allergens) if possible.

If you have asthma, try to avoid irritants and allergens that make your asthma worse. Take your asthma medicines as your doctor prescribes.

GERD occurs if acid from your stomach backs up into your throat. Your doctor may prescribe a medicine to reduce acid in your stomach. You also may be able to relieve GERD symptoms by waiting three to four hours after a meal before lying down, and by sleeping with your head raised.

Smoking also can cause a chronic cough. If you smoke, it's important to quit. Talk with your doctor about programs and products that can help you quit smoking. Also, try to avoid secondhand smoke.

Many hospitals have programs that help people quit smoking, or hospital staff can refer you to a program.

Other causes of a chronic cough include respiratory infections, chronic bronchitis, bronchiectasis, lung cancer, and heart failure. Treatments for these causes may include medicines, procedures, and other therapies. Treatment also may include avoiding irritants and allergens and quitting smoking.

If your chronic cough is due to a medicine you're taking, your doctor may prescribe a different medicine.

Treating The Cough Rather Than The Cause

Coughing is important because it helps clear your airways of irritants, such as smoke and mucus (a slimy substance). Coughing also helps prevent infections.

Cough medicines usually are used only when the cause of the cough is unknown and the cough causes a lot of discomfort.

Medicines can help control a cough and make it easier to cough up mucus. Your doctor may recommend medicines such as these:

- **Prescription Cough Suppressants** (also called antitussives): These medicines can help relieve a cough. However, they're usually used when nothing else works. No evidence shows that over-the-counter cough suppressants relieve a cough.

- **Expectorants:** These medicines may loosen mucus, making it easier to cough up.

- **Bronchodilators:** These medicines relax your airways.

Other treatments also may relieve an irritated throat and loosen mucus. Examples include using a cool-mist humidifier or steam vaporizer and drinking enough fluids. Examples of fluids are water, soup, and juice. Ask your doctor how much fluid you need.

Cough In Children

No evidence shows that cough and cold medicines help children recover more quickly from colds. These medicines can even harm children. Talk with your doctor about cough and how to treat it.

Living With Cough

If you have a cough, you can take steps to recover from the condition that's causing the cough. You also can take steps to relieve your cough. Ongoing care and lifestyle changes can help you.

Ongoing Care

Follow the treatment plan your doctor gives you for treating the cause of your cough. Take all medicines as your doctor prescribes. If you're using antibiotics, continue to take the medicine until it's all gone. You may start to feel better before you finish the medicine, but you should continue to take it.

Ask your doctor about ways to relieve your cough. He or she may recommend cough medicines. These medicines usually are used only when the cause of a cough is unknown and the cough is causing a lot of discomfort.

A cool-mist humidifier or steam vaporizer may help relieve an irritated throat and loosen mucus. Getting enough fluids (for example, water, soup, or juice) may have the same effect. Ask your doctor about how much fluid you need.

Your doctor will let you know when to schedule followup care.

Lifestyle Changes

If you smoke, quit. Ask your doctor about programs and products that can help you quit smoking.

Try to avoid irritants and allergens that make you cough. Examples of irritants include cigarette smoke, air pollution, paint fumes, and scented products like perfumes or air fresheners. Examples of allergens include dust, animal dander, mold, and pollens from trees, grasses, and flowers.

Follow a healthy diet and be as physically active as you can. A healthy diet includes a variety of fruits, vegetables, and whole grains. It also includes lean meats, poultry, fish, and fat-free or low-fat milk or milk products. A healthy diet also is low in saturated fat, trans fat, cholesterol, sodium (salt), and added sugar.

Chapter 12

Allergic Rhinitis

Allergic rhinitis is the body's response to outdoor or indoor allergens. Outdoor triggers of allergic rhinitis include ragweed, grass, tree pollen, and mold spores. Indoor triggers include dust mites, pet dander, or mold that grows in humid indoor places such as carpets. Outdoor allergens cause seasonal allergic rhinitis (also known as hay fever), which typically occurs during the spring and summer. Indoor allergens can cause perennial (year-round) allergic rhinitis.

Allergic rhinitis tends to run in families. If one or both parents have allergic rhinitis, there is a high likelihood that their children will also have allergic rhinitis. People with allergic rhinitis have an increased risk of developing asthma and other allergies. They are also at risk for developing sinusitis, sleep disorders (including snoring and sleep apnea), nasal polyps, and ear infections.

Introduction

The nose is separated into two passages by a wall of cartilage called the septum. The nasal passages are lined with a membrane that produces a clear liquid called mucus. Mucus is a one of the body's defense systems:

- Moisture from the mucus conditions the air before it reaches the lungs.

- The mucus traps small particles and bacteria, which may enter the nose as a person breathes.

- The trapped bacteria usually do not cause harm in healthy individuals.

- When one side of the nose is congested, air passes through the open (decongested) side. The sides normally alternate between being wide-open and partly or completely blocked.

If the congestion becomes severe or other changes occur that irritate the nasal passage, rhinitis develops. Rhinitis is inflammation of the nasal passages. To be diagnosed with rhinitis, a patient must experience at least two of the following symptoms for an hour or more on most days:

- Runny nose
- Nasal congestion
- Nasal itching
- Sneezing

These symptoms may occur as a result of colds or environmental irritants such as allergens, cigarette smoke, chemicals, changes in temperature, stress, exercise, or other factors.

- **Infectious Rhinitis:** If symptoms last fewer than six weeks, the condition is referred to as acute rhinitis and is usually caused by a cold or infection, or temporary overexposure to environmental chemicals or pollutants.

- **Chronic Rhinitis:** When rhinitis lasts for a longer period, the condition is called chronic rhinitis. Allergies are often the cause, but structural problems or chronic infections could also be to blame.

- **Allergic Rhinitis:** Allergic rhinitis is rhinitis caused by allergens, which are substances that trigger an allergic response. Allergens involved in allergic rhinitis come from either outdoor or indoor substances. Outdoor allergens such as pollen or mold spores are usually the cause of seasonal allergic rhinitis (also called hay fever). Indoor allergens such as animal dander or dust mites are common causes of perennial (year-round) allergic rhinitis.

Causes

The allergic process, called atopy, occurs when the body overreacts to a substance that it senses as a foreign "invader." The immune system works continuously to protect the body from potentially dangerous intruders such as bacteria, viruses, and toxins. However, for reasons not completely understood, some people are hypersensitive to substances that are typically harmless. When the immune system inaccurately identifies these substances (allergens) as harmful, an allergic reaction and inflammatory response occurs.

The antibody immunoglobulin E (IgE) is a key player in allergic reactions. When an allergen enters the body, the immune system produces IgE antibodies. These antibodies then attach themselves to mast cells, which are found in the nose, eyes, lungs, and digestive tract.

The mast cells release inflammatory chemical mediators, such as histamine, that cause atopic symptoms (sneezing, coughing, wheezing). The mast cells continue to produce more inflammatory chemicals that stimulate the production of more IgE, continuing the allergic process.

There are many types of IgE antibodies, and each are associated with a specific allergen. This is why some people are allergic to cat dander, while others are not bothered by cats yet are allergic to pollen. In allergic rhinitis, the allergic reaction begins when an allergen comes into contact with the mucous membranes in the lining of the nose.

Triggers Of Seasonal Allergic Rhinitis (Hay Fever)

Seasonal allergic rhinitis occurs only during periods of intense airborne pollen or spores. It is commonly, although inaccurately, called hay fever. No fever accompanies this condition, and the allergic response is not dependent on hay. In general, triggers of seasonal allergy in the U.S. include:

- **Ragweed:** Ragweed is the most dominant cause of allergic rhinitis in the U.S., affecting about 75% of allergy sufferers. One plant can release one million pollen grains a day. Ragweed occurs everywhere in the U.S., although it is less common in western coastal states, southern Florida, northern Maine, Alaska, and Hawaii. The effects of ragweed in the northern states are first felt in middle to late August and last until the first frost. Ragweed allergies tend to be most severe before midday.

- **Grasses:** Grasses affect people in mid-May to late June. Grass allergies are experienced more in the late afternoon.

- **Tree Pollen:** Small pollen grains from certain trees usually produce symptoms in late March and early April.

- **Mold Spores:** Mold spores that grow on dead leaves and release spores into the air are common allergens throughout the spring, summer, and fall. Mold spores may peak on dry windy afternoons or on damp or rainy days in the early morning.

Triggers Of Perennial (Year-Round) Allergic Rhinitis

Allergens In The House: Allergens in the house can trigger attacks in people with year-long allergic rhinitis, called perennial rhinitis. Household allergens include:

- House dust and mites. Dust mites, specifically mite feces, are coated with enzymes that contain a powerful allergen.

- Cockroaches

- Pet dander

- Molds growing on wallpaper, house plants, carpeting, and upholstery

Other Causes Of Chronic Nasal Congestion

Aging Process: The elderly are at risk for chronic rhinitis as the mucous membranes become dry with age. In addition, the cartilage supporting the nasal passages weakens, causing changes in airflow. In such cases, therapy involves avoiding possible allergens and airborne irritants as well as measures to keep the nasal passages moist. Decongestants are not helpful.

Irritative Rhinitis: Irritative rhinitis is caused by an overreaction to irritants, such as cigarette smoke, dozens of other air pollutants, strong odors, alcoholic beverages, and exposure to cold. The nasal passages become red and engorged. This reaction is not the same as an allergic reaction, although both are associated with increased numbers of white blood cells called eosinophils.

Vasomotor Rhinitis: Vasomotor rhinitis, another type of nonallergic rhinitis, is caused by oversensitive blood vessels and nerve cells in the nasal passages. It occurs in response to various triggers, including smoke, environmental toxins, changes in temperature and humidity, stress, and even sexual arousal. Symptoms of vasomotor rhinitis are similar to most of those caused by allergies, but eye irritation does not occur.

Blockage In The Nose From Polyps Or Structural Abnormalities: A number of conditions may block the nasal passages. Surgery may be helpful for certain cases.

- **Polyps:** These are soft tissues that develop off stalk-like structures on the mucous membrane. They impede mucus drainage and restrict airflow. Polyps usually develop from sinus infections that cause overgrowth of the mucus membrane in the nose. They do not regress on their own and may multiply and cause considerable obstruction.

- **Deviated Septum:** A common structural abnormality of the nose that causes problems with air flow is a deviated septum. The septum is the inner wall of cartilage and bone that separates the two sides of the nose. When deviated, it is not straight but shifted to one side, usually the left.

- **Other Causes Of Blockage:** Rarely, cleft palates, overgrowth of bones in the nose, or tumors cause nasal blockage.

Drugs: A number of drugs can cause rhinitis or worsen it in people with conditions such as deviated septum, allergies, or vasomotor rhinitis:

- Overuse of decongestant sprays used to treat nasal congestion can, over time (3–5 days), cause inflammation in the nasal passages and worsen rhinitis.

- Other medications that may cause rhinitis include oral contraceptives, hormone replacement therapy, anti-anxiety drugs (particularly alprazolam), some antidepressants, drugs used to treat erectile dysfunction, and some blood pressure medications, including beta-blockers and vasodilators.

- Sniffing cocaine damages nasal passages and can cause chronic rhinitis.

Estrogen In Women: Elevated levels of estrogen appear to increase mucus production and swelling in the nasal passages and can cause congestion. This effect is most apparent in women during pregnancy. In such cases the condition usually clears up after delivery. Oral contraceptives and hormone replacement therapies that contain estrogen have also been associated with nasal congestion in some women.

Risk Factors

Allergic rhinitis affects about 50 million Americans of all ages. Allergies most often appear first in childhood. Allergic rhinitis is the most common chronic condition in childhood, although it can develop at any age. About 20% of allergic rhinitis cases are due to seasonal allergies, 40% to perennial (chronic) rhinitis, and the rest are mixed.

Family History

Allergic rhinitis appears to have a genetic component. People with a parent who has allergic rhinitis have an increased risk of developing allergic rhinitis themselves. The risk increases significantly if both parents have allergic rhinitis.

Environmental Exposure

Home or workplace environments can increase the risk for exposure to allergens (mold spores, dust mites, animal dander) associated with allergic rhinitis.

Breastfeeding

Exclusively breastfeeding for the first four months of life can help prevent or delay wheezing and atopic dermatitis in high-risk infants. Some types of infant formulas that are made without cow's milk may possibly help prevent allergies. (There is no evidence that soy-based formulas are helpful.) Solid foods should not be introduced until an infant is four to six months old. Alterations in a mother's diet do not appear to affect her baby's risk for developing allergies.

Prognosis

Seasonal allergic rhinitis tends to diminish as a person ages. The earlier the symptoms start, the greater the chances for improvement. People who develop seasonal allergic rhinitis in early childhood tend not to have the allergy in adulthood. In some cases, allergies go into remission for years and then return later in life. People who develop allergies after age 20, however, tend to continue to have allergic rhinitis at least into middle age.

Complications

Quality Of Life

Although allergic rhinitis is not considered a serious condition, it can interfere with many important aspects of life. Surveys of nasal allergy sufferers report that symptoms such as feeling tired, miserable, or irritable are present in 50–75% of patients. Allergic rhinitis can interfere with work or school performance.

People with allergic rhinitis, particularly those with perennial allergic rhinitis, may experience sleep disorders and daytime fatigue. Often they attribute this to medication, but congestion may be the cause of these symptoms. Patients who have severe allergic rhinitis tend to have worse sleep problems, including snoring, than those with mild allergic rhinitis.

Higher Risk For Asthma And Other Allergies

Asthma and allergies often coexist. Patients with allergic rhinitis often have asthma or are increased risk of developing it. Allergic rhinitis is also associated with eczema (atopic dermatitis), an allergic skin reaction characterized by itching, scaling, and red swollen skin. Chronic uncontrolled allergic rhinitis can worsen asthma attacks and eczema.

Chronic Swelling In The Nasal Passages (Turbinate Hypertrophy)

Any chronic rhinitis, whether allergic or nonallergic, can cause swelling in the turbinates, which may become persistent (turbinate hypertrophy). The turbinates are tiny shelf-like bony structures that project into the nasal passageways. They help warm, humidify, and clean the air that passes over them. If turbinate hypertrophy develops, it causes persistent nasal congestion and, sometimes, pressure and headache in the middle of the face and forehead. This condition may require surgery.

Other Complications

Other possible complications of allergic rhinitis include:

- Sinusitis

- Middle ear infections (otitis media)

- Nasal polyps

- Sleep apnea

- Dental overbite

- Palate malformations caused by mouth breathing

Diagnosis

In most cases, a diagnosis of allergic rhinitis can be established on the basis of the patient's symptoms without any testing. The doctor will ask about:

- Time of day and year of rhinitis episodes. Rhinitis that appears seasonally is typically due to pollens and outdoor allergens. If symptoms occur throughout the year, the doctor will suspect perennial allergic or non-allergic rhinitis.

- Family history of allergies.

- History of medical problems.

- In women, if they are pregnant or taking drugs that contain estrogen (oral contraceptives, hormone replacement therapy).

- Use of other medications including decongestants, which can cause a rebound effect.

- Pets.

- Any additional unusual symptoms. As examples, bloody nasal discharge and obstruction in only one nasal passage could suggest a tumor. Fatigue, sensitivity to cold, weight gain, and depression may be signs of hypothyroidism.

Physical Examination

The doctor may examine the inside of the nose with an instrument called a speculum. This is a painless examination allowing the doctor to check for redness and other signs of inflammation. The doctor will also usually check the eyes, ears, and chest.

Possible physical findings may include:

- Redness and swelling of the eyes

- Swollen mucous membranes in the nose

- Swollen nasal turbinates or nasal polyps

- Evidence of fluid behind eardrum

- Skin rashes

- Wheezing

Allergy Skin Tests

A skin test is a simple method for detecting common allergens. Patients are usually tested for a panel of common allergens. Skin tests are rarely needed to diagnose milder seasonal allergic symptoms before a trial of treatment. The skin test is not appropriate for children younger than age three.

Laboratory Tests

Nasal Smear: The doctor may take a nasal smear. The nasal secretion is examined microscopically for factors that might indicate a cause, such as increased numbers of white blood cells, indicating infection, or high counts of eosinophils. High eosinophil counts indicate an allergic condition, but low counts do not rule out allergic rhinitis.

Tests For IgE: Blood tests for IgE immunoglobulin production may also be performed. One test, called the radioallergosorbent test (RAST), is used to detect increased levels of allergen-specific IgE in response to particular allergens. Blood tests for IgE may be less accurate than skin tests. They should be performed only on patients who cannot undergo skin testing or when skin test results are uncertain.

Imaging Tests

In people with chronic rhinitis, the doctor may also check for sinusitis. Imaging tests may be useful if other tests are ambiguous. Computed tomography (CT) scans may be useful for some cases of suspected sinusitis or sinus polyps.

Nasal Endoscopy

In certain cases of chronic or unresponsive seasonal rhinitis, a doctor may use endoscopy to examine for any irregularities in the nose structure. Endoscopy uses a tube inserted through the nose that contains a miniature camera to view the passageways.

Treatment

If rhinitis symptoms are caused by non-allergic conditions, particularly if there are accompanying symptoms indicating a serious problem, the doctor should treat any underlying disorders. If rhinitis is caused by medications, such as decongestants, the patient may need to stop taking them or find alternatives.

A variety of factors must be considered in selecting a treatment approach. These include:

- Severity of the symptoms

- Frequency (seasonal versus all year, how often during the week)

- Age of patient

- Presence of other related illnesses, such as asthma, atopic eczema, sinusitis, and polyps

- Patient preference regarding types of treatment

- Association with allergens

- Potential and known side effects of medications

- Patient's age

Treatment Options

Patients with allergic rhinitis have many treatment options available to them:

- Environmental control measures can help reduce exposure to allergens.

- Nasal washes may provide good symptomatic relief for some patients.

- Different nasal sprays, including nasal corticosteroid sprays, nasal antihistamine sprays, ipratropium bromide nasal spray (Atrovent), nasal cromolyn, and nasal decongestant sprays are available. Do not use decongestant sprays for more than three days at a time.

- Many brands of antihistamine pills are available by prescription and over-the-counter. Some are combined with decongestants. Decongestant pills may also be used by themselves. [Ed. Note: For more information about medications, see "Chapter 9—Medications Used To Treat Allergic Symptoms."]

- Other anti-inflammatory drugs, including leukotriene antagonists

- Immunotherapy ("allergy shots")

All drug treatments have side effects, some very unpleasant and, in rare cases, serious. Patients may need to try different drugs until they find one that relieves symptoms without producing excessively distressing side effects.

Treating Seasonal Allergies

Because seasonal allergies generally last only a few weeks, most doctors do not recommend the stronger prescription treatments for children.

- Prescription drugs are required only in severe cases. However, in children with both asthma and allergies, treatments for allergic rhinitis may also improve asthmatic symptoms.

- Patients with severe seasonal allergies should start medications a few weeks before the pollen season and continue taking them until the season is over.

- Immunotherapy ("allergy shots") may be considered for patients with severe seasonal allergies that do not respond to treatment.

Treating Mild Allergy Attacks: Treating mild allergy attacks usually involves little more than reducing exposure to allergens and using a nasal wash. Dozens of treatments are available for allergic rhinitis. Many are available over-the-counter, but some require a prescription. They include:

- Nasal washes

- Intermittent usage of second-generation, nonsedating antihistamines

- Decongestants that relieve nasal congestion and itchy eyes for children over the age of two and adults

- The second-generation, non-sedating antihistamines—such as cetirizine (Zyrtec, generic), loratadine (Claritin, generic), fexofenadine (Allegra, generic), or desloratadine (Clarinex)—cause less drowsiness than older antihistamines, such as diphenhydramine (Benadryl, generic). They are also available as decongestant/antihistamine combinations.

- Because seasonal allergies generally last only a few weeks, most doctors do not recommend the stronger prescription medications for children. However, in children with both asthma and allergies, treatments for allergic rhinitis may also improve asthma symptoms.

Treating Moderate-To-Severe Allergic Rhinitis: Patients with chronic allergic rhinitis or those who have bothersome symptoms that active during most of the year (particularly if they also have asthma) may require daily medications. These drugs include:

- Anti-inflammatory drugs. Nasal corticosteroids are recommended for patients with moderate-to-severe allergies, either alone or in combination with second-generation antihistamines.

- Antihistamines. The second-generation, non-sedating antihistamines—such as cetirizine (Zyrtec, generic), loratadine (Claritin, generic), fexofenadine (Allegra, generic), or desloratadine (Clarinex)—cause less drowsiness than older antihistamines, such as diphenhydramine (Benadryl, generic). They are recommended alone or in combination with nasal corticosteroids for treatment of moderate-to-severe allergic rhinitis. Nasal antihistamine sprays also work well.

- Leukotriene-antagonists and nasal cromolyn may be beneficial in specific cases of allergies.

- Immunotherapy ("allergy shots") works well for many patients with severe allergies who do not respond to other treatments. It is also proving to reduce asthma symptoms and the use of asthma medications in patients with known allergies.

Nasal Washes

For mild allergic rhinitis, a nasal wash can be helpful for removing mucus from the nose. You can purchase a saline solution at a drug store or make one at home (two cups of warm water, a teaspoon salt, pinch of baking soda). Over-the-counter saline nasal sprays that contain benzalkonium chloride as a preservative may actually worsen symptoms and infection.

Here is a simple method for administering a nasal wash:

- Lean over the sink head down.

- Pour some solution into the palm of the hand and inhale it through the nose, one nostril at a time.

- Spit the remaining solution out.

- Gently blow the nose.

Neti pots have also become popular in recent years for prevention and treatment of allergic rhinitis. Nasal irrigation with a saline solution through a neti pot involves:

- Lean over the sink with your head tilted to one side.

- Insert the spout of the neti pot in the upper nostril.

- Slowly pour the salt water into your nose while continuing to breathe through your mouth.

- The water will flow through the upper nostril and out through the lower nostril.

- When the water finishes dripping out, blow your nose.

- Reverse the tilt of your head and repeat the process with the other nostril.

Treating Itchy Eyes

Itching and redness in the eyes sometimes respond to antihistamine pills. Eye drops, however, provide faster relief, and a combination of the two may be best. Eye drops for itchy eyes include:

- Antihistamine eye drops: azelastine (Optivar, generic), olopatadine (Patanol), ketotifen (Zaditor, generic), levocabastine (Livostin) for relief of both nasal symptoms and itchy red eyes

- Decongestant eye drops: naphazoline (Naphcon, generic), tetrahydrozoline (Visine, Tyzine, generic)

- Combination decongestant/antihistamine: Visine-A, Opcon-A

- Corticosteroids: loteprednol (Lotemax, Alrex), pemirolast (Alamast)

- Non-steroidal antiinflammatory eye drops: ketorolac (Acular, generic)

General Side Effects And Warnings

- All eye drops can cause stinging, and some may result in headache and congestion.

- No one should continue taking eye drops if they experience pain, changes in vision, worsened redness, or irritation, or if the condition lasts more than three days.

- Do not touch the tip of the device to the eye or touch other surfaces with it. Replace the cap after using. Discard any solution that changes color or becomes cloudy.

- People who have heart disease, high blood pressure, an enlarged prostate gland, or glaucoma should talk to their doctor before taking these types of eye drops.

Immunotherapy

Immunotherapy (commonly called "allergy shots") is a safe and effective treatment for patients with allergies. It is based on the premise that people who receive injections of a specific allergen will lose sensitivity to that allergen. The most common allergens for which shots are given are house dust, cat dander, grass pollen, and mold.

Immunotherapy benefits include:

- Targeting the specific allergen

- Reducing sensitivity in airways in the lungs as well as in the upper airways

- Preventing the development of new allergies in children

- Reducing asthma symptoms and the use of asthma medications in patients with known allergies. Research suggests it may also help prevent the development of asthma in children with allergies.

The major downside to immunotherapy is that it requires a prolonged course of weekly injections. The use of an injection series is effective, but patients often fail to comply with the regimens. Some other schedules and delivery methods are being investigated that might make the program easier and less distressing.

Side Effects And Complications Of Immunotherapy: Injections for ragweed and, sometimes, dust mites have higher risks for side effects than other allergy shots. If complications or allergic reactions develop, they usually occur within 20 minutes, although some can develop up to two hours after the shot is given. Side effects of immunotherapy include:

- General itching, swelling, red eyes, hives, soreness at the injection site.

- Less common side effects are low blood pressure, asthma worsening, or difficulty breathing. This is due to an extreme hypersensitivity response called anaphylaxis. It can also occur if excessive doses are given.

- In rare cases, particularly because of excessive doses or if a patient has a serious lung problem, severe reactions can occur, which can be life threatening.

- Premedicating patients with antihistamines and corticosteroids may help reduce the risk of reactions to immunotherapy, although this could mask early warning signs.

Lifestyle Changes

People with existing allergies should avoid irritants or allergens. These triggers include:

- Pollen. This is the primary cause of allergic rhinitis.

- Dust mites, specifically mite feces, which are coated with enzymes that contain a powerful allergen. These are the primary allergens inside the home.

- Animal dander (flakes of skin) and hair from cats, house mice, and dogs. House mice are a significant source of allergens, particularly in urban children.

- Molds.

- Fungi.

- Cockroaches are major asthma triggers and may reduce lung function even in people without a history of asthma.

- Some studies suggest that early exposure to some of these allergens, including dust mites and pets, may actually prevent allergies from developing in children.

Indoor Protection Against Allergens

Controlling Pets: People who already have pets and are not allergic to them are probably at low risk for developing such allergies later on. When children are exposed to more than one dog or cat during their first year, they have a much lower risk for not only pet allergies but also seasonal allergies and asthma. (Pet exposure does not protect them from other allergens, notably dust mites and cockroaches).

For children who have an existing allergy to pets:

- If possible, pets should be given away or kept outside.

- If this isn't possible, they should at least be confined to carpet-free areas outside the bedroom. Cats harbor significant allergens, which can even be carried on clothing. Dogs usually present fewer problems.

- Washing animals once a week can reduce allergens. Dry shampoos, such as Allerpet, that remove allergens from skin and fur and are available for both cats and dogs and are easier to use than wet shampoos.

Preventing Exposure To Cigarette And Cooking Smoke: Parents who smoke should quit. Studies show that exposure to second-hand smoke in the home increases the risk for asthma and asthma-related emergency room visits in children.

Controlling Dust: Spray furniture polish is very effective for reducing both dust and allergens. Air cleaners, filters for air conditioners, and vacuum cleaners with high efficiency particulate air (HEPA) filters can help remove particles and small allergens found indoors. Neither vacuuming nor the use of anti-mite carpet shampoo, however, is effective in removing mites in house dust. Vacuuming actually stirs up both mites and cat allergens. People with these types of allergies should avoid having carpets or rugs in their homes. For children with allergies, vacuuming should be performed when the child is not around.

Bedding And Curtains: Replace curtains with shades or blinds, and wash bedding using the highest temperature setting. Encase mattress and pillows in special dust mite proof covers (however, washing is very important since impermeable covers alone do not help prevent allergies and studies have not proven benefit with these covers). Wash pillows in water hotter than 150° F, or in cooler water with detergent and bleach. Wash sheets and blankets weekly in hot water. Avoid sleeping or lying on cushions or furniture that is cloth covered.

Stuffed toys should be kept away from the bed and washed weekly as described above. Placing toys in a dryer or freezer may help but is not considered enough protection. Children should sleep as high off the floor as possible (avoid the bottom bunk of a bunk bed).

Reducing Humidity In The House: Living in a damp environment is counterproductive.

- Humidity levels should not exceed 30–50%.

- Fix all leaky faucets and pipes, and eliminate collections of water around the outside of the house.

- Dehumidify basements, but empty and clean humidifier daily with a vinegar solution.

- Clean often any moldy surfaces in basement or in other areas of the home.

Exterminating Pests (Cockroaches And Mice): Use professional exterminators to eliminate cockroaches. (Cleaning the house using standard housecleaning techniques may not eliminate the cockroach allergens themselves.) Exterminate mice and attempt to remove all dust, which might contain mouse urine and dander. Keep food and garbage in closed containers. Keep food out of bedrooms.

Outdoor Protection

Avoiding Outdoor Allergens: The following are some recommendations for avoiding allergens outside:

- Start taking allergy medications one to two weeks before ragweed season begins. Be sure to take allergy medications before going outside. If regular medications do not work, ask your doctor about allergy shots.

- Camping and hiking trips should not be scheduled during times of high pollen count (May and June for grass pollen and September to October for ragweed).

- Patients who are allergic should avoid barns, hay, raking leaves, and mowing grass. (A mask can be worn during outdoor chores to help reduce pollen exposure.)

- Sunglasses can help prevent pollen from getting into eyes.

- After being outdoors, clean off pollen residue by bathing, washing hair and clothes, and using a nasal salt water rinse.

- Keep doors and windows closed during pollen season.

Dietary Factors

Some evidence suggests that people with allergic rhinitis and asthma may benefit from a diet rich in omega-3 fatty acids (found in fish, almonds, walnuts, pumpkin, and flax seeds) and fruits and vegetables (at least five servings a day). Investigators are also studying probiotics—so-called good bacteria, such as lactobacillus and Bifidobacterium—which can be obtained in supplements. Some studies have found that probiotics may help reduce allergic rhinitis symptom severity and medication use.

Chapter 13

Sinusitis

What are the sinuses?

The paranasal sinuses are air-filled structures within the bony facial skeleton, located adjacent to the nasal cavity. There are four paired paranasal sinuses, eight in total: two maxillary, two ethmoid, two sphenoid, and two frontal sinuses. The bony cavities are lined with soft tissue called mucosa.

What is sinusitis?

Sinusitis is an inflammatory condition of the mucosa of the paranasal sinuses that results in symptoms such as thickened nasal drainage, nasal obstruction, and facial pain or pressure.

Viruses, bacteria, and nasal allergies are common causes of inflammation. The inflamed, swollen mucosa of the nasal and sinus cavities leads to obstruction of the openings of the sinuses, or ostia. Unable to circulate air and eliminate the secretions that are produced, the sinuses then become an ideal environment for bacterial infection. Because sinusitis is often preceded by, and almost always accompanied by, inflammation of the nasal mucosa (rhinitis), the term "rhinosinusitis" is used by otolaryngologists to replace the term "sinusitis".

Rhinosinusitis is categorized into types according to the duration of symptoms:

- **Acute:** Symptoms are present for four weeks or less.

- **Subacute:** Symptoms are present for more than four weeks, but less than 12 weeks.

- **Chronic:** Symptoms are present for 12 weeks or greater.

About This Chapter: "Sinusitis Q&A," by Lori Lemonnier, MD, revised September 2011. © American Rhinologic Society (www.american-rhinologic.org). Reprinted with permission.

- **Recurrent Acute:** Four or more acute episodes occurring within one year, with resolution of symptoms between episodes.

- **Acute Exacerbation Of Chronic Rhinosinusitis:** An acute episode occurring in a patient with chronic rhinosinusitis, producing a sudden worsening of baseline symptoms.

How common is sinusitis?

In the United States, more than 30 million people are diagnosed with sinusitis each year. Moreover, chronic rhinosinusitis affects approximately 15% of the U.S. population and is one of the most common chronic illnesses in America.

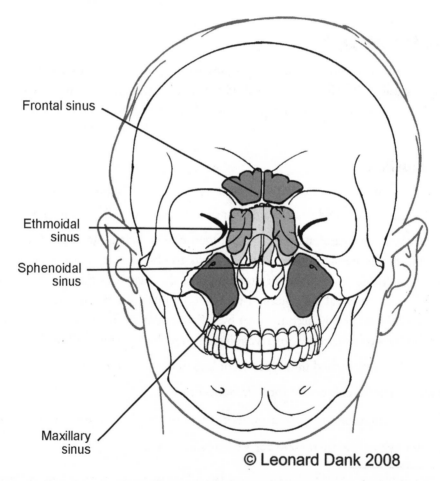

© Leonard Dank 2008

Figure 13.1. Paranasal Sinuses (Source: The Inner Man DVD, © Leonard Dank; reprinted with permission.)

What causes sinusitis?

The central event in sinusitis is blockage of the sinus openings, or ostia as a result of inflammation. Causes of sinonasal inflammation include:

- Viruses
- Bacteria
- Fungus
- Nasal allergy
- Reactive airway disease, such as asthma and Samter triad
- Congenital diseases, such as cystic fibrosis
- Inflammatory diseases, such as sarcoidosis and Wegener granulomatosis
- Immunodeficiencies, such as AIDS
- Previous surgery, resulting in scar tissue formation
- Trauma, resulting in facial fractures

Unable to circulate air and eliminate the secretions that are produced, obstructed sinuses then become an ideal environment for bacterial infection.

Many different types of bacteria can infect the paranasal sinuses. The bacteria most often cultured in acute rhinosinusitis are:

- *Streptococcus pneumoniae*
- *Haemophilus pneumoniae*
- *Moraxella catarrhalis*

In chronic rhinosinusitis, it is not uncommon to find multiple bacteria present in a single culture sample. In addition, these organisms may demonstrate drug resistance, responding to only select antibiotics. Bacteria commonly cultured in chronic rhinosinusitis include:

- *Staphylococcus aureus*
- Gram negative organisms, such as *Pseudomonas aeruginosa*

How can sinusitis be diagnosed?

The diagnosis of sinusitis, especially chronic sinusitis, can be difficult to make. Physicians rely upon patient history and physical examination to make the diagnosis. Your otolaryngologist will ask questions to determine exactly what symptoms you are experiencing and for how long.

Acute sinusitis is predominately caused by viruses and bacteria. Because viral and bacterial sinusitis are managed differently, it is important to distinguish between the two causes. Both produce thickened, discolored nasal drainage accompanied by the cardinal symptoms of nasal obstruction and/or facial pain/pressure/fullness. Initially, acute sinusitis is considered to be a viral event. According to the most recent clinical practice guidelines, only once symptoms are present for at least 10 days (but less than four weeks) is the diagnosis of acute bacterial sinusitis made. Double worsening, a phenomenon in which symptoms initially improve, but then subsequently increase in severity, is also considered diagnostic for acute bacterial sinusitis.

The clinical practice guidelines base the diagnosis of chronic rhinosinusitis (CRS) on a history of greater than 12 weeks of sinonasal signs/symptoms accompanied by evidence of nasal inflammation on examination and/or a CT scan of the paranasal sinuses.

Diagnostic signs and symptoms include:

- Nasal drainage that is thick and discolored, or purulent

- Facial pain, pressure, or fullness, that often affects the cheeks, teeth, or area around the eyes

- Nasal obstruction and/or congestion

- Decreased sense of smell

Additional symptoms that may be encountered include:

- Cough

- Postnasal drip

- Bad breath or halitosis

- Headache

- Ear pain, pressure, or fullness

If two or more signs/symptoms are present for a duration of 12 weeks or more, and evidence of inflammation is encountered on examination and/or CT scan, a diagnosis of CRS is made. Physical examination may be performed with a nasal speculum or nasal endoscope, depending on the severity of findings. Nasal endoscopes are thin telescopes designed to examine the nasal cavity and ostia of the paranasal sinuses. If purulent secretions are present, a culture can be taken to identify the causative organism(s). Inflammation is evidenced by findings of:

- Thickened, purulent secretions

- Edematous, swollen nasal mucosa

- Red, erythematous nasal mucosa
- Nasal polyps

A CT scan of the paranasal sinuses is typically ordered if medical therapy fails to improve the above signs/symptoms. CT scans provide details of the bony anatomy of the sinuses and are able to demonstrate thickening or abnormalities of the nasal and sinus mucosa.

How can sinusitis be treated?

Much like the common cold, acute viral sinusitis resolves without treatment. Because viruses do not respond to antibiotic therapy, viral sinusitis is primarily managed with supportive care such as nasal saline rinses. Medications, including antihistamines, decongestants and pain relievers may be offered by your physician to help decrease the severity of your symptoms.

The mainstay of treatment for acute bacterial sinusitis is an appropriate antibiotic. Your physician will base the choice of antibiotics on many factors, including:

- The most likely type of bacteria causing the infection
- Potential resistance of the bacteria to certain antibiotics
- Results of sinus cultures, if they are available
- Patient allergies
- Other medications that the patient is also taking
- The patient's other medical conditions
- Previous treatment

The physician will consider each of these factors prior to choosing an antibiotic. The duration of treatment is typically between 10–14 days. Pain relief should also be provided with either over-the-counter or prescription medications. As with acute viral sinusitis, additional medications, such as steroids, antihistamines, decongestants, and mucolytics may be offered by your physician to help decrease the severity and duration of your symptoms. Nasal saline rinses are also often recommended.

Because of the vast number of underlying, often multiple, causes, the treatment of chronic rhinosinusitis becomes more complicated. In general, however, CRS requires more prolonged durations of medical therapy. Antibiotics, when required, are often based on the results of sinonasal cultures and prescribed for 3–4 weeks' time.

Who treats sinusitis?

Primary care physicians, family practitioners, internists, allergists, and pulmonologists are all involved in the medical treatment of sinusitis. However, patients suffering from symptoms of recurrent acute or chronic rhinosinusitis are often referred to an otolaryngologist. Otolaryngologists, or ENT physicians, are specialists providing both medical and surgical treatment of disorders or the ears, nose and throat.

Some otolaryngologists choose to further subspecialize in rhinology; the management of diseases of the nose and paranasal sinuses. Patients with severe or complicated disease and those requiring revision surgery are often referred to rhinologists for evaluation and management.

When is surgery needed?

Sinus surgery is performed for chronic rhinosinusitis that does not resolve with medical treatment. It must be remembered that sinusitis is primarily a medical disease that needs to be treated aggressively with medication before considering surgery. Even after successful sinus surgery, many patients with CRS will continue to require medication to control the underlying cause(s) of inflammation and prevent the return of symptoms.

For patients who continue to have symptoms despite appropriate medical treatment, sinus surgery is an excellent option. Today, this surgery is typically performed using the principles of functional endoscopic sinus surgery (FESS). The goal of FESS is to restore normal function to the blocked sinuses. During a FESS procedure, the surgeon locates and enlarges the small natural drainage passageways of the sinuses. The entire operation is performed through the nostril using the nasal endoscope, with external incisions through the facial skin very rarely being required.

Sinus infections are capable of spreading to adjacent structures outside of the sinus cavities, such as the eye and brain. Such complications are quite rare, but considered medical and surgical emergencies, requiring immediate treatment. Typically, surgery will be required to drain the collection of infection and enlarge the ostia of the responsible sinuses.

Chapter 14

The Link Between Asthma And Allergies

Defining Asthma

Asthma is a chronic (long-term) lung disease that inflames and narrows the airways. Asthma causes recurring periods of wheezing (a whistling sound when you breathe), chest tightness, shortness of breath, and coughing. The coughing often occurs at night or early in the morning.

The airways are tubes that carry air into and out of your lungs. People who have asthma have inflamed airways. This makes the airways swollen and very sensitive. They tend to react strongly to certain inhaled substances.

When the airways react, the muscles around them tighten. This narrows the airways, causing less air to flow into the lungs. The swelling also can worsen, making the airways even narrower. Cells in the airways may make more mucus than normal. Mucus is a sticky, thick liquid that can further narrow your airways.

This chain reaction can result in asthma symptoms. Symptoms can happen each time the airways are inflamed.

Sometimes, asthma symptoms are mild and go away on their own or after minimal treatment with an asthma medicine. Other times, symptoms continue to get worse. When symptoms get more intense and/or more symptoms occur, you're having an asthma attack. Asthma attacks also are called flare-ups or exacerbations.

It's important to treat symptoms when you first notice them. This will help prevent the symptoms from worsening and causing a severe asthma attack. Severe asthma attacks may require emergency care, and they can be fatal.

Excerpted from "What Is Asthma," National Heart Lung and Blood Institute (www.nhlbi.nih.gov), February 2011.

Asthma can't be cured. Even when you feel fine, you still have the disease and it can flare up at any time.

However, with today's knowledge and treatments, most people who have asthma are able to manage the disease. They have few, if any, symptoms. They can live normal, active lives and sleep through the night without interruption from asthma.

You can take an active role in managing your asthma. For successful, thorough, and ongoing treatment, build strong partnerships with your doctor and other health care providers.

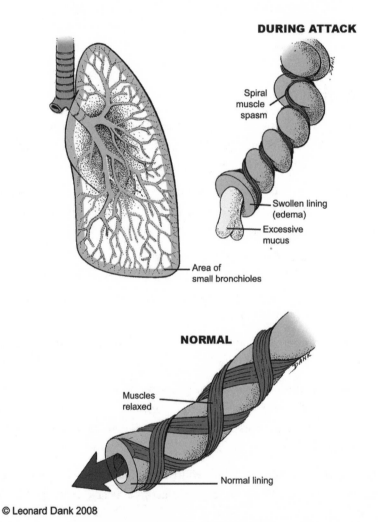

© Leonard Dank 2008

Figure 14.1. Asthma, Normal And During Attack (Source: The Inner Man DVD, © Leonard Dank; reprinted with permission.)

One Airway, One Disease

Asthma and seasonal allergies are related conditions linked by a common airway. The air we breathe in passes through our nose (at the start of our airway) and continues down the airway into the lungs. Asthma and seasonal allergies cause problems with our breathing by obstructing the free passage of air along this path.

With asthma, the breathlessness and wheezing is caused by a narrowing of the bronchioles (small branched airways in the lungs). Inflammation of the membranes of these small airways may cause an increase in the production of mucus, making the obstruction worse; the dry cough that develops is an attempt to clear the airways.

With seasonal allergies, the obstruction occurs in the upper section of the airway (in the nose). A blocked and runny nose occurs when the membranes of the nose become inflamed. In the same way as coughing is an attempt to clear the obstruction in the lower part of the airway, sneezing is an attempt to clear the mucus from the upper part.

Asthma Causes

The exact cause of asthma isn't known. Researchers think some genetic and environmental factors interact to cause asthma, most often early in life. These factors include an inherited tendency to develop allergies (called atopy), parents who have asthma, certain respiratory infections during childhood, and contact with some airborne allergens or exposure to some viral infections in infancy or in early childhood when the immune system is developing. If asthma or atopy runs in your family, exposure to irritants (for example, tobacco smoke) may make your airways more reactive to substances in the air.

Asthma Risk Factors

Asthma affects people of all ages, but it most often starts during childhood. In the United States, more than 22 million people are known to have asthma. Nearly six million of these people are children.

Young children who often wheeze and have respiratory infections—as well as certain other risk factors—are at highest risk of developing asthma that continues beyond six years of age. The other risk factors include having allergies, eczema (an allergic skin condition), or parents who have asthma.

Among children, more boys have asthma than girls. But among adults, more women have the disease than men. It's not clear whether or how sex and sex hormones play a role in causing asthma.

Most, but not all, people who have asthma have allergies.

Some people develop asthma because of contact with certain chemical irritants or industrial dusts in the workplace. This type of asthma is called occupational asthma.

Signs And Symptoms Of Asthma

- **Coughing:** Coughing from asthma often is worse at night or early in the morning, making it hard to sleep.

- **Wheezing:** Wheezing is a whistling or squeaky sound that occurs when you breathe.

- **Chest Tightness:** This may feel like something is squeezing or sitting on your chest.

- **Shortness Of Breath:** Some people who have asthma say they can't catch their breath or they feel out of breath. You may feel like you can't get air out of your lungs.

Not all people who have asthma have these symptoms. Likewise, having these symptoms doesn't always mean that you have asthma. The best way to diagnose asthma for certain is to use a lung function test, a medical history (including type and frequency of symptoms), and a physical exam.

The types of asthma symptoms you have, how often they occur, and how severe they are may vary over time. Sometimes your symptoms may just annoy you. Other times, they may be troublesome enough to limit your daily routine.

Severe symptoms can be fatal. It's important to treat symptoms when you first notice them so they don't become severe.

With proper treatment, most people who have asthma can expect to have few, if any, symptoms either during the day or at night.

Asthma Triggers

Many things can trigger or worsen asthma symptoms. Your doctor will help you find out which things (sometimes called triggers) may cause your asthma to flare up if you come in contact with them. Triggers may include:

- Allergens from dust, animal fur, cockroaches, mold, and pollens from trees, grasses, and flowers

Asthma And Allergies—The Symptoms

Asthma is a condition that affects the airways, the small tubes that carry the air in and out of the lungs. People with asthma have airways that are extra sensitive and react to substances (also known as "triggers") which irritate them.

Symptoms of asthma include difficulty breathing, wheezing, coughing, and chest tightness. Common triggers include colds or flu, cigarette smoke, exercise, and allergic responses to pollen, furry or feathery animals, or house dust mites.

Everyone's asthma manifests itself differently and can be brought on by different triggers. Your asthma may be brought on by a variety of triggers.

Allergies that affect the upper respiratory system cause inflammation in the nose—a condition called allergic rhinitis. The symptoms of allergic rhinitis include sneezing, itchy and runny nose, red and watery eyes, and a feeling of congestion that can lead to a headache.

Allergic reactions are caused by substances in the environment called allergens—some examples of the most common allergens are detailed here. For example, seasonal allergies, commonly referred to as hay fever, are common and caused by a reaction to pollen from grasses, trees and some other plants, or spores released at certain times of the year. Most cases of seasonal allergies are seasonal, but some people experience symptoms year-round. Other allergies may be triggered by a variety of allergens such as house dust mites, furry or feathery pets, or air pollution.

Source: "Asthma and Allergies: The Symptoms," © 2009 Allergy/Asthma Information Association. All rights reserved. Reprinted with permission. For additional information, visit http://aaia.ca/learnthelink or http://aaia.ca.

- Irritants such as cigarette smoke, air pollution, chemicals or dust in the workplace, compounds in home décor products, and sprays (such as hairspray)

- Medicines such as aspirin or other nonsteroidal anti-inflammatory drugs and nonselective beta-blockers

- Sulfites in foods and drinks

- Viral upper respiratory infections, such as colds

- Physical activity, including exercise

Other health conditions can make asthma harder to manage. Examples of these conditions include a runny nose, sinus infections, reflux disease, psychological stress, and sleep apnea. These conditions need treatment as part of an overall asthma care plan.

Asthma is different for each person. Some of the triggers listed above may not affect you. Other triggers that do affect you may not be on the list. Talk with your doctor about the things that seem to make your asthma worse.

Controlling Asthma

Asthma is a long-term disease that can't be cured. The goal of asthma treatment is to control the disease. Good asthma control will prevent chronic and troublesome symptoms, such as coughing and shortness of breath. It will also reduce your need for quick-relief medicines, help you maintain good lung function, and let you maintain your normal activity level and sleep through the night. Good control will help prevent asthma attacks that could result in an emergency room visit or hospital stay

To control asthma, partner with your doctor to manage your asthma. Children aged 10 or older—and younger children who are able—also should take an active role in their asthma care.

Taking an active role to control your asthma involves:

- Working with your doctor to treat other conditions that can interfere with asthma management.

- Avoiding things that worsen your asthma (asthma triggers). However, one trigger you should not avoid is physical activity. Physical activity is an important part of a healthy lifestyle. Talk with your doctor about medicines that can help you stay active.

- Working with your doctor and other health care providers to create and follow an asthma action plan.

Asthma Action Plans

An asthma action plan gives guidance on taking your medicines properly, avoiding asthma triggers (except physical activity), tracking your level of asthma control, responding to worsening asthma, and seeking emergency care when needed.

Asthma is treated with two types of medicines: long-term control and quick-relief medicines. Long-term control medicines help reduce airway inflammation and prevent asthma symptoms. Quick-relief, or "rescue," medicines relieve asthma symptoms that may flare up.

Your initial treatment will depend on the severity of your asthma. Followup asthma treatment will depend on how well your asthma action plan is controlling your symptoms and preventing asthma attacks.

Your level of asthma control can vary over time and with changes in your home, school, or work environments. These changes can alter how often you're exposed to the factors that can worsen your asthma.

Your doctor may need to increase your medicine if your asthma doesn't stay under control. On the other hand, if your asthma is well controlled for several months, your doctor may decrease your medicine. These adjustments to your medicine will help you maintain the best control possible with the least amount of medicine necessary.

Asthma treatment for certain groups of people—such as children, pregnant women, or those for whom exercise brings on asthma symptoms—will need to be adjusted to meet their special needs.

You can work with your doctor to create a personal asthma action plan. The plan will describe your daily treatments, such as which medicines to take and when to take them. The plan also will explain when to call your doctor or go to the emergency room.

On One End Of The Scale—Allergies

Avoiding allergens that trigger your allergic reaction will help to reduce or stop symptoms. If you suffer from seasonal allergies, where pollen and spores are the trigger, you should try to stay indoors when the pollen count is high, take steps to prevent pollen from getting into the house, and keep yourself and your clothes as free from the allergen as possible. For example, avoid drying your clothes outside during high pollen times, especially early morning and early evening , or avoid having flowers with so-called hairy stems in the house, such as geraniums or clematis.

Those with allergies need to avoid triggers as much as possible by staying away from furred and feathered pets, keeping the house free from dust mites, mold, and spores, and avoiding air pollution. For example, you can reduce the risk of dust mites by using an anti-allergy mattress cover, bed cover and pillows, and by avoiding padded headboards where dust mites can breed. The warmth of central heating also provides an ideal environment for dust mites.

In some cases, you may not even have identified exactly what causes your allergic reaction. It may be helpful to make a note of what the symptoms are and when they occur before discussing it with your doctor.

Use A Peak Flow Meter

This small, hand-held device shows how well air moves out of your lungs. You blow into the device and it gives you a score, or peak flow number. Your score shows how well your lungs are working at the time of the test.

Your doctor will tell you how and when to use your peak flow meter. He or she also will teach you how to take your medicines based on your score.

Your doctor and other health care providers may ask you to use your peak flow meter each morning and keep a record of your results. You may find it very useful to record peak flow scores for a couple of weeks before each medical visit and take the results with you.

When you're first diagnosed with asthma, it's important to find your "personal best" peak flow number. To do this, you record your score each day for a two- to three-week period when your asthma is well-controlled. The highest number you get during that time is your personal best. You can compare this number to future numbers to make sure your asthma is controlled.

Your peak flow meter can help warn you of an asthma attack, even before you notice symptoms. If your score shows that your breathing is getting worse, you should take your quick-relief medicines the way your asthma action plan directs. Then you can use the peak flow meter to check how well the medicine worked.

Asthma Medicines

Your doctor will consider many things when deciding which asthma medicines are best for you. Doctors usually use a stepwise approach to prescribing medicines. Your doctor will check to see how well a medicine works for you; he or she will adjust the dose or medicine as needed.

Asthma medicines can be taken in pill form, but most are taken using a device called an inhaler. An inhaler allows the medicine to go directly to your lungs.

Not all inhalers are used the same way. Ask your doctor or another health care provider to show you the right way to use your inhaler. Ask your doctor to review the way you use your inhaler at every visit.

Long-Term Control Medicines

Most people who have asthma need to take long-term control medicines daily to help prevent symptoms. The most effective long-term medicines reduce airway inflammation. These medicines are taken over the long term to prevent symptoms from starting. They don't give you quick relief from symptoms.

If your doctor prescribes a long-term control medicine, take it every day to control your asthma. Your asthma symptoms will likely return or get worse if you stop taking your medicine. Long-term control medicines can have side effects. Talk with your doctor about these side effects and ways to monitor or avoid them.

Inhaled Corticosteroids: Inhaled corticosteroids are the preferred medicines for long-term control of asthma. They're the most effective option for long-term relief of the inflammation and swelling that makes your airways sensitive to certain inhaled substances.

Reducing inflammation helps prevent the chain reaction that causes asthma symptoms. Most people who take these medicines daily find they greatly reduce the severity of symptoms and how often they occur.

Inhaled corticosteroids generally are safe when taken as prescribed. These medicines are different from the illegal anabolic steroids taken by some athletes. Inhaled corticosteroids aren't habit-forming, even if you take them every day for many years.

Like many other medicines, though, inhaled corticosteroids can have side effects. Most doctors agree that the benefits of taking inhaled corticosteroids and preventing asthma attacks far outweigh the risk of side effects.

One common side effect from inhaled corticosteroids is a mouth infection called thrush. You may be able to use a spacer or holding chamber on your inhaler to avoid thrush. These devices attach to your inhaler. They help prevent the medicine from landing in your mouth or on the back of your throat.

Work with your health care team if you have any questions about how to use a spacer or holding chamber. Rinsing your mouth out with water after taking inhaled corticosteroids also can lower your risk for thrush.

If you have severe asthma, you may have to take corticosteroid pills or liquid for short periods to get your asthma under control. If taken for long periods, these medicines raise your risk for cataracts and osteoporosis. A cataract is the clouding of the lens in your eye. Osteoporosis is a disorder that makes your bones weak and more likely to break.

Your doctor may have you add another long-term control asthma medicine so he or she can lower your dose of corticosteroids. Or, your doctor may suggest you take calcium and vitamin D pills to protect your bones.

Inhaled Long-Acting Beta2-Agonists: These medicines open the airways. They may be added to low-dose inhaled corticosteroids to improve asthma control. Inhaled long-acting beta2-agonists should never be used for long-term asthma control unless they're used with inhaled corticosteroids.

Leukotriene Modifiers: These medicines are taken by mouth. They help block the chain reaction that increases inflammation in your airways.

Theophylline: This medicine is taken by mouth. Theophylline helps open the airways.

Balancing Treatment

Managing symptoms of asthma and seasonal allergies can be a real task for people who suffer from both. While there is no cure for asthma or allergies—like seasonal allergies—there are treatments available that, in most cases, can help to control symptoms. Some of these treatments are detailed below.

Treating Seasonal Allergies

Antihistamines: These aim to provide quick relief of symptoms by lessening the effects of histamine which is one of the chemicals released by the body during an allergic reaction. They can reduce sneezing, runny noses, watery eyes, and itchy throats for a while. Newer antihistamines may reduce drowsiness while some may interact with certain medicines and foods. A doctor or pharmacist can advise regarding proper usage.

Decongestant Sprays: These can help relieve a blocked nose. They are generally recommended for use no longer than a few days at a time.

Preventer Treatments: These aim to prevent symptoms from developing by suppressing the allergic reaction. With seasonal allergies (hay fever), you need to begin treatment several weeks before the "high season" for your particular allergic reaction. Until now, these have been delivered with eye drops and nasal sprays, which you must use correctly if they are to be effective. Some preventer medications contain corticosteroids. If you need to take these long-term, you'll need to discuss this with your doctor.

Treating Asthma And Seasonal Allergies Together

There are treatments available for people with both mild to moderate asthma and seasonal allergies which are available by prescription from your doctor. They work by blocking the action of naturally occurring chemicals in the lungs which play a part in the normal inflammatory process of asthma and allergy symptoms and could lead to inflammation in both upper and lower airways.

Treating asthma and seasonal allergies together can help reduce the number of medications that you're taking, and may be more convenient for you in balancing your asthma and allergy treatments.

At your next check-up, talk to your doctor, nurse or pharmacist about how seasonal allergies affects your asthma and which treatment(s) may be suitable for you.

Quick-Relief Medicines

All people who have asthma need quick-relief medicines to help relieve asthma symptoms that may flare up. Inhaled short-acting beta2-agonists are the first choice for quick relief. These medicines act quickly to relax tight muscles around your airways when you're having a flare-up. This allows the airways to open up so air can flow through them.

You should take your quick-relief medicine when you first notice asthma symptoms. If you use this medicine more than two days a week, talk with your doctor about how well controlled your asthma is. You may need to make changes to your asthma action plan.

You shouldn't use quick-relief medicines in place of prescribed long-term control medicines. Quick-relief medicines don't reduce inflammation.

Emergency Care

Most people who have asthma, including many children, can safely manage their symptoms by following their asthma action plans. However, there may be times when you need medical attention.

Call your doctor for advice if:

- Your medicines don't relieve an asthma attack.
- Your peak flow is less than half of your personal best peak flow number.

Call 9-1-1 for emergency care if:

- You have trouble walking and talking because you're out of breath.
- You have blue lips or fingernails.

At the hospital, you'll be closely watched and given oxygen and more medicines, as well as medicines at higher doses than you take at home. Such treatment can save your life.

Get Asthma Checkups

When you first begin treatment, you'll see your doctor about every two to six weeks. Once your asthma is under control, your doctor may want to see you anywhere from once a month to twice a year.

During these checkups, your doctor or nurse will ask whether you've had an asthma attack since the last visit or any changes in symptoms or peak flow measurements. You also will be asked about your daily activities. This will help your doctor or nurse assess your level of asthma control.

Your doctor or nurse also will ask whether you have any problems or concerns with taking your medicines or following your asthma action plan. Based on your answers to these questions, your doctor may change the dose of your medicine or give you a new medicine.

If your control is very good, you may be able to take less medicine. The goal is to use the least amount of medicine needed to control your asthma.

Preventing Asthma

Currently, asthma can't be prevented. However, you can take steps to control the disease and prevent its symptoms.

- Learn about your asthma and how to control it.

- Follow your written asthma action plan.

- Use medicines as your doctor prescribes.

- Identify and try to avoid things that make your asthma worse (asthma triggers). However, one trigger you should not avoid is physical activity. Physical activity is an important part of a healthy lifestyle. Talk with your doctor about medicines that can help you stay active.

- Keep track of your asthma symptoms and level of control.

- Get regular checkups for your asthma.

Living With Asthma

Asthma is a long-term disease that requires long-term care. Successful asthma treatment requires you to take an active role in your care and follow your asthma action plan.

A New Way Of Looking At Asthma And Seasonal Allergies

International guidelines from the Seasonal Allergies and Its Impact on Asthma (ARIA) panel, in association with the World Health Organization, emphasize that because these related conditions are both caused by inflammation in the airways, they should be treated together. By managing the dual burden of asthma and seasonal allergies together, doctors can ensure an effective approach to alleviate the irritating symptoms of both diseases and administer an appropriate treatment.

Source: "A New Way of Looking at Asthma and Seasonal Allergies," © 2009 Allergy/Asthma Information Association. All rights reserved. Reprinted with permission. For additional information, visit http://aaia.ca/learnthelink or http://aaia.ca.

Learn How To Manage Your Asthma: Partner with your doctor to develop an asthma action plan. This plan will help you know when and how to take your medicines. The plan also will help you identify your asthma triggers and manage your disease if asthma symptoms worsen.

Children aged 10 or older—and younger children who can handle it—should be involved in developing and following their asthma action plans. For a sample plan, go to the National Heart, Lung, and Blood Institute's "Asthma Action Plan" (available online at http://www .nhlbi.nih.gov/health/public/lung/asthma/asthma_actplan.htm).

Most people who have asthma can successfully manage their symptoms at home by following their asthma action plans and having regular checkups. However, it's important to know when to seek emergency medical care.

Learn how to use your medicines correctly. If you take inhaled medicines, you should practice using your inhaler at your doctor's office. If you take long-term control medicines, take them daily as your doctor prescribes.

Record your asthma symptoms as a way to track how well your asthma is controlled. Also, your doctor may advise you to use a peak flow meter to measure and record how well your lungs are working.

Your doctor may ask you to keep records of your symptoms or peak flow results daily for a couple of weeks before an office visit. You'll bring these records with you to the visit.

These steps will help you keep track of how well you're controlling your asthma over time. This will help you spot problems early and prevent or relieve asthma attacks. Recording your symptoms and peak flow results to share with your doctor also will help him or her decide whether to adjust your treatment.

Ongoing Care: Have regular asthma checkups with your doctor so he or she can assess your level of asthma control and adjust your treatment as needed. Remember, the main goal of asthma treatment is to achieve the best control of your asthma using the least amount of medicine. This may require frequent adjustments to your treatments.

If it's hard to follow your asthma action plan or the plan isn't working well, let your health care team know right away. They will work with you to adjust your plan to better suit your needs.

Get treatment for any other conditions that can interfere with your asthma management.

Watch For Signs That Your Asthma Is Getting Worse: Your asthma may be getting worse if your symptoms start to occur more often, are more severe, and/or bother you at night and cause you to lose sleep. Other signs that your asthma is getting worse include the following:

- You're limiting your normal activities and missing school or work because of your asthma.

- Your peak flow number is low compared to your personal best or varies a lot from day to day.

- Your asthma medicines don't seem to work well anymore.

- You have to use your quick-relief inhaler more often. If you're using quick-relief medicine more than two days a week, your asthma isn't well controlled.

- You have to go to the emergency room or doctor because of an asthma attack.

If you have any of these signs, see your doctor. He or she may need to change your medicines or take other steps to control your asthma.

Partner with your health care team and take an active role in your care. This can help you better control your asthma so it doesn't interfere with your activities and disrupt your life.

Asthma And Allergies—Learn The Link

Research by expert groups reveals:

- 75% of asthma patients also have seasonal allergies.
- Asthma and seasonal allergies are related conditions—both diseases of the airway that are caused by inflammation.
- The two conditions frequently overlap, as several of the same allergens are known to trigger asthma and seasonal allergy exacerbations.
- Seasonal allergies tend to make asthma worse and may be a risk factor for the development of asthma.
- Effective treatment of seasonal allergies can reduce asthma symptoms and may even help prevent the development of asthma.

Because asthma and seasonal allergies are so closely linked, it makes sense to treat them together, and when possible, with one approach—this is known as the "one airway, one disease" concept.

Source: "Asthma and Allergies: Learn the Link," © 2009 Allergy/Asthma Information Association. All rights reserved. Reprinted with permission. For additional information, visit http://aaia.ca/learnthelink or http://aaia.ca.

Chapter 15

Hypersensitivity Pneumonitis

Understanding Hypersensitivity Pneumonitis

Hypersensitivity pneumonitis, or HP, is a disease in which the lungs become inflamed from breathing in foreign substances, such as molds, dusts, and chemicals. These substances also are known as antigens.

People are exposed to antigens at home, while at work, and in other settings. However, most people who breathe in these substances don't develop HP.

To understand HP, it helps to understand how the lungs work. When you breathe, air passes through your nose and mouth into your windpipe. The air then travels to your lungs' air sacs. These sacs are called alveoli.

Small blood vessels called capillaries run through the walls of the air sacs. When air reaches the air sacs, the oxygen in the air passes through the air sac walls into the blood in the capillaries. The capillaries connect to a network of arteries and veins that move blood through your body.

In HP, the air sacs become inflamed and may fill with fluid. This makes it harder for oxygen to pass through the air sacs and into the bloodstream.

The two main types of HP are acute (short-term) and chronic (ongoing). Both types can develop as a result of repeatedly breathing in an antigen.

Over time, your lungs can become sensitive to that antigen. If this happens, they'll become inflamed, which can lead to symptoms and may even cause long-term lung damage.

About This Chapter: From "Explore Hypersensitivity Pneumonitis?" National Heart Lung and Blood Institute (www.nhlbi.nih.gov), October 2010.

With acute HP, symptoms usually occur within two to nine hours of exposure to an antigen you're sensitive to. Acute HP can cause chills, body aches, coughing, and chest tightness. After hours or days of no contact with the antigen, symptoms usually go away.

If acute HP isn't found and treated early, chronic HP may develop. Symptoms of chronic HP occur slowly, over months. Chronic HP can cause a worsening cough, shortness of breath with physical activity, fatigue (tiredness), and weight loss. Severe HP may cause clubbing (a widening and rounding of the tips of the fingers or toes).

With chronic HP, symptoms may continue and/or worsen, even after avoiding the antigen. Sometimes, chronic HP can cause long-term lung damage, such as pulmonary fibrosis. This is a condition in which tissue deep in your lungs becomes scarred over time.

Avoiding or reducing your contact with antigens can help prevent and treat HP. For example, cleaning heating and ventilation filters can help reduce your contact with mold. Wetting compost prior to handling it can reduce contact with harmful dust.

If HP is caught early, avoiding the antigen that caused it may be the only treatment you need. If you have chronic HP, your doctor may prescribe medicines to reduce lung inflammation.

Researchers continue to study why some people develop HP after being exposed to antigens, while others don't. They're also looking for better ways to quickly pinpoint which antigens are causing HP in people who are believed to have the disease.

Other Names For Hypersensitivity Pneumonitis

- Bird fancier's lung
- Extrinsic allergic alveolitis
- Farmer's lung
- Hot tub lung
- Humidifier lung
- Mushroom picker's disease

Causes Of Hypersensitivity Pneumonitis

Repeatedly breathing in foreign substances can cause hypersensitivity pneumonitis (HP). Examples of these substances include molds, dusts, and chemicals. (Mold often is the cause of HP.) These substances also are known as antigens.

Over time, your lungs can become sensitive to antigens. If this happens, your lungs will become inflamed, which can lead to symptoms and may even cause long-term lung damage.

Antigens may be found in the home, workplace, or in other settings. Antigens can come from many sources, such as:

- Bird droppings

- Humidifiers, heating systems, and hot tubs

- Liquid chemicals used in the landscaping and florist industries

- Moldy hay, straw, and grain

- Chemicals released during the production of plastics and electronics, and chemicals released during painting

- Mold released during lumber milling, construction, and wood stripping

Risk Factors For Hypersensitivity Pneumonitis

People who repeatedly breathe in foreign substances are at risk for hypersensitivity pneumonitis (HP). However, most people who breathe in these substances don't develop HP. People at increased risk include the following:

- Farm and dairy cattle workers

- People who use hot tubs often

- People who are exposed to molds or dusts from humidifiers, heating systems, or wet carpeting

- Bird fanciers (people who keep pet birds) and poultry handlers

- Florists and landscapers, especially those who use liquid chemicals on lawns and gardens

- People who work in grain and flour processing and loading

- Lumber milling, construction, wood stripping, and paper and wallboard workers

- People who make plastics or electronics, and people who paint or work with other chemicals

Signs And Symptoms Of Hypersensitivity Pneumonitis

Signs and symptoms of hypersensitivity pneumonitis (HP) depend on whether the disease is acute (short-term) or chronic (ongoing).

Acute Hypersensitivity Pneumonitis

With acute HP, symptoms usually occur within two to nine hours of exposure to an antigen you're sensitive to. Acute HP can cause chills, body aches, coughing, and chest tightness. After hours or days of no contact with the antigen, symptoms usually go away.

Chronic Hypersensitivity Pneumonitis

If acute HP isn't found and treated early, chronic HP may develop. With chronic HP, symptoms occur slowly, over months. Chronic HP can cause a worsening cough, shortness of breath with physical activity, fatigue (tiredness), and weight loss.

Some symptoms may continue and/or worsen, even after avoiding the antigen. Chronic HP can cause long-term lung damage, such as pulmonary fibrosis. This is a condition in which tissue deep in your lungs becomes scarred over time.

Clubbing also may occur if HP is severe. Clubbing is the widening and rounding of the tips of the fingers or toes. A low level of oxygen in the blood causes this condition.

Diagnosing Hypersensitivity Pneumonitis

To diagnose hypersensitivity pneumonitis (HP), your doctor must pinpoint the antigen that's causing the disease and its source. Your doctor will ask you detailed questions about these items:

- Your current and past jobs
- Your hobbies and leisure activities
- The types of places where you spend time
- Your exposure to damp and moldy places

Your doctor also will do a physical exam and look at test results to diagnose HP.

Physical Exam

During the physical exam, your doctor will ask about your signs and symptoms, such as coughing and weight loss. Your doctor also will look for signs of HP. For example, he or she will listen to your lungs with a stethoscope for abnormal breathing sounds. HP can cause a crackling sound when you breathe.

Your doctor also may look for signs of pulmonary fibrosis, a possible complication of chronic (ongoing) HP. Pulmonary fibrosis is a condition in which tissue deep in your lungs becomes scarred over time.

Your doctor also may check for clubbing.

Diagnostic Tests And Procedures

To help diagnose HP, your doctor may recommend or more of the following tests or procedures.

Chest X-Ray Or Chest Computed Tomography (CT) Scan: A chest x-ray and chest CT scan create pictures of the structures inside your chest, such as your heart, lungs, and blood vessels. These pictures can show signs of HP.

Lung Function Tests: Lung function tests measure how much air you can breathe in and out, how fast you can breathe air out, and how well your lungs can deliver oxygen to your blood. One of these tests is spirometry.

During this test, a technician will ask you to take a deep breath. Then, you'll blow as hard as you can into a tube connected to a small machine. The machine is called a spirometer. The machine measures how much air you breathe out. It also measures how fast you can blow air out.

Pulse Oximetry: This test measures the amount of oxygen in your blood. A small sensor is attached to your finger or ear. The sensor uses light to estimate how much oxygen is in your blood.

Precipitin Test: This blood test looks for antibodies (proteins) that your body creates in response to antigens. The presence of these proteins may suggest HP.

Challenge Test: During this test, you're re-exposed to the suspected antigen. Then, you'll be watched for signs and symptoms of HP.

Bronchoscopy: For bronchoscopy, your doctor passes a thin, flexible tube through your nose (or sometimes your mouth), down your throat, and into your airways. At the tip of the tube are a light and mini-camera. This allows your doctor to see your windpipe and airways.

Your doctor may insert forceps (a device used to grab or hold things) through the tube to collect a tissue sample. You'll be given medicine to make you relaxed and sleepy during the procedure.

Bronchoalveolar Lavage: During bronchoscopy, your doctor may inject a small amount of salt water (saline) through the tube into your lungs. This method is called bronchoalveolar lavage. This fluid washes the lungs and helps bring up cells from the airways and the area around the air sacs. Your doctor will look at these cells under a microscope.

Surgical Lung Biopsy: To confirm a diagnosis of HP, your doctor may do a surgical lung biopsy. Your doctor can use a biopsy to rule out other causes of symptoms and check the condition of your lungs. For a surgical lung biopsy, your doctor takes samples of lung tissue from several places in your lungs. He or she then looks at them under a microscope.

Treating Hypersensitivity Pneumonitis

The best way to treat hypersensitivity pneumonitis (HP) is to avoid the antigen that caused it. In acute (short-term) HP, symptoms usually go away once you're no longer in contact with the antigen. In chronic (ongoing) HP, you may need medicines to relieve your symptoms.

People who have chronic HP may develop pulmonary fibrosis. People who have this condition may need further treatment, such as oxygen therapy and pulmonary rehabilitation (rehab).

Avoiding Antigens

Once the antigen that caused the HP and its source are found, you can take steps to avoid it. If HP is caught early, avoiding the antigen may be the only treatment you need.

Avoiding an antigen may be easier at home than at school or other places. For example, if your pet bird, moldy carpet, or hot tub is the source of the antigen, you can remove it from your home. If your heating system is the source of the antigen, your parents can have the system properly serviced.

However, if the antigen is at school or work, you may need to talk with officials about your condition and ways to protect yourself. For example, masks or personal respirators may help protect you from antigens in the air. (A personal respirator is a device that helps filter the air you breathe in.)

Some people who have HP may need to move to a different home or change jobs to avoid antigens. After hurricanes, for example, some people have to move from their homes to avoid molds that could harm their lungs. However, moving and changing jobs sometimes isn't possible.

Medicines And Other Treatments

If you have chronic HP, your doctor may prescribe medicines called corticosteroids. These medicines reduce lung inflammation. Prednisone is an example of a corticosteroid. Long-term use of prednisone, especially at high doses, can cause serious side effects. Thus, if your doctor prescribes this medicine, he or she may reduce the dose over time. Examples of side effects from corticosteroids are increased risk of infections, high blood pressure, high blood sugar, and osteoporosis (thinning of the skin and bones).

People who develop pulmonary fibrosis may need medicines, oxygen therapy, and/or pulmonary rehab.

Smoking can make HP symptoms worse and lead to other lung diseases. If you smoke, try to quit. Talk with your doctor about programs and products that can help you quit. Also, try to avoid secondhand smoke. Ask family members, friends, and coworkers not to smoke in front of you or in your home, car, or workplace.

Chapter 16

Oral Allergy Syndrome

Recent research into food allergen structures and their function within plants has been focused especially on allergens in foods that cross-react with those in botanically unrelated trees and grasses. The reason for the interest in these particular allergens is because of increasing numbers of persons reporting the symptoms of oral allergy syndrome (OAS).

Oral allergy syndrome is a complex of clinical symptoms in the mouth and throat that result from direct contact with food allergens in a sensitized individual who also exhibits respiratory allergy to inhaled allergen. The inhaled (air-borne) allergens are usually tree, weed, or grass pollens that cause hay-fever symptoms in the allergic individual. It seems that after several years, oral tissues, which are closely positioned to the mucous membranes of the upper respiratory tract, also become sensitized to these antigens.

However, the symptoms in the mouth do not occur in contact with the tree pollens, but after exposure to structurally identical antigens in unrelated plant foods such as fruits, vegetables, and sometimes nuts. Oral symptoms following ingestion of specific fruits, vegetables, and nuts have been described in patients with co-existing allergy to trees of the birch/alder group, weeds such as mugwort and ragweed, and grasses.

Symptoms Of OAS

Symptoms of oral allergy syndrome include itching and irritation of oral tissues, swelling of the lips and tongue, and sometimes papules or blistering of these tissues. Persons who have this allergy show immediate-type symptoms, which usually begin within a few minutes after eating the offending food. Most patients exhibit symptoms within five minutes, and almost all patients within 30 minutes after contact with the food. Swelling and "tightening" in the throat (glottic edema) is probably the most severe local reaction.

An interesting variation of oral allergy syndrome occurred in a patient of the Allergy Nutrition Clinic at Vancouver Hospital some years ago. She complained of watery, itchy, swollen eyes while peeling potatoes and apples. She had also recently experienced irritation of oral tissues and throat tightening while eating a raw apple and milder symptoms in the mouth after consuming a raw carrot. She had a twenty-year history of hay fever to alder and birch pollens but had only been experiencing the eye, mouth, and throat symptoms for the past year. The important association here is that raw potato, apple, and carrot contain structurally similar antigens to the birch and alder trees to which she is allergic. She remains free from these symptoms as long as she carefully avoids contact with raw potato, carrot, and apple. The association to oral allergy syndrome is that in peeling raw potato and raw apple, the antigens become aerosolized in small droplets, which spray the eyes, and can also be conveyed to the eyes on contaminated hands.

Nature Of The Allergens Associated With OAS

All allergens are components of the living organism in which they occur. Some are part of the structure, others are regulatory factors of the plant or animal. When one considers that some components (for example, cytochrome c) are present and active in many different, unrelated organisms, it is not surprising that the same factor, with the same function, even in unrelated organisms, should invoke the same antibody when it enters the animal system.

Function Of Some Plant Allergens

When an allergen has been isolated, its characteristics often suggest a probable function within the plant. For example: The birch pollen component named Bet v 2 and the 15 kd antigen in celery have been identified as profilins, which are regulatory proteins associated with the reproductive processes in plants, hence their association with pollens.

The birch antigen Bet v 1 and the apple antigen Mal d 1 are proteins that are made by the plants when they are under conditions of environmental stress. Various stresses can stimulate the expression of these proteins, which implies that allergens increase in plants under stressful conditions like severe growing situations and exposure to some kinds of chemicals. It has been suggested that some of these proteins are made by the plants in response to environmental pollution. This might explain the apparent surge of patients exhibiting oral allergy syndrome in the past few years as pollution levels, especially in cities, increase. Furthermore, because defense-related proteins usually provide a plant with resistance to stresses, varieties that are apt to intensively induce such proteins are agriculturally valuable and are often selected for cultivation, thus increasing the number of plants that produce the potentially allergenic proteins.

Definitions

- **Antigen:** Protein molecule, foreign to the body, which induces the immune system to respond by producing antibodies specifically designed to neutralize the antigen. Most antigens elicit a protective response of the immune system.
- **Allergen:** Antigen that induces the immune system to respond with an allergic rather than protective reaction.

All allergens are antigens. Not all antigens are allergens

All antigens contain a protein molecule that is unique in structure and specific to the plant, animal or microorganism that produced it.

The allergen Pru p3 in peach is a lipid transfer protein (LTP). LTPs are a family of 9kda polypeptides, widely found in the vegetable kingdom and implicated in cuticle formation and defense against pathogens. They are heat-stable and resistant to pepsin digestion, which makes them potent food allergens.

Other antigens such the allergen named Art v 1 from mugwort, which shows antigenic relatedness to antigens in a number of pollens and food plants (birch, timothy grass, celery), is described as trypsin resistant, but its function in the plant has not been identified.

As we become more informed about the nature of the antigens that can elicit the production of IgE and induce allergy, it may be possible to predict the potential for cross-reactions between similar antigenic proteins within unrelated plant species. However, since allergy is an individual characteristic, potential allergenicity will not necessarily predict the effect of the food when consumed by any given person. Statistical methods have been utilized in an attempt to measure the probability that a person sensitized to one edible plant will demonstrate significant cross-reactivity to other, unrelated plants.

However, elimination and challenge still remains the only reliable method of demonstrating individual reactivity to each suspect plant food.

Management Of Pollen And Associated Plant Food Allergy

Frequently, high temperatures will destroy the antigen in the plant food that is responsible for oral allergy syndrome. People demonstrating oral allergy syndrome after eating raw fruits and vegetables often can eat the same food with impunity when it is cooked.

There are reported indications that the ripeness of the fruit or vegetable may influence its allergenicity, the riper the fruit or more mature the vegetable, the greater the potential that it might incite an allergic response compared to the unripe form.

When a person has evidence of an IgE-mediated allergy (for example, rhinitis, allergic conjunctivitis, asthma) to pollens of plants usually associated with oral allergy syndrome (birch, mugwort, ragweed, timothy grass, other grasses), it is wise for them to avoid the foods known to possess identical antigens when:

- the foods have been demonstrated to cause immediate reactions in the oral cavity;

- there are positive indications of allergy to the foods, based on skin tests or immunological analysis such as RAST or ELISA.

Table 16.1. Cross-Reacting Foods, Pollens, And Other Allergens

Non-Food Allergens	Fruits And Vegetables	Legumes And Grains	Nuts And Seed	Other Foods
Birch pollen Mugwort pollen Grass pollens Timothy grass Ragweed	Apple Apricot Carrot Celery Cherry Fennel Kiwi fruit Melon Nectarine Orange Peach Potato Tomato Watermelon	Peanut	Hazelnut "Tree nuts" (unspecified)	Spice (unspecified)
Ragweed	Banana Cantaloupe Cucumber Honeydew Melon Watermelon			

When pollen-allergic individuals do not have oral symptoms and in addition, skin tests and/or immunological teats are negative for the associated foods, it is probably unnecessary to avoid the foods. However, some practitioners feel that as a precautionary measure it is wise to provide the patient who has demonstrated signs of allergy to the pollens known to share common allergens with foods in OAS with information on the types of foods likely to trigger OAS (see Table 16.1). The observation that the longer the duration of birch pollinosis, the higher the level of birch-specific IgE tends to become, and the greater the risk for a more severe reaction, which are predisposing factors for the onset of OAS, suggests that such precautions might be advisable.

Table 16.1 provides a chart of potential allergenic cross-reactivity between plant species, based on current published reports that can be used as the basis of an elimination diet for detecting the specific triggers of allergic reactions. However, hypersensitivity to these plants is an individual idiosyncrasy. Even if species are shown to have common antigens, persons who are allergic to one species in an antigenically related group do not necessarily experience an adverse reaction to others in the same group. As in all allergy management, demonstration of triggering of the allergic response when the food is reintroduced in a controlled fashion (challenge) is the only reliable way to identify the allergen responsible for the reaction.

Chapter 17

Eye Allergies

Allergies Of The Eye

Definition

Allergies of the eye, like all allergies, are overreactions of the immune system to foreign substances, which might otherwise be harmless. In people without allergies, the immune response that occurs following exposure to an allergen is controlled, and produces few if any symptoms. In people with allergies, activation of the immune response results in the release of inappropriate, high quantities of chemical mediators—the most common is histamine. These mediators are responsible for the symptoms of allergic reactions. The different types of allergies affecting the eye—atopic (vernal keratoconjunctivitis, atopic keratoconjunctivitis, and hayfever conjunctivitis), medication reactions, toxic papillary reactions, and contact lens-related allergies are covered below.

Different Types Of Allergies

Atopic

Vernal keratoconjunctivitis: A seasonally recurring conjunctivitis which can also affect the peripheral cornea, generally occurring in children and young adults.

About This Chapter: This chapter begins with "Allergies of the Eye," reprinted with permission from the University of Michigan Kellogg Eye Center, www.kellogg.umich.edu. © 2012 Regents of the University of Michigan. All rights reserved. Text under the heading "Allergic Conjunctivitis," is excerpted from "Conjunctivitis (Pink Eye)," Centers for Disease Control and Prevention (www.cdc.gov), June 4, 2010.

Atopic keratoconjunctivitis: A similar entity to vernal keratoconjunctivitis, but occurs mainly in older patients who have had a history of atopic eczematoid dermatitis, is not seasonal, and can cause more extensive corneal and conjunctival scarring if untreated.

Hayfever conjunctivitis: A sudden intense response to an (usually) airborne allergen, this type tends to be short-lived and episodic. Also known as "seasonal allergic conjunctivitis."

Adverse Or Allergic Reactions to Medications

IgE mediated (anaphylactoid): A sudden, intense reaction which often includes chemosis (conjunctival swelling) and an urticarial response (intense itching). Common offenders include topical penicillin, bacitracin, sulfacetamide, and anesthetics.

Toxic (irritative) papillary reactions: Very common and result in a chronic red eye. Can occur any time after one week of medication use, and are due to some antibiotic and antiviral drops, as well as certain preservatives.

Allergic contact reactions: Slower and more gradual in onset than the above two, caused by many topical medications, and easily treated by discontinuing the offending agent.

Contact Lens Related Allergy

Contact allergic conjunctivitis: Occurs when the contact lenses themselves or the proteins in tear film that bind to the surface of the lens can cause an irritative response of the conjunctiva, resulting in redness, itching, mucous discharge, and lens discomfort. A more severe form, known as giant papillary conjunctivitis, has been recognized, typified by large swellings of the mucous membranes of the upper lid and may result ultimately in the inability to wear lenses. Symptoms:

- Swelling or puffiness of the eyes
- Redness
- Itching
- Tearing
- Mucous discharge
- Contact lens discomfort
- Foreign body sensation

The symptoms described above may not necessarily mean that you have allergies of the eye. However, if you experience one or more of these symptoms, contact your eye doctor for a complete exam.

Treatment

Atopic Allergies: Cool compresses and artificial tears are often helpful; topical vaso-constrictors and antihistamines are useful to counteract the histamine-induced leakiness and dilation of blood vessels. Many of these are now available as over-the-counter preparations. Topical steroids may be used in severe cases. Mast cell stabilizers (cromolyn sodium, lodoxamide) can be used in seasonal cases and are most effective if instituted before or soon after the onset of symptoms. These agents limit the body's sensitivity to an allergen, resulting in less of an immune response.

Medication Allergies: Discontinue the offending agent; topical vasoconstrictors and anti-histamines provide relief, and artificial tears may help remove any remaining medication and lubricate the corneal surface if irritated.

Contact Lens Allergy: Decreasing lens wear time, insuring proper cleaning of lenses, and perhaps changing the cleaning regimen may improve this condition. In addition, recognition of early symptoms is essential in limiting this problem, e.g., if eight hours of wear feels fine, but then the eyes get red and irritated, it is wise to remove the lenses then, and not to continue to wear them for hours more. If these measures are not helpful or if there is already moderate to severe disease, one may add mast cell stabilizers and a short course of mild steroids to help "put out the fire" and limit the body's response. If still not helpful, consider changing the lens type. A period of weeks to months without any lens wear is often helpful in controlling this entity.

Allergic Conjunctivitis (Pink Eye)

Conjunctivitis is a common eye condition worldwide. It causes inflammation (swelling) of the conjunctiva—the thin layer that lines the inside of the eyelid and covers the white part of the eye. Conjunctivitis is often called "pink eye" or "red eye" because it can cause the white of the eye to take on a pink or red color.

The most common causes of conjunctivitis are viruses, bacteria, and allergens. But there are other causes, including chemicals, fungi, certain diseases, and contact lens use (especially the extended-wear type). The conjunctiva can also become irritated by foreign bodies in the eye and by indoor and outdoor air pollution caused, for example, by chemical vapors, fumes, smoke, or dust.

Allergic conjunctivitis is caused by the body's reaction to certain substances to which it is allergic, such as pollen from trees, plants, grasses, and weeds; dust mites; molds; dander from animals; contact lenses and lens solution; and cosmetics. Allergic conjunctivitis has these characteristics:

- Occurs more frequently among people with other allergic conditions, such as hay fever, asthma, and eczema

- Usually occurs in both eyes

- Can occur seasonally, when pollen counts are high

- Can occur year-round due to indoor allergens, such as dust mites and animal dander

- May result, in some people, from exposure to certain drugs and cosmetics

- Clears up once the allergen or irritant is removed or after treatment with allergy medications

Signs And Symptoms

It can be hard to determine the exact cause of every case of conjunctivitis. This is because some signs and symptoms of the condition can differ depending on the cause, and other signs and symptoms are similar no matter what caused the conjunctivitis.

Symptoms of conjunctivitis can include the following:

- Pink or red color in the white of the eye(s) (often one eye for bacterial and often both eyes for viral or allergic conjunctivitis)

- Swelling of the conjunctiva (the thin layer that lines the white part of the eye and the inside of the eyelid) and/or eyelids

- Increased tearing

- Discharge of pus, especially yellow-green (more common in bacterial conjunctivitis)

- Itching, irritation, and/or burning

- Feeling like a foreign body is in the eye(s) or an urge to rub the eye(s)

- Crusting of eyelids or lashes sometimes occurs, especially in the morning

- Symptoms of a cold, flu, or other respiratory infection may also be present

- Sensitivity to bright light sometimes occurs

- Enlargement and/or tenderness, in some cases, of the lymph node in front of the ear. This enlargement may feel like a small lump when touched. (Lymph nodes act as filters in the body, collecting and destroying viruses and bacteria.)

- Symptoms of allergy, such as an itchy nose, sneezing, a scratchy throat, or asthma may be present in cases of allergic conjunctivitis

Sometimes there are situations that can help your healthcare provider determine what is causing the conjunctivitis. For example, if a person with allergies develops conjunctivitis when the pollen count increases in the spring, this would be a sign that he or she might have allergic conjunctivitis. And if someone develops conjunctivitis during an outbreak of viral conjunctivitis, this would be a sign that he or she might have viral conjunctivitis.

Diagnosing Allergic Conjunctivitis

Allergic conjunctivitis can be diagnosed from signs and symptoms, and patient history; for example, allergic conjunctivitis may occur seasonally when pollen counts are high, and it can cause the patient's eyes to itch intensely. This type of conjunctivitis is a common occurrence in people who have other signs of allergic disease, such as hay fever, asthma, or eczema. Allergic conjunctivitis results from a person's reaction to substances they are allergic to, such as pollen, dust mites, animal dander, medications, cosmetics, and other allergy-provoking substances.

Treating Allergic Conjunctivitis

The treatment for conjunctivitis depends on the cause. It is not always necessary to see a healthcare provider for conjunctivitis. But, as noted below, there are times when it is important to seek medical care.

Conjunctivitis caused by an allergy usually improves when the allergen (such as pollen or animal dander) is removed. Allergy medications and certain eye drops (topical antihistamine and vasoconstrictors), including some prescription eye drops, can also provide relief from allergic conjunctivitis. In some cases, a combination of drugs may be needed to improve symptoms. Your doctor can help if you have conjunctivitis caused by an allergy.

When To Seek Medical Care For Conjunctivitis

A healthcare provider should be seen in these situations:

- Conjunctivitis is accompanied by moderate to severe pain in the eye(s).

- Conjunctivitis is accompanied by vision problems, such as sensitivity to light or blurred vision, that does not improve when any discharge that is present is wiped from the eye(s).

- Conjunctivitis is accompanied by intense redness in the eye(s).

- Conjunctivitis symptoms become worse or persist when a patient is suspected of having a severe form of viral conjunctivitis—for example, a type caused by herpes simplex virus or varicella-zoster virus (the cause of chickenpox and shingles).

- Conjunctivitis occurs in a patient who is immunocompromised (has a weakened immune system) from HIV infection, cancer treatment, or other medical conditions or treatments.

- Bacterial conjunctivitis is being treated with antibiotics and does not begin to improve after 24 hours of treatment.

Chapter 18

Contact Dermatitis

What is contact dermatitis?

If you develop redness, heat, swelling, and pain on your skin when you come in contact with certain substances, you may have what is known as *contact dermatitis*.

Contact dermatitis is caused either by an allergy or a sensitivity (a non-allergic response) to common substances. About 80% of skin reactions are caused by direct contact with an irritating, harsh, or dangerous chemical. Household cleaners, dish detergent, and soap are everyday examples of products that also can cause irritant contact dermatitis in many people, especially with longtime use. Battery acid, drain cleaner, and turpentine are chemicals that cause irritant contact dermatitis in everyone.

What is allergic contact dermatitis?

Your skin is one of the first places where allergy symptoms can appear. In people who have a skin allergy—allergic contact dermatitis—the immune system overreacts to normally harmless substances that come in direct contact with the skin. These substances are referred to as *allergens*.

What causes allergic contact dermatitis?

An allergic response on the skin may be the result of exposure to chemicals found in many different products and plants, including:

- Dye for your hair, clothing, leather, furs

About This Chapter: "Contact Dermatitis," reprinted with permission from the Asthma and Allergy Foundation of America (www.aafa.org), © 2005. Reviewed by David A. Cooke, MD, FACP, September 2012.

- Nail care products, cosmetics, sunscreen

- Fragrances, perfumes

- Rubber compounds

- Topical medications

- Poison ivy, other plants

- Detergents, cleaning products

- Metals, especially nickel

Allergic contact dermatitis occurs when you become sensitized to a specific substance. If you are allergic to something, you may have an allergic response to it on first contact and allergy symptoms will appear within 10 days. At this point, you have become sensitized to that particular substance. Once you develop a specific sensitivity, even brief contact with that allergen may cause your allergic contact dermatitis to reappear within 24–48 hours.

What are the signs and symptoms of contact dermatitis?

Symptoms of allergic contact dermatitis and irritant contact dermatitis are similar and can range from mild to severe. Telltale signs are a red, itchy, swollen area or rash that may or may not have blisters. Cracking or peeling skin may follow. Symptoms usually appear on the area of the skin that has been exposed.

How is allergic contact dermatitis diagnosed?

A skin patch test is used to determine the most likely substances that are causing you to have an allergic response on your skin. A complete physical and history, along with test results, will assist your doctor in making a diagnosis. To help your doctor make the most accurate diagnosis, keep a log with details related to your skin reactions such as:

Is eczema the same as allergic contact dermatitis?

No. Eczema—also called atopic dermatitis—is a skin disorder in which an allergic response, especially to foods, has a role in some people, especially children. Eczema is most common in infants and children. Although all eczema is not allergy-related, people with eczema usually have a family history of one or more allergic conditions such as asthma, hay fever, hives, or allergic rhinitis (runny, stuffy nose). Nonallergic factors also play a role in eczema.

- What you were doing in the 24–48 hours prior to your skin outbreak?

- Where the activity occurred (In a wooded area? Working on a hobby or handicraft project? At the beach? After cleaning the house?)

- How much of a product were you using? How often?

- Where did the substance touch your skin (even places with no signs of outbreak)?

- What are your usual symptoms?

- Any previous skin reactions? To what products or situations?

How is contact dermatitis treated?

You can treat milder cases of contact dermatitis yourself. Over-the-counter medications such as calamine lotion, antihistamines, or cortisone creams and ointments usually will relieve your discomfort. Talk with the pharmacist about recommended products.

If you have frequent and/or severe outbreaks of contact dermatitis, consult a physician. A proper diagnosis along with identification of key allergens and stronger prescription medications will help you manage your skin allergy effectively.

Are there common sources for contact dermatitis?

Thousands of common products contain substances that can trigger an allergic response on your skin. Many times these substances can be "hidden" components of a product you are using, so be sure to read labels.

Here is a list of materials that often cause allergic contact dermatitis, along with tips to help protect against an outbreak if you have a known allergy.

Fragrances And Perfumes are found in soaps, deodorants, body creams, cosmetics, tissues (scented toilet paper), and products whose contents include the word "fragrance." To avoid problems, use fragrance-free products. Hypoallergenic products may be helpful, but could still contain fragrance. Unscented products also may contain small amounts of fragrance, which is used to mask natural odors found in the product.

Nickel is an element in many metal alloys. Nickel is used to coat hundreds of everyday objects such as buttons, costume jewelry, and kitchen utensils. Even 14k and 18k gold contains nickel that can be drawn out by sweating, water, or detergent.

- To help manage nickel allergies, cover nickel-containing objects that touch your skin with clear nail polish or special sprays available from your health care provider. Your dermatologist also can provide you with a kit that allows you to test items for nickel.

- Ear piercing (and body piercing) that employs earrings with nickel posts actually can set off a lifetime of nickel sensitivity. For nickel-sensitive individuals, new rashes can appear in other areas of the body whenever objects containing nickel are touched. Always use surgical steel posts to avoid developing nickel sensitivity.

- People who are highly allergic to nickel should not eat foods containing traces of nickel: nuts, chocolate, beer, tea, coffee and apricots all contain nickel.

Latex is the stretchy material used in hundreds of items that come in direct contact with the body. Waistbands, bras, condoms, surgical gloves, toys, and radial tire dust particles are some of the most common places where latex is found. Because latex is used in so many products today, there are increasing reports of latex sensitivity. Besides irritating the skin, latex exposure can trigger hives, hay fever, or asthma symptoms, and even life-threatening anaphylactic shock.

- If you are sensitive to latex, avoid or cover clothes that have exposed rubber. Use a lambskin and a latex condom together: layer the condoms so that the partner sensitive to latex is only exposed to lambskin. (Remember: Lambskin condoms do not protect against HIV.) Be sure to tell your health care providers if you have a serious allergy to latex before they put on gloves or use other rubber and latex products.

- Some fruits cross-react to latex. If you have an allergic reaction to latex or rubber, you could also react to certain fruits, including banana, avocado or chestnuts.

Nail Care Products usually contain a formaldehyde resin, and many people are allergic to it. Nail polishes, nail hardeners, and artificial nails can all set off an allergic reaction when hands with the wet nail product come in contact with skin. Many women experience contact dermatitis on their eyelids, face, and neck because their hands touch these areas before the nail product is dry. If you use nail care products, be sure to keep your hands away from your face and neck until your nails are completely dry; use a nail-drying machine to speed up drying time.

The Sun can be a culprit in causing skin allergies. Harmless chemicals applied to the skin are converted into *photocontact allergens* by ultraviolet rays. Alone, neither the sun nor the substance cause a reaction. But together, they produce an allergic response. Photocontact allergens often are found in topical antibiotics, cosmetics, perfumes, and even sunscreen products.

- You can confirm sun sensitivity with a photopatch test. Also ask your physician if any medications you are taking could cause photosensitivity. If you are allergic to sunscreen products themselves, you need to find a substitute. Look for non-PABA containing products if you are allergic to PABA or its derivatives; chemical-free sunscreens also are available.

Chapter 19

Atopic Dermatitis (Eczema)

Defining Atopic Dermatitis

Atopic dermatitis is a chronic (long-lasting) disease that affects the skin. It is not contagious; it cannot be passed from one person to another. The word *dermatitis* means inflammation of the skin. *Atopic* refers to a group of diseases in which there is often an inherited tendency to develop other allergic conditions, such as asthma and hay fever. In atopic dermatitis, the skin becomes extremely itchy. Scratching leads to redness, swelling, cracking, "weeping" clear fluid, and finally, crusting and scaling. In most cases, there are periods of time when the disease is worse (called exacerbations or flares) followed by periods when the skin improves or clears up entirely (called remissions). As some children with atopic dermatitis grow older, their skin disease improves or disappears altogether, although their skin often remains dry and easily irritated. In others, atopic dermatitis continues to be a significant problem in adulthood.

Atopic dermatitis is often referred to as *eczema*, which is a general term for the several types of inflammation of the skin. Atopic dermatitis is the most common of the many types of eczema. Several have very similar symptoms.

Atopic dermatitis is very common. It affects males and females at about the same rate. Although atopic dermatitis may occur at any age, it most often begins in infancy and childhood. Scientists estimate that 65 percent of patients develop symptoms in the first year of life, and 85 percent develop symptoms before the age of five. Onset after age 30 is less common and is often caused by exposure of the skin to harsh or wet conditions.

About This Chapter: Excerpted from "Handout on Health: Atopic Dermatitis," National Institute of Arthritis and Musculoskeletal and Skin Diseases (www.niams.nih.gov), August 2011.

Causes Of Atopic Dermatitis

The cause of atopic dermatitis is not known, but the disease seems to result from a combination of genetic (hereditary) and environmental factors.

Children are more likely to develop this disorder if a parent has had it or another atopic disease like asthma or hay fever. If both parents have an atopic disease, the likelihood increases. Although some people outgrow skin symptoms, approximately half of children with atopic dermatitis go on to develop hay fever or asthma. Environmental factors can bring on symptoms of atopic dermatitis at any time in individuals who have inherited the atopic disease trait.

Atopic dermatitis is also associated with malfunction of the body's immune system: the system that recognizes and helps fight bacteria and viruses that invade the body. Scientists have found that people with atopic dermatitis have a low level of a cytokine (a protein) that is essential to the healthy function of the body's immune system and a high level of other cytokines that lead to allergic reactions. The immune system can become misguided and create inflammation in the skin even in the absence of a major infection. This can be viewed as a form of autoimmunity, where a body reacts against its own tissues.

In the past, doctors thought that atopic dermatitis was caused by an emotional disorder. We now know that emotional factors, such as stress, can make the condition worse, but they do not cause the disease.

Skin Features Associated With Atopic Dermatitis

Atopic Pleat (Dennie-Morgan Fold): An extra fold of skin that develops under the eye.

Cheilitis: Inflammation of the skin on and around the lips.

Hyperlinear Palms: Increased number of skin creases on the palms.

Hyperpigmented Eyelids: Eyelids that have become darker in color from inflammation or hay fever.

Ichthyosis: Dry, rectangular scales on the skin.

Keratosis Pilaris: Small, rough bumps, generally on the face, upper arms, and thighs.

Lichenification: Thick, leathery skin resulting from constant scratching and rubbing.

Papules: Small raised bumps that may open when scratched and become crusty and infected.

Urticaria: Hives (red, raised bumps) that may occur after exposure to an allergen, at the beginning of flares, or after exercise or a hot bath.

Types Of Eczema (Dermatitis)

Allergic Contact Eczema (Dermatitis): A red, itchy, weepy reaction where the skin has come into contact with a substance that the immune system recognizes as foreign, such as poison ivy or certain preservatives in creams and lotions.

Atopic Dermatitis: A chronic skin disease characterized by itchy, inflamed skin.

Contact Eczema: A localized reaction that includes redness, itching, and burning where the skin has come into contact with an allergen (an allergy-causing substance) or with an irritant such as an acid, a cleaning agent, or other chemical.

Dyshidrotic Eczema: Irritation of the skin on the palms of hands and soles of the feet characterized by clear, deep blisters that itch and burn.

Neurodermatitis: Scaly patches of the skin on the head, lower legs, wrists, or forearms caused by a localized itch (such as an insect bite) that become intensely irritated when scratched.

Nummular Eczema: Coin-shaped patches of irritated skin—most common on the arms, back, buttocks, and lower legs—that may be crusted, scaling, and extremely itchy.

Seborrheic Eczema: Yellowish, oily, scaly patches of skin on the scalp, face, and occasionally other parts of the body.

Stasis Dermatitis: A skin irritation on the lower legs, generally related to circulatory problems.

Symptoms Of Atopic Dermatitis

Symptoms (signs) vary from person to person. The most common symptoms are dry, itchy skin and rashes on the face, inside the elbows and behind the knees, and on the hands and feet. Itching is the most important symptom of atopic dermatitis. Scratching and rubbing in response to itching irritates the skin, increases inflammation, and actually increases itchiness. Itching is a particular problem during sleep when conscious control of scratching is lost.

The appearance of the skin that is affected by atopic dermatitis depends on the amount of scratching and the presence of secondary skin infections. The skin may be red and scaly, be thick and leathery, contain small raised bumps, or leak fluid and become crusty and infected.

Atopic dermatitis may also affect the skin around the eyes, the eyelids, and the eyebrows and lashes. Scratching and rubbing the eye area can cause the skin to redden and swell. Some people with atopic dermatitis develop an extra fold of skin under their eyes. Patchy loss of eyebrows and eyelashes may also result from scratching or rubbing.

Researchers have noted differences in the skin of people with atopic dermatitis that may contribute to the symptoms of the disease. The outer layer of skin, called the epidermis, is divided into two parts: an inner part containing moist, living cells, and an outer part, known as the horny layer or stratum corneum, containing dry, flattened, dead cells. Under normal conditions the stratum corneum acts as a barrier, keeping the rest of the skin from drying out and protecting other layers of skin from damage caused by irritants and infections. When this barrier is damaged, irritants act more intensely on the skin.

The skin of a person with atopic dermatitis loses moisture from the epidermal layer, allowing the skin to become very dry and reducing its protective abilities. Thus, when combined with the abnormal skin immune system, the person's skin is more likely to become infected by bacteria or viruses, such as those that cause warts and cold sores.

Stages Of Atopic Dermatitis

When atopic dermatitis occurs during infancy and childhood, it affects each child differently in terms of onset and severity of symptoms. In infants, atopic dermatitis typically begins around 6–12 weeks of age. It may first appear around the cheeks and chin as a patchy facial rash, which can progress to red, scaling, oozing skin. The skin may become infected. Once the infant becomes more mobile and begins crawling, exposed areas, such as the inner and outer parts of the arms and legs, may also be affected. An infant with atopic dermatitis may be restless and irritable because of the itching and discomfort of the disease.

In childhood, the rash tends to occur behind the knees and inside the elbows; on the sides of the neck; around the mouth; and on the wrists, ankles, and hands. Often, the rash begins with papules that become hard and scaly when scratched. The skin around the lips may be inflamed, and constant licking of the area may lead to small, painful cracks in the skin around the mouth.

In some children, the disease goes into remission for a long time, only to come back at the onset of puberty when hormones, stress, and the use of irritating skin care products or cosmetics may cause the disease to flare.

Although a number of people who developed atopic dermatitis as children also experience symptoms as adults, it is also possible for the disease to show up first in adulthood. The pattern in adults is similar to that seen in children; that is, the disease may be widespread or limited to only a few parts of the body. For example, only the hands or feet may be affected and become dry, itchy, red, and cracked. Sleep patterns and work performance may be affected, and long-term use of medications to treat the atopic dermatitis may cause complications. Adults with atopic dermatitis also have a predisposition toward irritant contact dermatitis, where the skin becomes red and inflamed from contact with detergents, wool, friction from clothing, or other potential irritants. It is more likely to occur in occupations involving frequent hand washing or exposure to chemicals. Some people develop a rash around their nipples. These localized symptoms are difficult to treat. Because adults may also develop cataracts, the doctor may recommend regular eye exams.

Diagnosing Atopic Dermatitis

Each person experiences a unique combination of symptoms, which may vary in severity over time. The doctor will base a diagnosis on the symptoms the patient experiences and may need to see the patient several times to make an accurate diagnosis and to rule out other diseases and conditions that might cause skin irritation. In some cases, the family doctor or pediatrician may refer the patient to a dermatologist (doctor specializing in skin disorders) or allergist (allergy specialist) for further evaluation.

A medical history may help the doctor better understand the nature of a patient's symptoms, when they occur, and their possible causes. The doctor may ask about family history of allergic disease; whether the patient also has diseases such as hay fever or asthma; and about exposure to irritants, sleep disturbances, any foods that seem to be related to skin flares, previous treatments for skin-related symptoms, and use of steroids or other medications. A preliminary diagnosis of atopic dermatitis can be made if the patient has three or more features from each of two categories: major features and minor features. Currently, there is no single test to diagnose atopic dermatitis. However, there are some tests that can give the doctor an indication of allergic sensitivity.

Factors That Make Atopic Dermatitis Worse

Many factors or conditions can make symptoms of atopic dermatitis worse, further triggering the already overactive immune system, aggravating the itch-scratch cycle, and increasing damage to the skin. These factors can be broken down into two main categories: irritants and allergens. Emotional factors and some infections and illnesses can also influence atopic dermatitis.

Irritants are substances that directly affect the skin and, when present in high enough concentrations with long enough contact, cause the skin to become red and itchy or to burn. Specific irritants affect people with atopic dermatitis to different degrees. Over time, many patients and their family members learn to identify the irritants causing the most trouble. For example, frequent wetting and drying of the skin may affect the skin barrier function. Also, wool or synthetic fibers and rough or poorly fitting clothing can rub the skin, trigger inflammation, and cause the itch-scratch cycle to begin. Soaps and detergents may have a drying effect and worsen itching, and some perfumes and cosmetics may irritate the skin. Exposure to certain substances, such as solvents, dust, or sand, may also make the condition worse. Cigarette smoke may irritate the eyelids. Because the effects of irritants vary from one person to another, each person can best determine what substances or circumstances cause the disease to flare.

Allergens are substances from foods, plants, animals, or the air that inflame the skin because the immune system overreacts to the substance. Inflammation occurs even when the person is exposed to small amounts of the substance for a limited time. Although it is known that allergens in the air, such as dust mites, pollens, molds, and dander from animal hair or skin, may worsen the symptoms of atopic dermatitis in some people, scientists aren't certain whether inhaling these allergens or their actual penetration of the skin causes the problems. When people with atopic dermatitis come into contact with an irritant or allergen they are sensitive to, inflammation producing cells become active. These cells release chemicals that cause itching and redness. As the person responds by scratching and rubbing the skin, further damage occurs.

Major And Minor Features Of Atopic Dermatitis

Major Features

- Intense itching
- Characteristic rash in locations typical of the disease
- Chronic or repeatedly occurring symptoms
- Personal or family history of atopic disorders (eczema, hay fever, asthma)

Some Minor Features

- Early age of onset
- Dry skin that may also have patchy scales or rough bumps
- High levels of immunoglobulin E (IgE), an antibody, in the blood
- Numerous skin creases on the palms
- Hand or foot involvement
- Inflammation around the lips
- Nipple eczema
- Susceptibility to skin infection
- Positive allergy skin tests

Children with atopic disease tend to have a higher prevalence of food allergy than those in the general population. An allergic reaction to food can cause skin inflammation (generally an itchy red rash), gastrointestinal symptoms (abdominal pain, vomiting, diarrhea), and/or upper respiratory tract symptoms (congestion, sneezing, and wheezing). The most common allergenic (allergy-causing) foods are eggs, milk, peanuts, wheat, soy, tree nuts, shellfish, and fish. A recent analysis of a large number of studies on allergies and breastfeeding indicated that breastfeeding an infant, although preferable for many reasons, has little effect on protecting the infant from developing atopic dermatitis.

In addition to irritants and allergens, emotional factors, skin infections, and temperature and climate play a role in atopic dermatitis. Although the disease itself is not caused by emotional factors, it can be made worse by stress, anger, and frustration. Interpersonal problems or major life changes, such as divorce, job changes, or the death of a loved one, can also make the disease worse.

Bathing without proper moisturizing afterward is a common factor that triggers a flare of atopic dermatitis. The low humidity of winter or the dry year-round climate of some geographic areas can make the disease worse, as can overheated indoor areas and long or hot baths and showers. Alternately sweating and chilling can trigger a flare in some people. Bacterial infections can also trigger or increase the severity of atopic dermatitis. If a patient experiences a sudden flare of illness, the doctor may check for infection.

Treatment Of Atopic Dermatitis

Treatment is more effective when a partnership develops that includes the patient, family members, and doctor. The doctor will suggest a treatment plan based on the patient's age, symptoms, and general health. The patient or family member providing care plays a large role in the success of the treatment plan by carefully following the doctor's instructions and paying attention to what is or is not helpful. Most patients will notice improvement with proper skin care and lifestyle changes.

The doctor has two main goals in treating atopic dermatitis: healing the skin and preventing flares. These may be assisted by developing skin care routines and avoiding substances that lead to skin irritation and trigger the immune system and the itch-scratch cycle. It is important for the patient and family members to note any changes in the skin's condition in response to treatment, and to be persistent in identifying the treatment that seems to work best.

Medications

New medications known as immunomodulators have been developed that help control inflammation and reduce immune system reactions when applied to the skin. They can be used in patients older than two years of age and have few side effects (burning or itching the first few days of application). They not only reduce flares, but also maintain skin texture and reduce the need for long-term use of corticosteroids.

Corticosteroid creams and ointments have been used for many years to treat atopic dermatitis and other autoimmune diseases affecting the skin. Sometimes over-the-counter preparations are used, but in many cases the doctor will prescribe a stronger corticosteroid cream or ointment. When prescribing a medication, the doctor will take into account the patient's age, location of the skin to be treated, severity of the symptoms, and type of preparation (cream or ointment) that will be most effective. Sometimes the base used in certain brands of corticosteroid creams and ointments irritates the skin of a particular patient. Side effects of repeated or long-term use of topical corticosteroids can include thinning of the skin, infections, growth suppression (in children), and stretch marks on the skin.

When topical corticosteroids are not effective, the doctor may prescribe a systemic corticosteroid, which is taken by mouth or injected instead of being applied directly to the skin. Typically, these medications are used only in resistant cases and only given for short periods of time. The side effects of systemic corticosteroids can include skin damage, thinned or weakened bones, high blood pressure, high blood sugar, infections, and cataracts.

It can be dangerous to suddenly stop taking corticosteroids, so it is very important that the doctor and patient work together in changing the corticosteroid dose.

Antibiotics to treat skin infections may be applied directly to the skin in an ointment, but are usually more effective when taken by mouth. If viral or fungal infections are present, the doctor may also prescribe specific medications to treat those infections.

Certain antihistamines that cause drowsiness can reduce nighttime scratching and allow more restful sleep when taken at bedtime. This effect can be particularly helpful for patients whose nighttime scratching makes the disease worse.

In adults, drugs that suppress the immune system may be prescribed to treat severe cases of atopic dermatitis that have failed to respond to other forms of therapy. These drugs block the production of some immune cells and curb the action of others. The side effects of drugs like these can include high blood pressure, nausea, vomiting, kidney problems, headaches, tingling or numbness, and a possible increased risk of cancer and infections. There is also a risk of relapse after the drug is stopped. Because of their toxic side effects, systemic corticosteroids and immunosuppressive drugs are used only in severe cases and then for as short a period of time as possible. Patients requiring systemic corticosteroids should be referred to dermatologists or allergists specializing in the care of atopic dermatitis to help identify trigger factors and alternative therapies.

In rare cases, when home-based treatments have been unsuccessful, a patient may need a few days in the hospital for intense treatment.

Phototherapy

Use of ultraviolet A or B light waves, alone or combined, can be an effective treatment for mild to moderate dermatitis in older children (over 12 years old) and adults. A combination of ultraviolet light therapy and a drug called psoralen can also be used in cases that are resistant to ultraviolet light alone. Possible long-term side effects of this treatment include premature skin aging and skin cancer. If the doctor thinks that phototherapy may be useful to treat the symptoms of atopic dermatitis, he or she will use the minimum exposure necessary and monitor the skin carefully.

Skin Care

Healing the skin and keeping it healthy are important to prevent further damage and enhance quality of life. Developing and sticking with a daily skin care routine is critical to preventing flares.

A lukewarm bath helps to cleanse and moisturize the skin without drying it excessively. Because soaps can be drying to the skin, the doctor may recommend use of a mild bar soap or nonsoap cleanser. Bath oils are not usually helpful.

After bathing, a person should air-dry the skin, or pat it dry gently (avoiding rubbing or brisk drying), and then apply a lubricant to seal in the water that has been absorbed into the skin during bathing. A lubricant increases the rate of healing and establishes a barrier against further drying and irritation. Lotions that have a high water or alcohol content evaporate more quickly, and alcohol may cause stinging. Therefore, they generally are not the best choice. Creams and ointments work better at healing the skin.

Another key to protecting and restoring the skin is taking steps to avoid repeated skin infections. Signs of skin infection include tiny pustules (pus-filled bumps), oozing cracks or sores, or crusty yellow blisters. If symptoms of a skin infection develop, the doctor should be consulted and treatment should begin as soon as possible.

Protection from allergen exposure: The doctor may suggest reducing exposure to a suspected allergen. For example, the presence of the house dust mite can be limited by encasing mattresses and pillows in special dust-proof covers, frequently washing bedding in hot water, and removing carpeting. However, there is no way to completely rid the environment of airborne allergens.

Changing the diet may not always relieve symptoms of atopic dermatitis. A change may be helpful, however, when the medical history, laboratory studies, and specific symptoms strongly suggest a food allergy. It is up to the patient and his or her family and physician to decide whether the dietary restrictions are appropriate. Unless properly monitored by a physician or dietitian, diets with many restrictions can contribute to serious nutritional problems, especially in children.

Atopic Dermatitis And Quality Of Life

Despite the symptoms caused by atopic dermatitis, it is possible for people with the disorder to maintain a good quality of life. The keys to quality of life lie in being well-informed; awareness of symptoms and their possible cause; and developing a partnership involving the patient or caregiving family member, medical doctor, and other health professionals. Good communication is essential.

When a child has atopic dermatitis, the entire family may be affected. It is helpful if families have additional support to help them cope with the stress and frustration associated with the disease. A child may be fussy and difficult and unable to keep from scratching and rubbing the skin. Distracting the child and providing activities that keep the hands busy are helpful but require much effort on the part of the parents or caregivers. Another issue families face is the social and emotional stress associated with changes in appearance caused by atopic dermatitis. The child may face difficulty in school or with social relationships and may need additional support and encouragement from family members.

Adults with atopic dermatitis can enhance their quality of life by caring regularly for their skin and being mindful of the effects of the disease and how to treat them. Adults should develop a skin care regimen as part of their daily routine, which can be adapted as circumstances and skin conditions change. Stress management and relaxation techniques may help decrease the likelihood of flares. Developing a network of support that includes family, friends, health professionals, and support groups or organizations can be beneficial. Chronic anxiety and depression may be relieved by short-term psychological therapy.

Controlling Atopic Dermatitis

- Prevent scratching or rubbing whenever possible.
- Protect skin from excessive moisture, irritants, and rough clothing.
- Maintain a cool, stable temperature and consistent humidity levels.
- Limit exposure to dust, cigarette smoke, pollens, and animal dander.
- Recognize and limit emotional stress.

Atopic Dermatitis And Vaccination Against Smallpox

Although scientists are working to develop safer vaccines, individuals diagnosed with atopic dermatitis (or eczema) should not receive the current smallpox vaccine. According to the Centers for Disease Control and Prevention (CDC), a U.S. government organization, individuals who have ever been diagnosed with atopic dermatitis, even if the condition is mild or not presently active, are more likely to develop a serious complication if they are exposed to the virus from the smallpox vaccine.

People with atopic dermatitis should exercise caution when coming into close physical contact with a person who has been recently vaccinated, and make certain the vaccinated person has covered the vaccination site or taken other precautions until the scab falls off (about three weeks). Those who have had physical contact with a vaccinated person's unhealed vaccination site or to their bedding or other items that might have touched that site should notify their doctor, particularly if they develop a new or unusual rash.

During a smallpox outbreak, these vaccination recommendations may change. People with atopic dermatitis who have been exposed to smallpox should consult their doctor about vaccination.

Recognizing the situations when scratching is most likely to occur may also help. For example, many patients find that they scratch more when they are idle, and they do better when engaged in activities that keep the hands occupied. Counseling also may be helpful to identify or change career goals if a job involves contact with irritants or involves frequent hand washing, such as work in a kitchen or auto machine shop.

Current Research

Researchers supported by the National Institute of Arthritis and Musculoskeletal and Skin Diseases and other institutes of the National Institutes of Health are gaining a better understanding of what causes atopic dermatitis and how it can be managed, treated, and, ultimately, prevented. Some promising avenues of research are described below.

Genetics

Although atopic dermatitis runs in families, the role of genetics (inheritance) remains unclear. It does appear that more than one gene is involved in the disease.

Research has helped shed light on the way atopic dermatitis is inherited. Studies show that children are at increased risk for developing the disorder if there is a family history of other atopic disease, such as hay fever or asthma. The risk is significantly higher if both parents have an atopic disease. In addition, studies of identical twins (who have the same genes) show that a person whose identical twin has atopic dermatitis is seven times more likely to have atopic dermatitis than someone in the general population. A person whose fraternal (nonidentical) twin has atopic dermatitis is three times more likely to have atopic dermatitis than someone in the general population. These findings suggest that genes play an important role in determining who gets the disease.

Also, scientists have discovered mutations in a certain gene that plays a role in the production of a protein called filaggrin. The filaggrin protein is normally found in the outermost layer of the skin and functions as a component of the skin barrier. The gene mutation disrupts filaggrin's ability to maintain a normal skin barrier and appears to be a genetic factor that predisposes people to develop atopic dermatitis and other diseases in which the skin barrier is compromised.

Biochemical Abnormalities

Scientists suspect that changes in the skin's protective barrier make people with atopic dermatitis more sensitive to irritants. Such people have lower levels of fatty acids (substances that provide moisture and elasticity) in their skin, which causes dryness and reduces the skin's ability to control inflammation. Researchers continue to search for treatments that help keep the skin intact and prevent flares.

Other research points to a possible defect in a type of white blood cell called a monocyte. In people with atopic dermatitis, monocytes appear to play a role in the decreased production of an immune system hormone called interferon gamma (IFN-γ), which helps regulate allergic reactions. This defect may cause exaggerated immune and inflammatory responses in the blood and tissues of people with atopic dermatitis.

Faulty Regulation Of Immunoglobulin E (IgE)

As already described in the section on diagnosis, IgE is a type of antibody that controls the immune system's allergic response. An antibody is a special protein produced by the immune system that recognizes and helps fight and destroy viruses, bacteria, and other foreign substances that invade the body. Normally, IgE is present in very small amounts, but levels are high in about 80 percent of people with atopic dermatitis.

In allergic diseases, IgE antibodies are produced in response to different allergens. When an allergen comes into contact with IgE on specialized immune cells, the cells release various chemicals, including histamine. These chemicals cause the symptoms of an allergic reaction, such as wheezing, sneezing, runny eyes, and itching. The release of histamine and other chemicals alone cannot explain the typical long-term symptoms of the disease. Research is underway to identify factors that may explain why too much IgE is produced and how it plays a role in the disease.

Immune System Imbalance

Researchers also think that an imbalance in the immune system may contribute to the development of atopic dermatitis. It appears that the part of the immune system responsible for stimulating IgE is overactive, and the part that handles skin viral and fungal infections is underactive. Indeed, the skin of people with atopic dermatitis shows increased susceptibility to skin infections. This imbalance appears to result in the skin's inability to prevent inflammation, even in areas of skin that appear normal. In one project, scientists are studying the role of the infectious bacterium *Staphylococcus aureus* in atopic dermatitis.

Researchers believe that one type of immune cell in the skin, called a Langerhans cell, may be involved in atopic dermatitis. Langerhans cells pick up viruses, bacteria, allergens, and other foreign substances that invade the body and deliver them to other cells in the immune defense system. Langerhans cells appear to be hyperactive in the skin of people with atopic diseases. Certain Langerhans cells are particularly potent at activating white blood cells called T cells in atopic skin, which produce proteins that promote allergic response. This function results in an exaggerated response of the skin to tiny amounts of allergens.

Drug Research

Some researchers are focusing on new treatments for atopic dermatitis, including biologic agents, fatty acid supplements, and phototherapy. For example, they are studying how ultraviolet light affects the skin's immune system in healthy and diseased skin. They are also investigating biologic response modifiers, or biologics, which are a new family of genetically engineered drugs that block specific molecular pathways of the immune system that are involved in the inflammatory process. A clinical trial is underway to test a drug to see if it can help control the itching associated with atopic dermatitis.

Researchers also continue to look for drugs that suppress the immune system. Also, anti-inflammatory drugs have been developed that affect multiple cells and cell functions, and may prove to be an effective alternative to corticosteroids in the treatment of atopic dermatitis.

Other Research

Several experimental treatments are being evaluated that attempt to replace substances that are deficient in people with atopic dermatitis. Evening primrose oil is a substance rich in gamma-linolenic acid, one of the fatty acids that is decreased in the skin of people with atopic dermatitis. Studies to date using evening primrose oil have yielded contradictory results. In addition, dietary fatty acid supplements have not proven highly effective. There is also a great deal of interest in the use of herbs and plant extracts to treat the disease. Studies to date show some benefit, but not without concerns about toxicity and the risks involved in suppressing the immune system without close medical supervision.

Hope For The Future

Although the symptoms of atopic dermatitis can be difficult and uncomfortable, the disease can be successfully managed. People with atopic dermatitis can lead healthy, productive lives. As scientists learn more about atopic dermatitis and what causes it, they continue to move closer to effective treatments, and perhaps, ultimately, a cure.

Chapter 20

Urticaria (Hives)

Hives are a common occurrence, affecting up to 25% of the population at least once in their lives. They can be short term, lasting only a few days to six weeks, but they can be chronic and last for months or years. Chronic hives can be especially frustrating for patients. They may or not be related to an allergy. In some cases the cause is never identified.

There are three principal classifications:

Type 1: Acute Urticaria

Acute hives can appear at any age, but they are most commonly seen in young adults. The rash has very itchy red areas with white raised central circles that resemble mosquito bites. If the welts grow very large, spreading and joining together or swelling downward deep into body tissue, then they are known as giant hives or angioedema. Angioedema is painful and unsightly, but it is not as itchy. With angioedema the eruptions become large enough to cause swelling of the eyelids, tongue, mouth, hands, or feet. In severe cases, hives can be accompanied by other symptoms such as difficulty in breathing, difficulty swallowing, digestive upsets, and fever. Hives can occur internally to produce swelling of internal organs.

Hives can be caused by an allergic reaction to foods, drugs, insect bites, infections, or substances which can cause other allergic reactions. However not all cases are caused by allergy; frequently they are caused by viruses. It can sometimes be extremely difficult to find the cause. Triggers include medications, food, viruses, latex, heat, cold, and direct exposure to sun. If the cause is known, the trigger should be avoided.

Since hives can come and go so swiftly, a very significant percentage of cases are never accurately diagnosed. The hives can appear and disappear without any explanation of what caused them or cured them. Skin testing may be used in finding the source of infrequent hives; a detailed history is usually more rewarding. The patient can record everything that was ingested or touched for the 24 hours prior to the outbreak and bring this to the physician.

Treatment Of Acute Hives

- **Avoidance:** If the cause is found, then it should be removed from the environment or diet.

- **Medications:** Topical ointments can be applied to the skin to relieve the itch. Antihistamines will reduce the itching and swelling. Cortisone drugs used as an ointment or given by mouth may be needed.

- **Immunotherapy:** Allergy shots help only if a person has hives because of what they breathe. These people can be successfully desensitized. Cross reacting proteins from inhalants that are also found in foods can help drop the degree of reactivity to those foods.

Hives can look ugly and are unbelievably itchy, but they are not in themselves dangerous. However, if you have hives and other symptoms such as dizziness, vomiting, diarrhea, difficulty in breathing, difficulty swallowing, or faintness, these are signs and symptoms of a much more serous reaction—anaphylaxis. Anaphylaxis is life-threatening! If you experience hives plus one or more of these other symptoms soon after eating or being injected with a substance that you do not usually use, OBTAIN MEDICAL HELP IMMEDIATELY.

Type 2: Chronic Urticaria

When a person has had hives for over six weeks, they are termed chronic urticaria. Many experts believe that acute and chronic urticaria are no different except for duration. Some studies indicate that allergy is less likely to be an underlying factor in chronic urticaria. Since in 80 percent of the cases of chronic urticaria the underlying cause is never found, not many conclusions can be made.

Discovering the exact cause of chronic urticaria is often extremely difficult. If the hives occur daily, they are most likely caused by something that you are exposed to daily. In that case, it is easier to see the cause/effect relationship. Sometimes it is several hours after exposure before the itching begins. In that case, some real detective work will be needed to find the culprit. These are the things to consider in order of importance: foods, drugs, infections, inhalants, and psychological factors.

To diagnose chronic hives the doctor will first make sure that the hives are not caused by infection or an underlying disease state. However, in the evaluation of patients with chronic urticaria, it is their history which is the most important diagnosis tool. The physician will look for clues regarding drug or chemical exposure, changes in dietary habits, changes in personal habits, or alterations in residence or place of employment. She/he will also look for a pattern such as: Is there a relationship to eating? Does the patient wake-up with hives? Are they as likely to occur at home as at work/school? Are weekends or weekdays different in any way? The physician will often place a patient with chronic urticaria on a diet to see if elimination of the hive-trigger will bring relief. It is important to see a doctor before going on an elimination diet. Systemic diseases should be ruled out with this appointment. Sometimes these diseases can cause hives that are painful or burning in nature.

Type 3: Physical Urticaria

Typically, acute and chronic display round or oval hives, occur over virtually any part of the body and last for hours or days. There are others forms of urticaria which show up in lines or odd shapes, appear on specific parts of the body, and appear then disappear within two hours. This is urticaria which is triggered by a physical cause. There are several possible causes:

Pressure Urticaria: Pressure hives produces deep and painful local swelling. The swelling can occur immediately or several hours later. This type of urticaria can be triggered by prolonged sitting. It is also triggered by the wearing of tight clothing and consequently is seen in areas such as the waist/belt line, under elastic bands such as panties, socks, or wristbands. Choosing appropriate clothing and/or taking regular breaks from sitting, usually controls pressure urticaria. If medication is needed, steroids are usually administered for a short time.

Cold-Induced Urticaria: Cold-induced urticaria is a disorder in which hives occur within minutes of being exposed to the cold or appear as a result of the effects of warming. Total body exposure to cold, such as swimming in frigid water can result in a drop in blood pressure, fainting, shock, and drowning.

Dermographism: Dermographism literally means skin writing. Scratching the skin will produce a raised mark and redden the surrounding skin. It is easy to test. Simply use a moderately sharp object, such as a fingernail or a key, and run it over the skin. If a recognizable pattern is used in testing, such as a name or the game of X's and O's, it is a form of physical urticaria which is easily identified.

This phenomenon usually occurs only in young adults and gradually disappears. An antihistamine will alleviate any associated itchiness.

Solar Urticaria: In this rare form of physical urticaria, hives occur after exposure to the sun or to certain artificial light sources. It is believed that the condition is an allergic reaction to an antigen formed by the interaction of light waves on the skin. Antihistamines are helpful to relieve the itch.

Heat Urticaria: There are two forms of heat urticaria. The more common form is also called cholinergic urticaria or generalized heat urticaria. In this form, it occurs when the body temperature is raised such as in a hot bath or shower, from a fever or exercise. The outbreak begins with a few small hives and gradually become more widespread. If the reaction is very severe, the wheals will run together, leading to a drop in blood pressure and loss of consciousness. Cholinergic urticaria is helped by antihistamines given regularly in severe cases or intermittently upon exposure to milder cases.

The other form of heat urticaria is a very rare form in which welts develop within minutes at the site of locally applied heat, such as a hot water bottle or heating pad. Allergy does not appear to be a factor in this form of urticaria. Elimination of exposure to such items should control condition.

Conclusion

There are many patterns of hives with different underlying causes. In order to cope with urticaria, it is important to understand exactly which form of urticaria exists because the treatment is directly affected by the diagnosis. It is important to note that there are other skin conditions due to allergy, one of the most common being eczema or dermatitis. Moreover, allergic skin conditions are common and plague people the world over, but not all skin problems are allergic in origin. See a qualified medical physician for diagnosis and treatment.

Chapter 21

Anaphylaxis

Anaphylaxis is a serious allergic reaction that involves more than one organ system (for example, skin and respiratory tract and/or gastrointestinal tract), can begin very rapidly, and can cause death.

Causes

The leading cause of anaphylaxis is food allergy, especially allergy to peanut and tree nuts. However, medications like penicillin, insect stings, and latex can also cause an allergic reaction that leads to anaphylaxis.

Symptoms

Anaphylaxis includes a wide range of symptoms that can occur in many combinations and be difficult to recognize. Some symptoms are not life-threatening, but the most severe ones restrict breathing and blood circulation.

Many different organs of your body can be affected:

- **Skin:** Itching, hives, redness, swelling
- **Nose:** Sneezing, stuffy nose, runny nose
- **Mouth:** Itching, swelling of lips or tongue
- **Throat:** Itching, tightness, difficulty swallowing, swelling of the back of the throat

About This Chapter: "Allergic Diseases: Anaphylaxis," National Institute of Allergy and Infectious Diseases (www .niaid.nih.gov), June 7, 2012.

- **Chest:** Shortness of breath, cough, wheeze, chest pain, tightness
- **Heart:** Weak pulse, passing out, shock
- **Gastrointestinal (GI) Tract:** Vomiting, diarrhea, cramps
- **Nervous System:** Dizziness or fainting

How soon after exposure will symptoms occur?

Symptoms can begin within several minutes to several hours after exposure to the allergen. Sometimes the symptoms go away, only to return later—anywhere from 8–72 hours later. When you begin to experience symptoms, seek immediate medical attention because anaphylaxis can be life-threatening.

How do you know if a person is having an anaphylactic reaction?

Anaphylaxis is highly likely if at least one of the following three conditions occurs:

1. Your symptoms appear within minutes to several hours and involve skin, mucosal tissue (such as tissues lining the respiratory and GI tracts), or both. You also have trouble breathing or have a drop in blood pressure (pale, weak pulse, confusion, loss of consciousness).

2. You have two or more of the following symptoms that occur within minutes to several hours after exposure to the allergen:

   - Hives, itchiness, or redness all over your body and swelling of the lips, tongue, or the back of the throat
   - Trouble breathing in the upper and/or lower part of your airways
   - Drop in blood pressure
   - Long-lasting GI symptoms such as abdominal cramps or vomiting

3. Your blood pressure drops, leading to dizziness or fainting, within minutes to several hours after exposure to a substance to which you know you have an allergy.

If you are experiencing symptoms of anaphylaxis, seek immediate treatment and tell your healthcare professional if you have a history of allergic reactions.

Can anaphylaxis be predicted?

Anaphylaxis caused by an allergic reaction is highly unpredictable. The severity of a given attack does not predict the severity of subsequent attacks. The response will vary depending on several factors, including the following:

- Your sensitivity to the allergen
- How much of the allergen you are exposed to
- How the allergen entered your body

Any anaphylactic reaction can become dangerous quickly and must be evaluated immediately by a healthcare professional.

Timing

An anaphylactic reaction can occur as any of the following:

- A single reaction that occurs immediately after exposure to the allergen and gets better with or without treatment within the first minutes to hours. Symptoms do not recur later in relation to that episode.
- Two reactions. The first reaction includes an initial set of symptoms that seem to go away but then reappear. The second reaction most typically occurs eight hours after the first reaction but may occur as much as 72 hours later.
- A single, long-lasting reaction that continues for hours or days following the initial reaction.

Treatment

If you or someone you know is having an anaphylactic episode, health experts advise using an auto-injector, if available, to inject epinephrine (a hormone that increases heart rate, constricts the blood vessels, and opens the airways) into the thigh muscle, and calling 9-1-1 if you are not in a hospital. If you are in a hospital, summon a resuscitation team.

If epinephrine is not given promptly, rapid decline and death could occur within 30 to 60 minutes. Epinephrine acts immediately, but it may be necessary to give repeat doses.

After epinephrine has been given, the patient can be placed in a reclining position with feet elevated to help restore normal blood flow.

A healthcare professional also may give the patient any of the following secondary treatments:

- Medications to open the airways
- Antihistamines to relieve itching and hives
- Corticosteroids (a class of drugs used to treat inflammatory diseases) to prevent prolonged inflammation and long-lasting reactions

- Additional medications to constrict blood vessels and increase heart rate

- Supplemental oxygen therapy

- Intravenous fluids

Conditions such as asthma, chronic lung disease, and cardiovascular disease may increase the risk of death from anaphylaxis. Medications such as those that treat high blood pressure also may worsen symptom severity and limit response to treatment.

Antihistamines should be used only as a secondary treatment. Giving antihistamines instead of epinephrine may increase the risk of a life-threatening allergic reaction.

Management

Before leaving emergency medical care, your healthcare professional should provide the following:

- An epinephrine auto-injector or a prescription for two doses and training on how to use the auto-injector

- A follow-up appointment or an appointment with a clinical specialist such as an allergist or immunologist

- Information on where to get medical identification jewelry or an anaphylaxis wallet card that alerts others of the allergy

- Education about allergen avoidance, recognizing the symptoms of anaphylaxis, and giving epinephrine

- An anaphylaxis emergency action plan (You can download a sample plan from the American Academy of Allergy, Asthma and Immunology at http://www.aaaai.org/ Aaaai/media/MediaLibrary/PDF%20Documents/Libraries/New-ANAPHYLAXIS -EMERGENCY-ACTION-PLAN-2010-New.pdf.)

If you or someone you know has a history of severe allergic reactions or anaphylaxis, your healthcare professional should remember to keep you S.A.F.E.

- **Seek Support:** Your healthcare professional should tell you the following: Anaphylaxis is a life-threatening condition. The symptoms of the current episode may occur again (sometimes up to three days later). You are at risk for anaphylaxis in the future. At the first sign of symptoms, give yourself epinephrine and then immediately call an ambulance or go to the nearest emergency facility.

- **Allergen Identification And Avoidance:** Before you leave the hospital, your healthcare professional should have done the following: Made efforts to identify the allergen by taking your medical history. Explained the importance of getting additional testing to confirm what triggered the reaction, so you can successfully avoid it in the future.

- **Follow-Up With Specialty Care:** Your healthcare professional should encourage you to consult a specialist for an allergy evaluation.

- **Epinephrine For Emergencies:** Your healthcare professional should give you the following: An epinephrine auto-injector or a prescription and training on how to use an auto-injector. Advice to routinely check the expiration date of the auto-injector.

Research

Research funded by the National Institute of Allergy and Infectious Diseases (NIAID) focuses on anaphylaxis induced by food allergens. NIAID supports basic research in allergy and immunology to understand how, in certain people, foods elicit allergic reactions that can range from mild to severe.

NIAID also conducts clinical trials of therapies that may alter the body's immune response so that it no longer triggers an allergic response to food. Learn more about NIAID-funded research programs in food allergy at http://www.niaid.nih.gov/topics/foodAllergy/research/Pages/funding.aspx.

The NIAID Laboratory of Allergic Diseases (LAD) supports basic, translational, and clinical research on anaphylaxis. Researchers in LAD seek to better understand the various immune system components that are involved in anaphylaxis; identify molecular events that cause and characterize anaphylactic reactions to understand their triggers; and discover diagnostic markers or reveal targets for new therapies to help prevent and treat life-threatening allergic reactions. Read more about LAD online at http://www.niaid.nih.gov/LabsAndResources/labs/aboutlabs/lad/Pages/default.aspx.

In December 2010, comprehensive guidelines for the diagnosis and management of food allergy were published. The guidelines provide healthcare professionals with recommendations on the best ways to identify food allergy and help people manage this condition, even its most severe forms. NIAID helped lead the guidelines effort, working with 34 professional organizations, patient advocacy groups, and federal agencies. Read about the Guidelines for the Diagnosis and Management of Food Allergy in the United States at http://www.niaid.nih.gov/topics/foodAllergy/clinical/Pages/default.aspx.

Part Three
Food Allergies And Intolerances

Chapter 22

Distinguishing Between Food Allergies And Intolerances

An Allergic Reaction To Food

A food allergy occurs when the immune system responds to a harmless food as if it were a threat. The first time a person with food allergy is exposed to the food, no symptoms occur; but the first exposure primes the body to respond the next time. When the person eats the food again, an allergic response can occur.

A First Exposure

Usually, the way you are first exposed to a food is when you eat it. But sometimes a first exposure or subsequent exposure can occur without your knowledge.

This may be true in the case of peanut allergy. A person who experiences anaphylaxis on the first known exposure to peanut may have previously touched peanuts, used a peanut-containing skin care product, or breathed in peanut dust in the home or when close to other people eating peanuts.

The Allergic Reaction Process

An allergic reaction to food is a two-step process.

Step 1: The first time you are exposed to a food allergen, your immune system reacts as if the food were harmful and makes specific IgE antibodies to that allergen. The antibodies circulate through your blood and attach to mast cells and basophils. Mast cells are found in all

About This Chapter: Excerpted from "Food Allergy: An Overview," National Institute of Allergy and Infectious Diseases (www.niaid.nih.gov), November 2010.

body tissues, especially in areas of your body that are typical sites of allergic reactions. Those sites include your nose, throat, lungs, skin, and gastrointestinal (GI) tract. Basophils are found in your blood and also in tissues that have become inflamed due to an allergic reaction.

Step 2: The next time you are exposed to the same food allergen, it binds to the IgE antibodies that are attached to the mast cells and basophils. The binding signals the cells to release massive amounts of chemicals such as histamine. Depending on the tissue in which they are released, these chemicals will cause you to have various symptoms of food allergy. The symptoms can range from mild to severe. A severe allergic reaction can include a potentially life-threatening reaction called anaphylaxis.

Generally, you are at greater risk for developing a food allergy if you come from a family in which allergies are common. These allergies are not necessarily food allergies but perhaps other allergic diseases, such as asthma or eczema (atopic dermatitis). If you have two parents who have allergies, you are more likely to develop food allergy than someone with one parent who has allergies.

An allergic reaction to food usually takes place within a few minutes to several hours after exposure to the allergen. The process of eating and digesting food and the location of mast cells both affect the timing and location of the reaction.

Symptoms Of Food Allergy

If you are allergic to a particular food, you may experience all or some of the following symptoms:

- Itching in your mouth
- Swelling of lips and tongue
- GI symptoms, such as vomiting, diarrhea, or abdominal cramps and pain
- Hives
- Worsening of eczema
- Tightening of the throat or trouble breathing
- Drop in blood pressure

Eosinophilic Esophagitis

Eosinophilic esophagitis (EoE) is a newly recognized chronic disease that can be associated with food allergies. It is increasingly being diagnosed in children and adults.

Symptoms of EoE include nausea, vomiting, and abdominal pain after eating. A person may also have symptoms that resemble acid reflux from the stomach. In older children and adults, it can cause more severe symptoms, such as difficulty swallowing solid food or solid food sticking in the esophagus for more than a few minutes. In infants, this disease may be associated with failure to thrive.

If you are diagnosed with EoE, you will probably be tested for allergies. In some situations, avoiding certain food allergens will be an effective treatment for EoE.

Cross-Reactive Food Allergies

If you have a life-threatening reaction to a certain food, your healthcare professional will show you how to avoid similar foods that may trigger this reaction. For example, if you have a history of allergy to shrimp, allergy testing will usually show that you are also allergic to other shellfish, such as crab, lobster, and crayfish. This is called cross-reactivity.

Food Allergy Versus Food Intolerance

Food allergy is sometimes confused with food intolerance. To find out the difference between food allergy and food intolerance, your healthcare professional will go through a list of possible causes for your symptoms.

Types Of Food Intolerance

Lactose Intolerance: Lactose is a sugar found in milk and most milk products. Lactase is an enzyme in the lining of the gut that breaks down or digests lactose. Lactose intolerance occurs when lactase is missing. Instead of the enzyme breaking down the sugar, bacteria in the gut break it down, which forms gas, which in turn causes symptoms of bloating, abdominal pain, and sometimes diarrhea.

Lactose intolerance is uncommon in babies and young children under the age of five years. Because lactase levels decline as people get older, lactose intolerance becomes more common with age. Lactose intolerance also varies widely based on racial and ethnic background. Your healthcare professional can use laboratory tests to find out whether your body can digest lactose.

Food Additives: Another type of food intolerance is a reaction to certain products that are added to food to enhance taste, add color, or protect against the growth of microbes. Several compounds such as MSG (monosodium glutamate) and sulfites are tied to reactions that can be confused with food allergy.

- MSG is a flavor enhancer. When taken in large amounts, it can cause some of the following: flushing; sensations of warmth; headache; and chest discomfort. These passing reactions occur rapidly after eating large amounts of food to which MSG has been added.

- Sulfites are found in food for several reasons: They have been added to increase crispness or prevent mold growth. They occur naturally in the food. They have been generated during the wine-making process. Sulfites can cause breathing problems in people with asthma. The Food and Drug Administration (FDA) has banned sulfites as spray-on preservatives for fresh fruits and vegetables. When sulfites are present in foods, they are listed on ingredient labels.

Gluten Intolerance: Gluten is a part of wheat, barley, and rye. Gluten intolerance is associated with celiac disease, also called gluten-sensitive enteropathy. This disease develops when the immune system responds abnormally to gluten. This abnormal response does not involve IgE antibody and is not considered a food allergy.

Food Poisoning: Some of the symptoms of food allergy, such as abdominal cramping, are common in food poisoning. However, food poisoning is caused by microbes, such as bacteria, and bacterial products, such as toxins, that can contaminate meats and dairy products.

Histamine Toxicity: Fish, such as tuna and mackerel that are not refrigerated properly and become contaminated by bacteria, may contain very high levels of histamine. A person who eats such fish may show symptoms that are similar to food allergy. However, this reaction is not a true allergic reaction. Instead, the reaction is called histamine toxicity or scombroid food poisoning.

Other: Several other conditions, such as ulcers and cancers of the GI tract, cause some of the same symptoms as food allergy. These symptoms, which include vomiting, diarrhea, and cramping abdominal pain, become worse when you eat.

Diagnosing Food Allergy

Detailed History

Your healthcare professional will begin by taking a detailed medical history to find out whether your symptoms are caused by an allergy to specific foods, a food intolerance, or other health problems.

A detailed history is the most valuable tool for diagnosing food allergy. Your healthcare professional will ask you several questions and listen to your history of food reactions to decide whether the facts fit a diagnosis of food allergy.

Your healthcare professional is likely to ask some of the following questions:

- Did your reaction come on quickly, usually within minutes to several hours after eating the food?

- Is your reaction always associated with a certain food?

- How much of this potentially allergenic food did you eat before you had a reaction?

- Have you eaten this food before and had a reaction?

- Did anyone else who ate the same food get sick?

- Did you take allergy medicines, and if so, did they help? (Antihistamines should relieve hives, for example.)

Diet Diary

Sometimes your healthcare professional can't make a diagnosis based only on your history. In that case, you may be asked to keep a record of what you eat and whether you have a reaction. This diet diary contains more details about the foods you eat than your history. From the diary, you and your healthcare professional may be able to identify a consistent pattern in your reactions.

Elimination Diet

The next step some healthcare professionals use is a limited elimination diet, in which the food that is suspected of causing an allergic reaction is removed from your diet. For example, if you suspect you are allergic to egg, your healthcare professional will instruct you to eliminate this one food from your diet. The limited elimination diet is done under the direction of your healthcare professional.

Skin Prick Test

If your history, diet diary, or elimination diet suggests a specific food allergy is likely, then your healthcare professional will use the skin prick test to confirm the diagnosis.

With a skin prick test, your healthcare professional uses a needle to place a tiny amount of food extract just below the surface of the skin on your lower arm or back. If you are allergic, there will be swelling or redness at the test site. This is a positive result. It means that there are IgE molecules on the skin's mast cells that are specific to the food being tested.

The skin prick test is simple and relatively safe, and results are ready in minutes.

You can have a positive skin prick test to a food, however, without having an allergic reaction to that food. A healthcare professional often makes a diagnosis of food allergy when someone has both a positive skin prick test to a specific food and a history of reactions that suggests an allergy to the same food.

Blood Test

Instead of the skin prick test, your healthcare professional can take a blood sample to measure the levels of food-specific IgE antibodies.

As with skin prick testing, positive blood tests do not necessarily mean that you have a food allergy. Your healthcare professional must combine these test results with information about your history of reactions to food to make an accurate diagnosis of food allergy.

Oral Food Challenge

Caution: Because oral food challenges can cause a severe allergic reaction, they should always be conducted by a healthcare professional who has experience performing them.

An oral food challenge is the final method healthcare professionals use to diagnose food allergy. This method includes the following steps:

- Your healthcare professional gives you individual doses of various foods (masked so you do not know what food is present), some of which are suspected of starting an allergic reaction.

- Initially, the dose of food is very small, but the amount is gradually increased during the challenge.

- You swallow the individual dose.

- Your healthcare professional watches you to see whether a reaction occurs.

To prevent bias, oral food challenges are often done double blinded. In a true double-blind challenge, neither you nor your healthcare professional knows whether the substance you eat contains the likely allergen. Another medical professional has made up the individual doses. In a single-blind challenge, your healthcare professional knows what you are eating but you do not.

A reaction only to suspected foods and not to the other foods tested confirms the diagnosis of a food allergy.

Chapter 23

Peanut And Tree Nut Allergies

Peanut Allergy

Peanut allergy is one of the most common food allergies. Unfortunately, it also is one of the most dangerous, since peanuts tend to cause particularly severe reactions (anaphylaxis). Some people are very sensitive and have reactions from eating trace amounts of peanut. Non-ingestion contact (touching peanuts or inhaling airborne peanut allergens, such as dust from the shells) is less likely to trigger a severe reaction.

Peanut allergies seem to be on the rise in children. In the United States, the number of children with peanut allergy doubled between 1997 and 2002. Subsequent studies in the United Kingdom and Canada also showed a high prevalence of peanut allergy in schoolchildren. Unlike egg and cow's milk allergies, which most children outgrow, peanut allergies tend to be life-long. Recent studies, however, indicate that approximately 20% of peanut-allergic children do eventually outgrow their allergy.

The peanut (*Arachis hypogaea*) is not really a nut, but a kind of legume. It is related to other beans, such as peas, lentils, and soybeans. People with peanut allergy are not necessarily allergic to other legumes (even soy, another of the "big eight" food allergens), so be sure to speak with your doctor before assuming that you have to avoid these protein-rich foods. A person with a peanut allergy may also be allergic to tree nuts (almonds, walnuts, hazelnuts, cashews, etc.). In fact, some 30–40% of people who have peanut allergy also are allergic to tree nuts. Not surprisingly, allergists usually tell their peanut-allergic patients to avoid tree nuts.

Researchers have isolated three major peanut allergens. They are trying to learn why peanuts cause such severe reactions and why the number of people who suffer from peanut allergy is increasing. Investigators also are trying to develop therapies that would prevent anaphylaxis in people with peanut allergies.

How To Avoid Peanuts*

The federal Food Allergen Labeling and Consumer Protection Act (FALCPA) requires that any packaged food product that contains peanuts as an ingredient must list the word "Peanut" on the label. Please be sure to read all product labels carefully before purchasing and consuming any item. Remember, also, that ingredients change from time to time, so check labels every time you shop. If you are still not sure whether or not a product contains peanuts, call the manufacturer. Always take extra precaution when dining in restaurants or eating foods prepared by others. If you are in doubt about any product or dish, don't eat it.

- The following ingredients indicate the presence of peanut protein: Beer nuts, ground nuts, mixed nuts, and peanut (including peanut flour and peanut butter).

- Peanut protein is found in *Arachis* oil, and in cold pressed, expressed, expelled, and extruded peanut oils. Highly processed peanut oil has been shown to be safe for the vast majority of individuals allergic to peanut. As the degree of processing of commercial peanut oil may be difficult to determine, avoidance is prudent.

- Nu-Nuts and other artificial flavored nuts contain peanut protein.

- Ethnic restaurants (such as Chinese, African, Indonesian, Thai, and Vietnamese), bakeries, and ice cream parlors are considered high-risk for individuals with peanut allergy due to the common use of peanut and the risk of cross contamination—even if you order a peanut-free item.

- Peanut butter and/or peanut flour have been used in chili and spaghetti sauce as thickeners. Always ask if peanut was in the recipe.

- Many candies and chocolates contain peanut or run the risk of cross contact with peanut protein.

- Lupine or lupin is a legume that may cause an allergic reaction in those with peanut allergy. Lupine is used in this country in many gluten-free and high-protein products. In many European countries, particularly Italy and France, lupine flour and/or peanut flour may be mixed with wheat flour in baked goods.

- Many tree nuts are processed with peanuts and therefore may contain trace amounts of peanut protein. Extreme caution is advised.

*The Food Allergy Initiative (FAI) wishes to thank the Jaffe Food Allergy Institute at Mount Sinai School of Medicine (New York, NY) for providing the allergen avoidance information in this article.

Tree Nut Allergy

Tree nut allergy is one of the most common food allergies in children and adults. Like peanuts, tree nuts (almonds, cashews, walnuts, etc.) tend to cause particularly severe reactions, even if a person is exposed to only a tiny amount.

In a registry of 5,149 people who had peanut or tree nut allergy, the median age of reaction to tree nuts was 36 months. Sixty-eight percent of the tree nut-allergic participants were not aware of any previous exposure to tree nuts before their first reaction. This allergy tends to be life-long; recent studies have shown that approximately 9% of tree nut-allergic children eventually outgrow their allergy.

People seldom are allergic to just one type of tree nut, so allergists usually will tell patients to avoid all tree nuts.

How To Avoid Tree Nuts*

The federal Food Allergen Labeling and Consumer Protection Act (FALCPA) requires that any packaged food product that contains tree nuts as an ingredient must list the specific tree nut on the label. Please be sure to read all product labels carefully before purchasing and consuming any item. Remember, also, that ingredients change from time to time, so check labels every time you shop. If you are still not sure whether or not a product contains tree nuts, call the manufacturer. Always take extra precaution when dining in restaurants or eating foods prepared by others. If you are in doubt about any product or dish, don't eat it.

The following common nuts are considered tree nuts under U.S. law: Almond; Brazil nut; cashew; chestnut; filbert/hazelnut; macadamia nut; pecan; pine nut (pignolia nut); pistachio; walnut.

The following are uncommon, additional tree nuts that require disclosure by U.S. law. However, the risk of an allergic reaction to these nuts is unknown: Beechnut; ginkgo; shea nut; butternut; hickory; chinquapin; lychee nut; pili nut; coconut. The American Academy of Allergy, Asthma and Immunology (AAAAI) states: "There is conflicting information on whether or not coconut must be avoided by tree nut allergic individuals. In the past,

A New Form Of Immunotherapy Holds Promise

A new treatment may be a safe and effective form of immunotherapy for children with peanut allergy, according to researchers at Duke University Medical Center and Massachusetts General Hospital. Currently, there are no treatments available for people with peanut allergy. The double-blind, placebo-controlled study, funded in part by the National Center for Complementary and Alternative Medicine (NCCAM) and published in *The Journal of Allergy and Clinical Immunology*, investigated the safety, clinical effectiveness, and immunologic changes with sublingual immunotherapy—a treatment that involves administering very small amounts of the allergen extract under a person's tongue.

Researchers randomly assigned 18 children (ages 1–11 years) with known peanut allergy to receive either peanut sublingual immunotherapy or placebo. Participants in the peanut group received increased doses of peanut extract every two weeks for six months. Following each dose increase, participants continued the same daily dose at home. Once a maximum dose of 2,000 micrograms of peanut protein was reached, participants continued to take this daily maintenance dose at home for approximately six more months.

After a total of 12 months of sublingual immunotherapy, participants underwent a food challenge, which involved taking increasing doses of peanut protein in the form of peanut flour mixed with food. The food-challenge placebo consisted of oat flour mixed with food given in the same increments. Allergy skin prick tests were performed, and participants' blood samples were taken at different points throughout the study.

The researchers found that the participants who had received peanut sublingual immunotherapy could safely consume 20 times more peanut protein than those who had received the placebo (1710 mg vs. 85 mg). This level of desensitization is clinically significant because it represents protection from accidental ingestion of peanut, which is often less than 100 mg (or one peanut). In addition, allergy skin prick tests showed a decreased allergic response to peanut in the treatment group. The blood tests showed immunologic changes in the treatment group, suggesting a significant change in allergic response.

The researchers concluded that these findings are promising, but more study is needed to determine whether sublingual immunotherapy can increase long-term tolerance to peanuts in children with peanut allergy.

Reference

Kim EH, Bird JA, Kulis M, et al. Sublingual immunotherapy for peanut allergy: clinical and immunologic evidence of desensitization. *The Journal of Allergy and Clinical Immunology*. 2011.

Source: "New Approach for Peanut Allergy in Children Holds Promise," National Center for Complementary and Alternative medicine (http://nccam.nih.gov), July 28, 2011.

coconut has not been considered a tree nut and typically has not been restricted in the diets of people with a tree nut allergy. Coconut is in the palm family and it is actually the seed of a drupaceous fruit, not a tree nut. It does not cross-react with tree nuts. However, in October 2006, the FDA began to define coconut as a tree nut. There are a small number of documented cases of allergic reactions to coconut. However, most occurred in individuals who were not allergic to other tree nuts. Thus, it is possible to be allergic to coconut, although coconut does not cross-react with tree nuts. It is important to discuss this issue with your allergist/immunologist who can instruct you on whether or not you need to avoid coconut if you are tree nut allergic."

- Tree nut proteins may be found in cereals, crackers, cookies, candy, chocolates, energy bars, flavored coffee, frozen desserts, marinades, barbeque sauces, and some cold cuts, such as mortadella.

- Tree nut protein will be found in foods such as gianduja (a creamy mixture of chocolate and chopped almonds and hazelnuts, although other nuts may be used); marzipan (almond paste); nougat; Nu-Nuts artificial nuts; pesto; and nut meal.

- Tree nut oils may contain nut protein and should be avoided.

- Ethnic restaurants (for example, Chinese, African, Indian, Thai, and Vietnamese), ice cream parlors, and bakeries are considered high-risk for people with tree nut allergy due to the common use of nuts and the possibility of cross contamination, even if you order a tree-nut-free item.

- Avoid natural extracts, such as pure almond extract and natural wintergreen extract (for the filbert/hazelnut allergy). Imitation or artificially flavored extracts generally are safe.

- The following are not considered nuts: nutmeg, water chestnuts, and butternut squash.

- Tree nut oils are sometimes used in lotions and soaps. Shea nut, although not usually found in food products, is often used in lotions.

- Some alcoholic beverages may contain nut flavoring and should be avoided [Ed. Note: And, all teens should avoid drinking alcoholic beverages irrespective of allergy-related concerns]. Since these beverages are not currently regulated by FALCPA, you may need to call the manufacturer to determine the safety of ingredients such as natural flavoring.

* FAI wishes to thank the Jaffe Food Allergy Institute at Mount Sinai School of Medicine (New York, NY) for providing the allergen avoidance information in this article.

Chapter 24

Wheat, Soy, And Seed Allergies

Wheat Allergy

Wheat allergy most commonly affects children and often is outgrown by age three. Wheat, a type of grain, contains four major proteins that can cause an allergy: albumin, globulin, gliadin, and gluten. Gluten is also found in barley, rye, and oats. You or your child may not necessarily have to avoid foods that contain grains other than wheat. However, about 20% of wheat-allergic children also are allergic to other grains. Be sure to ask your doctor whether foods containing barley, rye, or oats are safe for you or your child to eat.

A wheat allergy should not be confused with "gluten intolerance" or celiac disease. Celiac disease (also known as celiac sprue), which affects the small intestine, is caused by an abnormal immune reaction to gluten. Usually diagnosed by a gastroenterologist, it is a digestive disease that can cause serious complications, including malnutrition and intestinal damage, if left untreated.

How To Avoid Wheat*

The federal Food Allergen Labeling and Consumer Protection Act (FALCPA) requires that any packaged food product that contains wheat as an ingredient must list the word "Wheat" on the label. The law states that any species in the genus *Triticum* is considered wheat. Please be sure to read all product labels carefully before purchasing and consuming any item. Remember, also, that ingredients change from time to time, so check labels every time you

About This Chapter: This chapter includes "Wheat Allergy," "Soy Allergy," and "Seed Allergy," © 2012 Food Allergy Initiative (www.faiusa.org). All rights reserved. Reprinted with permission. Although some of the information in this chapter addresses parents, the facts are still beneficial for teens.

shop. If you are still not sure whether or not a product contains wheat, call the manufacturer. Always take extra precaution when dining in restaurants or eating foods prepared by others. If you are ever in doubt about any product or dish, don't eat it.

The following ingredients indicate the presence of wheat protein:

- Bread crumbs
- Bulgur
- Cereal extract
- Couscous
- Durum, durum flour, durum wheat
- Emmer
- Einkorn
- Farina
- Flour (all wheat types, such as all-purpose, cake, enriched, graham, high protein or high gluten, pastry)
- Kamut
- Semolina
- Spelt
- Sprouted wheat
- Triticale
- Vital wheat gluten
- Wheat (bran, germ, gluten, grass, malt, starch)
- Whole-wheat berries

Wheat may be found in ale, baking mixes, baked products, batter-fried foods, beer, breaded foods, breakfast cereals, candy, crackers, frankfurters and processed meats, ice cream products, salad dressings, sauces, soups, soy sauce, and surimi.

The following flour substitutes are available and may be used by people with wheat allergies if tolerated: amaranth, arrowroot, buckwheat, corn, millet, oat, potato, rice, soybean, tapioca, and quinoa flour. Please check with your doctor before including these in your diet.

*The Food Allergy Initiative (FAI) wishes to thank the Jaffe Food Allergy Institute at Mount Sinai School of Medicine (New York, NY) for providing the allergen avoidance information in this article.

Soy Allergy

Like peanuts, soybeans are legumes. In fact, soy and peanut proteins are similar in structure. Nevertheless, a person who is allergic to soy won't necessarily be allergic to peanuts, and vice versa. Soy is widely used in many food products, so if you have a soy allergy, it is especially important to read ingredient labels with care.

Comparatively little research has been done on soy allergy, but studies indicate that it generally occurs early in childhood and often is outgrown by age three.

How To Avoid Soy*

The federal Food Allergen Labeling and Consumer Protection Act (FALCPA) requires that any packaged food product that contains soy as an ingredient must list the word "Soy" on the label. Please be sure to read all product labels carefully before purchasing and consuming any item. Remember, also, that ingredients change from time to time, so check labels every time you shop. If you are still not sure whether or not a product contains soy, call the manufacturer. Always take extra precaution when dining in restaurants or eating foods prepared by others. If you are ever in doubt about any product or dish, don't eat it.

The following ingredients indicate the presence of soy protein:

- Edamame

- Miso

- Natto

- Shoyu sauce

- Soy (fiber, flour, grits, nuts, sprouts)

- Soy (milk, yogurt, ice cream, cheese)

- Soy protein (concentrate, hydrolyzed, isolate)

- Soy sauce

- Tamari

- Tempeh

- Textured vegetable protein
- Tofu

Soy protein may be found in numerous products, such as breads, cookies, crackers, canned broth and soups, canned tuna and meat, breakfast cereals, high-protein energy bars and snacks, low-fat peanut butters, and processed meats.

Asian cuisines are considered high-risk for people with soy allergy due to the common use of soy as an ingredient and the possibility of cross-contamination, even if a soy-free item is ordered.

Studies show that most people with soy allergy may safely eat products containing soy oil and soy lecithin. Soy oil is exempt from U.S. labeling laws.

*FAI wishes to thank the Jaffe Food Allergy Institute at Mount Sinai School of Medicine (New York, NY) for providing the allergen avoidance information in this article.

Seed Allergy

Sesame seed allergy appears to be on the rise in many countries, including the United States. These seeds are capable of causing severe allergic reactions. Canada and the European Commission have added sesame to the list of ingredients that must be reported on food labels, although the U.S. has not yet done so.

The more widely an allergenic food is consumed in a particular country, the more likely the population is to report an allergy to that food. In the Middle East, where sesame seeds and oil are dietary staples, the incidence of sesame seed allergy is very high. In fact, sesame is the third most common allergy in Israeli children, after cow's milk allergy and egg allergy. Researchers theorize that the growing popularity of snacks and ethnic foods that contain sesame in Europe, North America, Australia, and New Zealand accounts for the increase in sesame seed allergy in these parts of the world.

Allergies to other seeds (for example, poppy, sunflower, pumpkin, rapeseed, and flaxseed, also known as linseed) are much less common, so they are not discussed in detail here. People who are allergic to one type of seed don't necessarily have to avoid all others, so you should discuss this matter with your doctor.

How To Avoid Seeds

The federal Food Allergen Labeling and Consumer Protection Act (FALCPA) currently does not require that manufacturers list sesame or any other type of seed on ingredient labels. That means that if you have a seed allergy, you will have to be especially vigilant. Always read all product labels carefully before purchasing and consuming any item. Be on the lookout for vague language (for example, "spices") and call the manufacturer to find out whether or not the product contains sesame. Remember, also, that ingredients change from time to time, so check labels every time you shop. Sesame and other seeds are found in a wide array of foods, so always take extra precaution when dining in restaurants or eating foods prepared by others. If you are ever in doubt about any product or dish, don't eat it.

The following ingredients and foods indicate the presence of sesame seed protein:

- Benne/benne seed/benniseed
- Gomasio (sesame salt)
- Halvah
- Hummus
- Tahini
- Seeds
- Sesame oil (also known as gingelly or til oil)
- Sesamol/sesamolina
- Sesamum indicum
- Sim sim
- Vegetable oil

Baked goods (breads, buns, rolls, crackers, cookies, pastries, bagels, etc.) and certain cereals (for example, muesli) often contain sesame and other seeds (for example, poppy, sunflower).

Many snack foods (for example, trail mix, granola bars, protein bars, candy, rice cakes, pretzels, bagel chips or pita chips) contain sesame seeds.

Sesame seeds may be found in a wide variety of other foods, including margarine, sauces, dips, soups, salad dressing, processed meats, and vegetarian burgers.

Bakeries and ethnic restaurants (such as Middle Eastern and Asian) are considered high-risk for people with sesame allergy due to the common use of sesame and the risk of cross-contamination, even if a sesame-free item is ordered.

Non-food sources of sesame seeds include health and beauty aids (cosmetics, soaps, hair care products, etc.), certain drugs and ointments, pet food, and livestock feed.

Chapter 25

Milk And Egg Allergies

Milk Allergy

Cow's milk allergy is the most common food allergy in infants and young children. It occurs more frequently in infants who are fed cow's milk formula than in babies who are breast-fed or who are fed hypoallergenic or a less allergenic infant formula. Sensitivity to cow's milk varies greatly from person to person. Some people have a severe reaction after exposure to a tiny amount of milk. Others have only a mild reaction after ingesting a moderate amount of milk or dairy products.

Most children outgrow eventually outgrow cow's milk allergy. The allergy is most likely to persist in children who have high levels of cow's milk antibodies in their blood. Blood tests that measure these antibodies can help your allergist determine whether or not your child is likely to outgrow a milk allergy.

Some people confuse milk allergy with lactose intolerance. Unlike food allergies, food intolerances do not involve the immune system. People who are lactose intolerant are missing the enzyme lactase, which breaks down lactose, a sugar found in milk and dairy products. As a result, lactose-intolerant patients are unable to digest these foods, and may experience symptoms such as nausea, cramps, gas, bloating, and diarrhea. While lactose intolerance can cause great discomfort, it is not life-threatening.

About This Chapter: This chapter includes "Milk Allergy" and "Egg Allergy," © 2012 Food Allergy Initiative (www .faiusa.org). All rights reserved. Reprinted with permission. Although some of the information in this chapter addresses parents, the facts are still beneficial for teens.

How To Avoid Cow's Milk*

The federal Food Allergen Labeling and Consumer Protection Act (FALCPA) requires that any packaged food product that contains milk as an ingredient must list the word "Milk" on the label. Please be sure to read all product labels carefully before purchasing and consuming any item. Remember, also, that ingredients change from time to time, so check labels every time you shop. If you are still not sure whether or not a product contains milk, call the manufacturer. Always take extra precaution when dining in restaurants or eating foods prepared by others. If you are in doubt about any product or dish, don't eat it.

Milk protein is found in all dairy products, including milk, butter, cheese, cream, custard, yogurt, ice cream, and puddings. The following ingredients indicate the presence of milk protein: Artificial butter flavor, butter fat, and butter oil; Casein and caseinates (in all forms); Cheese flavor; Curds; Ghee; Hydrolysates (casein, milk protein, protein, whey, whey protein); Lactalbumin, lactalbumin phosphate, lactoglobulin, lactoferrin, lactulose; Nougat; Rennet, rennet casein; Recaldent, used in tooth-whitening chewing gums; Simplesse; and Whey (in all forms).

Milk protein may be found in numerous manufactured products, including many margarines, breads, cookies, cakes, chewing gum, cold cuts, crackers, cereals, non-dairy products, processed and canned meats, and frozen and refrigerated soy products.

Many frozen and refrigerated soy-based products are manufactured on dairy equipment and run the risk of cross-contact with milk protein.

Sheep's and goat's milk are not considered safe for people with cow's milk allergy, as most cow's milk-allergic individuals are also allergic to these milks.

Shellfish is occasionally dipped in milk to reduce the fishy odor. Please ask if there is any risk of milk contact when purchasing shellfish.

Kosher Dairy: A "D" or the word "dairy" following the circled K or U on a product label indicates the presence of milk protein or a risk of milk protein contamination. These products should be avoided.

Nutrition

Milk is an important dietary source of protein, calcium, vitamin D, and vitamin B12. Please discuss a safe dietary alternative to cow's milk with your doctor or dietitian.

Source: From "Milk Allergy," © 2012 Food Allergy Initiative (www.faiusa.org).

Kosher Pareve: A product labeled "pareve" is considered milk-free under kosher dietary law. However, a food product may be considered pareve even if it contains a very small amount of milk protein—potentially enough to cause an allergic reaction in susceptible individuals. Do not assume that pareve products are always safe.

Ingredients That Do Not Contain Milk Are: Cocoa butter, coconut milk, calcium lactate, calcium stearoyl lactylate, oleoresein, cream of tartar, sodium stearoyl lactylate, and lactic acid (although lactic acid starter culture may contain milk).

*The Food Allergy Initiative (FAI) wishes to thank the Jaffe Food Allergy Institute at Mount Sinai School of Medicine (New York, NY) for providing the allergen avoidance information in this article.

Egg Allergy

Hen's egg allergy is one of the most common allergies in children, second only to cow's milk. Most children eventually outgrow this allergy.

People who are allergic to hen's eggs must completely avoid both the white and the yolk. The white contains the allergenic proteins, but since it is impossible to separate it completely from the yolk, cross-contamination is likely to occur. Even a small amount of egg may be enough to cause an allergic reaction. Other bird eggs also are likely to cause a reaction, although limited research has been done on this topic.

If you are on an egg-restricted diet, your intake of grain may be limited because many commercially prepared grain products, such as breads and pastas, contain eggs. A diet that is limited in eggs and grains may be low in some of the B vitamins and possibly iron. Read ingredient labels to find egg-free pastas and grain products. You can also substitute rice in some recipes that call for pasta and make your own homemade bread products.

How To Avoid Eggs*

The federal Food Allergen Labeling and Consumer Protection Act (FALCPA) requires that any packaged food product that contains egg as an ingredient must list the word "Egg" on the label. Please be sure to read all product labels carefully before purchasing and consuming any item. Remember, also, that ingredients change from time to time, so check labels every time you shop. If you are still not sure whether or not a product contains eggs, call the manufacturer. Always take extra precaution when dining in restaurants or eating foods prepared by others. If you are ever in doubt about any product or dish, don't eat it.

The following ingredients indicate the presence of egg protein:

- Albumin
- Egg (white, yolk, dried, powdered, solids)
- Egg substitutes
- Eggnog
- Globulin
- Lecithin
- Lysozyme
- Mayonnaise
- Meringue
- Ovalbumin
- Ovovitellin

Egg protein may be found in numerous products, such as baked goods, breaded foods, cream fillings, custards, candies, canned soups, casseroles, frostings, ice creams, lollipops, marshmallows, marzipan, pastas, salad dressings, and meat-based dishes, such as meatballs or meatloaf.

Egg whites and shells also may be used as a clarifying agent in soup stocks, consommés, wine, and alcohol-based and coffee drinks.

For each egg, one of the following may be substituted in recipes:

- 1 teaspoon baking powder, 1 Tablespoon water, and 1 Tablespoon vinegar
- 1 teaspoon yeast dissolved in ¼ cup warm water
- ½ Tablespoon water, ½ Tablespoon oil, and 1 teaspoon baking powder
- 1 packet gelatin and two Tablespoons warm water (mix just prior to use)
- 2 Tablespoons fruit puree may be used for binding, but not leavening.

*FAI wishes to thank the Jaffe Food Allergy Institute at Mount Sinai School of Medicine (New York, NY) for providing the allergen avoidance information in this article.

Measles-Mumps-Rubella Vaccine

Several vaccines contain egg protein (MMR, influenza, yellow fever). The American Academy of Pediatrics has stated that egg allergy is not a contraindication for the MMR (measles-mumps-rubella) vaccine. Several studies have indicated that the MMR vaccine can be safely administered to all patients with egg allergy. Please be sure to consult with your physician before receiving any other vaccine that contains egg protein.

Source: From "Egg Allergy," © 2012 Food Allergy Initiative (www.faiusa.org).

Chapter 26

Fish And Shellfish Allergies

Fish Allergy

Finned fish can cause severe allergic reactions. This allergy is usually life-long. The protein in the flesh of fish most commonly causes the allergic reaction; however, it is also possible to have a reaction to fish gelatin, made from the skin and bones of fish. Although fish oil does not contain protein from the fish from which it was extracted, it is likely to be contaminated with small molecules of protein and therefore should be avoided.

More than half of all people who are allergic to one type of fish also are allergic to other fish, so allergists often advise their patients to avoid all fish. However, many people with fish allergies are able to eat canned tuna or salmon, which are less allergenic than fresh fish. Finned fish and shellfish do not come from related families of foods, so being allergic to one does not mean that you will not be able to tolerate the other. Be sure to talk to your doctor about which kinds of fish you can eat and which to avoid.

When eating out, people with fish allergies should be particularly alert to cross-contamination. Always check with the chef to make sure that the fish is not cooked on the same skillet or in the same oil as other food. You also should make sure that your dishes are not prepared with the same utensils or on the same work surfaces as fish.

How To Avoid Fish*

The federal Food Allergen Labeling and Consumer Protection Act (FALCPA) requires that any packaged food product that contains fish as an ingredient must list the name of the

About This Chapter: This chapter includes "Fish Allergy" and "Shellfish Allergy," © 2012 Food Allergy Initiative (www.faiusa.org). All rights reserved. Reprinted with permission.

specific fish on the label. Please be sure to read all product labels carefully before purchasing and consuming any item. Remember, also, that ingredients change from time to time, so check labels every time you shop. If you are still not sure whether or not a product contains fish, call the manufacturer. Always take extra precaution when dining in restaurants or eating foods prepared by others. If you are ever in doubt about any product or dish, don't eat it.

The term "fish" encompasses all species of finned fish, including (but not limited to): Anchovies; bass; catfish; cod; flounder; grouper; haddock; hake; herring; mahi mahi; perch; pike; pollock; salmon; scrod; sole; snapper; swordfish; tilapia; trout; and tuna.

- Some sensitive individuals may react to aerosolized fish protein through cooking vapors.

- Seafood restaurants are considered high-risk due to the possibility of cross-contamination, even if you do not order fish.

- Ethnic restaurants (for example, Chinese, African, Indonesian, Thai, and Vietnamese) are considered high-risk because of the common use of fish and fish ingredients and the possibility of cross-contamination, even if you do not order fish.

- Worcestershire sauce, Caesar salad, and Caesar dressing usually contain fish ingredients (anchovies).

- Caponata, a Sicilian eggplant relish, may contain anchovies.

- Surimi, an artificial crabmeat (also known as "sea legs" or "sea sticks"), is made from fish.

- Carrageen is a marine algae, not a fish, and is considered safe for those avoiding fish and shellfish.

*The Food Allergy Initiative (FAI) wishes to thank the Jaffe Food Allergy Institute at Mount Sinai School of Medicine (New York, NY) for providing the allergen avoidance information in this article.

Shellfish Allergy

Shellfish allergy usually develops in young adults. In fact, it is the most common significant food allergy reported by adults and is considered life-long. Along with peanuts and tree nuts, shellfish are the most frequent triggers of anaphylactic reactions.

There are two kinds of shellfish: crustacea (such as shrimp, crab, and lobster) and mollusks (such as clams, mussels, oysters, and scallops). Reactions to crustacean shellfish tend to be particularly severe. If you are allergic to one group of shellfish, you might be able to eat some varieties from the other group. Since most people who are allergic to one kind of shellfish usually are allergic to other types, however, allergists usually advise their patients to avoid all varieties. If you have been diagnosed with a shellfish allergy, never eat any kind of shellfish without consulting your doctor first.

When eating out, people with shellfish allergies should be particularly alert to cross-contamination. Always check with the chef to make sure that shellfish are not cooked on the same skillet or in the same oil as other food. You also should make sure that your dishes are not prepared with the same utensils or on the same work surfaces as shellfish.

How To Avoid Shellfish*

The federal Food Allergen Labeling and Consumer Protection Act (FALCPA) requires that any packaged food product that contains shellfish as an ingredient must list the name of the specific shellfish on the label. Please be sure to read all product labels carefully before purchasing and consuming any item. Remember, also, that ingredients change from time to time, so check labels every time you shop. If you are still not sure whether or not a product contains shellfish, call the manufacturer. Always take extra precaution when dining in restaurants or eating foods prepared by others. If you are ever in doubt about any product or dish, don't eat it.

Crustaceans

- Shrimp (prawns, crevette)
- Crab
- Crawfish (crayfish, ecrevisse)
- Lobster (langouste, langoustine, scampo, coral, tomalley)

Mollusks

- Abalone
- Clam
- Cockle
- Mussel
- Oyster
- Octopus
- Scallop

- Snail (escargot)

- Squid (calamari)

The following ingredients may indicate the presence of a shellfish protein:

- Bouillabaisse

- Fish stock

- Flavoring

- Seafood flavoring

- Surimi

Some sensitive individuals may react to aerosolized shellfish protein through cooking vapors. It is wise to stay away from steam tables or stovetops when shellfish are being cooked.

Seafood restaurants are considered high-risk due to the possibility of cross-contamination, even if a non-shellfish item is ordered.

Carrageen is a marine algae, not a fish, and is considered safe for those avoiding fish and shellfish.

Chapter 27

Lactose Intolerance

What is lactose intolerance?

Lactose intolerance is the inability or insufficient ability to digest lactose, a sugar found in milk and milk products. Lactose intolerance is caused by a deficiency of the enzyme lactase, which is produced by the cells lining the small intestine. Lactase breaks down lactose into two simpler forms of sugar called glucose and galactose, which are then absorbed into the bloodstream.

Not all people with lactase deficiency have digestive symptoms, but those who do may have lactose intolerance. Most people with lactose intolerance can tolerate some amount of lactose in their diet.

People sometimes confuse lactose intolerance with cow milk allergy. Milk allergy is a reaction by the body's immune system to one or more milk proteins and can be life threatening when just a small amount of milk or milk product is consumed. Milk allergy most commonly appears in the first year of life, while lactose intolerance occurs more often in adulthood.

What causes lactose intolerance?

The cause of lactose intolerance is best explained by describing how a person develops lactase deficiency.

Primary lactase deficiency develops over time and begins after about age two when the body begins to produce less lactase. Most children who have lactase deficiency do not experience symptoms of lactose intolerance until late adolescence or adulthood.

About This Chapter: From "Lactose Intolerance," National Digestive Diseases Information Clearinghouse, a service of the National Institute of Diabetes and Digestive and Kidney Diseases (digestive.niddk.nih.gov), April 23, 2012.

Researchers have identified a possible genetic link to primary lactase deficiency. Some people inherit a gene from their parents that makes it likely they will develop primary lactase deficiency. This discovery may be useful in developing future genetic tests to identify people at risk for lactose intolerance.

Secondary lactase deficiency results from injury to the small intestine that occurs with severe diarrheal illness, celiac disease, Crohn disease, or chemotherapy. This type of lactase deficiency can occur at any age but is more common in infancy.

Who is at risk for lactose intolerance?

Lactose intolerance is a common condition that is more likely to occur in adulthood, with a higher incidence in older adults. Some ethnic and racial populations are more affected than others, including African Americans, Hispanic Americans, American Indians, and Asian Americans. The condition is least common among Americans of northern European descent.

Infants born prematurely are more likely to have lactase deficiency because an infant's lactase levels do not increase until the third trimester of pregnancy.

What are the symptoms of lactose intolerance?

People with lactose intolerance may feel uncomfortable 30 minutes to two hours after consuming milk and milk products. Symptoms range from mild to severe, based on the amount of lactose consumed and the amount a person can tolerate. Common symptoms include abdominal pain, abdominal bloating, gas, diarrhea, and nausea.

How is lactose intolerance diagnosed?

Lactose intolerance can be hard to diagnose based on symptoms alone. People may think they suffer from lactose intolerance because they have digestive symptoms; however, other conditions such as irritable bowel syndrome can cause similar symptoms. After taking a medical history and performing a physical examination, the doctor may first recommend eliminating all milk and milk products from the person's diet for a short time to see if the symptoms resolve. Tests may be necessary to provide more information.

Two tests are commonly used to measure the digestion of lactose.

Hydrogen Breath Test: The person drinks a lactose-loaded beverage and then the breath is analyzed at regular intervals to measure the amount of hydrogen. Normally, very little hydrogen is detectable in the breath, but undigested lactose produces high levels of hydrogen. Smoking and some foods and medications may affect the accuracy of the results. People should check with their doctor about foods and medications that may interfere with test results.

Stool Acidity Test: The stool acidity test is used for infants and young children to measure the amount of acid in the stool. Undigested lactose creates lactic acid and other fatty acids that can be detected in a stool sample. Glucose may also be present in the stool as a result of undigested lactose.

Because lactose intolerance is uncommon in infants and children younger than two, a health professional should take special care in determining the cause of a child's digestive symptoms.

How is lactose intolerance managed?

Although the body's ability to produce lactase cannot be changed, the symptoms of lactose intolerance can be managed with dietary changes. Most people with lactose intolerance can tolerate some amount of lactose in their diet. Gradually introducing small amounts of milk or milk products may help some people adapt to them with fewer symptoms. Often, people can better tolerate milk or milk products by taking them with meals.

The amount of change needed in the diet depends on how much lactose a person can consume without symptoms. For example, one person may have severe symptoms after drinking a small glass of milk, while another can drink a large glass without symptoms. Others can easily consume yogurt and hard cheeses, such as cheddar and Swiss, but not milk or other milk products.

The *Dietary Guidelines for Americans* recommend that people with lactose intolerance choose milk products with lower levels of lactose than regular milk, such as yogurt and hard cheese.

Lactose-free and lactose-reduced milk and milk products, available at most supermarkets, are identical to regular milk except that the lactase enzyme has been added. Lactose-free milk remains fresh for about the same length of time or longer than regular milk if it is ultra-pasteurized. Lactose-free milk may have a slightly sweeter taste than regular milk. Soy milk and other products may be recommended by a health professional.

People who still experience symptoms after dietary changes can take over-the-counter lactase enzyme drops or tablets. Taking the tablets or a few drops of the liquid enzyme when consuming milk or milk products may make these foods more tolerable for people with lactose intolerance.

Parents and caregivers of a child with lactose intolerance should follow the nutrition plan recommended by the child's doctor or dietitian.

What should I know about lactose intolerance and calcium intake?

Milk and milk products are a major source of calcium and other nutrients. Calcium is essential for the growth and repair of bones at all ages. A shortage of calcium intake in children and adults may lead to fragile bones that can easily fracture later in life, a condition called osteoporosis.

The amount of calcium a person needs to maintain good health varies by age. Recommendations are shown in Table 27.1.

Women who are pregnant or breastfeeding need between 1,000 and 1,300 mg of calcium daily.

Getting enough calcium is important for people with lactose intolerance when the intake of milk and milk products is limited. Many foods can provide calcium and other nutrients the body needs. Non-milk products that are high in calcium include fish with soft bones such as salmon and sardines and dark green vegetables such as spinach.

Table 27.2 lists foods that are good sources of dietary calcium.

Yogurt made with active and live bacterial cultures is a good source of calcium for many people with lactose intolerance. When this type of yogurt enters the intestine, the bacterial cultures convert lactose to lactic acid, so the yogurt may be well-tolerated due to a lower lactose content than yogurt without live cultures. Frozen yogurt does not contain bacterial cultures, so it may not be well-tolerated.

Table 27.1. Recommended Calcium Intake By Age Group

Age group	Amount of calcium to consume daily, Age group in milligrams (mg)
0–6 months	210 mg
7–12 months	270 mg
1–3 years	500 mg
4–8 years	800 mg
9–18 years	1,300 mg
19–50 years	1,000 mg
51–70+ years	1,200 mg

Source: Adapted from Dietary Reference Intakes, 2004, Institute of Medicine, National Academy of Sciences.

Table 27.2. Calcium Content In Common Foods

Non-milk Products	Calcium Content
Rhubarb, frozen, cooked, 1 cup	348 mg
Sardines, with bone, 3 oz.	325 mg
Spinach, frozen, cooked, 1 cup	291 mg
Salmon, canned, with bone, 3 oz.	181 mg
Soy milk, unfortified, 1 cup	61 mg
Orange, 1 medium	52 mg
Broccoli, raw, 1 cup	41 mg
Pinto beans, cooked, ½ cup	40 mg
Lettuce greens, 1 cup	20 mg
Tuna, white, canned, 3 oz.	12 mg
Milk and Milk Products	
Yogurt, with active and live cultures, plain, low-fat, vitamin D-fortified, 1 cup	415 mg
Milk, reduced fat, vitamin D-fortified, 1 cup	285 mg
Swiss cheese, 1 oz.	224 mg
Cottage cheese, ½ cup	87 mg
Ice cream, ½ cup	84 mg

Source: Adapted from U.S. Department of Agriculture, Agricultural Research Service. 2008. USDA National Nutrient Database for Standard Reference, Release 21.

Calcium is absorbed and used in the body only when enough vitamin D is present. Some people with lactose intolerance may not be getting enough vitamin D. Vitamin D comes from food sources such as eggs, liver, and vitamin D-fortified milk and yogurt. Regular exposure to sunlight also helps the body naturally absorb vitamin D. Talking with a doctor or registered dietitian may be helpful in planning a balanced diet that provides an adequate amount of nutrients—including calcium and vitamin D—and minimizes discomfort. A health professional can determine whether calcium and other dietary supplements are needed.

What other products contain lactose?

Milk and milk products are often added to processed foods—foods that have been altered to prolong their shelf life. People with lactose intolerance should be aware of the many food products that may contain even small amounts of lactose, such as these:

- Bread and other baked goods

- Waffles, pancakes, biscuits, cookies, and mixes to make them

- Processed breakfast foods such as doughnuts, frozen waffles and pancakes, toaster pastries, and sweet rolls

- Processed breakfast cereals

- Instant potatoes, soups, and breakfast drinks

- Potato chips, corn chips, and other processed snacks

- Processed meats, such as bacon, sausage, hot dogs, and lunch meats

- Margarine

- Salad dressings

- Liquid and powdered milk-based meal replacements

- Protein powders and bars

- Candies

- Non-dairy liquid and powdered coffee creamers

- Non-dairy whipped toppings

Checking the ingredients on food labels is helpful in finding possible sources of lactose in food products. If any of the following words are listed on a food label, the product contains lactose:

- Milk

- Lactose

- Whey

- Curds

- Milk by-products

- Dry milk solids

- Non-fat dry milk powder

Lactose is also used in some prescription medicines, including birth control pills, and over-the-counter medicines like products to treat stomach acid and gas. These medicines most often cause symptoms in people with severe lactose intolerance.

Chapter 28

Gluten Intolerance (Celiac Disease)

What is celiac disease?

Celiac disease is a digestive disease that damages the small intestine and interferes with absorption of nutrients from food. People who have celiac disease cannot tolerate gluten, a protein in wheat, rye, and barley. Gluten is found mainly in foods but may also be found in everyday products such as medicines, vitamins, and lip balms.

When people with celiac disease eat foods or use products containing gluten, their immune system responds by damaging or destroying villi—the tiny, fingerlike protrusions lining the small intestine. Villi normally allow nutrients from food to be absorbed through the walls of the small intestine into the bloodstream. Without healthy villi, a person becomes malnourished, no matter how much food one eats.

Villi on the lining of the small intestine help absorb nutrients.

Celiac disease is both a disease of malabsorption—meaning nutrients are not absorbed properly—and an abnormal immune reaction to gluten. Celiac disease is also known as celiac sprue, nontropical sprue, and gluten-sensitive enteropathy. Celiac disease is genetic, meaning it runs in families. Sometimes the disease is triggered—or becomes active for the first time—after surgery, pregnancy, childbirth, viral infection, or severe emotional stress.

What are the symptoms of celiac disease?

Symptoms of celiac disease vary from person to person. Symptoms may occur in the digestive system or in other parts of the body. Digestive symptoms are more common in

About This Chapter: From "Celiac Disease," National Digestive Diseases Information Clearinghouse, a service of the National Institute of Diabetes and Digestive and Kidney Diseases (digestive.niddk.nih.gov), January 27, 2012.

infants and young children and may include abdominal bloating and pain, chronic diarrhea, vomiting, constipation, pale, foul-smelling, or fatty stool, and weight loss.

Irritability is another common symptom in children. Malabsorption of nutrients during the years when nutrition is critical to a child's normal growth and development can result in other problems such as failure to thrive in infants, delayed growth and short stature, delayed puberty, and dental enamel defects of the permanent teeth.

Adults are less likely to have digestive symptoms and may instead have one or more of the following:

- Unexplained iron-deficiency anemia

- Fatigue

- Bone or joint pain

- Arthritis

- Bone loss or osteoporosis

- Depression or anxiety

- Tingling numbness in the hands and feet

- Seizures

- Missed menstrual periods

- Infertility or recurrent miscarriage

- Canker sores inside the mouth

- An itchy skin rash called dermatitis herpetiformis

People with celiac disease may have no symptoms but can still develop complications of the disease over time. Long-term complications include malnutrition—which can lead to anemia, osteoporosis, and miscarriage, among other problems—liver diseases, and cancers of the intestine.

Why are celiac disease symptoms so varied?

Researchers are studying the reasons celiac disease affects people differently. The length of time a person was breastfed, the age a person started eating gluten-containing foods, and the amount of gluten-containing foods one eats are three factors thought to play a role in when and how celiac disease appears. Some studies have shown, for example, that the longer a person was breastfed, the later the symptoms of celiac disease appear.

Symptoms also vary depending on a person's age and the degree of damage to the small intestine. Many adults have the disease for a decade or more before they are diagnosed. The longer a person goes undiagnosed and untreated, the greater the chance of developing long-term complications.

What other health problems do people with celiac disease have?

People with celiac disease tend to have other diseases in which the immune system attacks the body's healthy cells and tissues. The connection between celiac disease and these diseases may be genetic. They include the following:

- Type 1 diabetes

- Autoimmune thyroid disease

- Autoimmune liver disease

- Rheumatoid arthritis

- Addison disease, a condition in which the glands that produce critical hormones are damaged

- Sjögren syndrome, a condition in which the glands that produce tears and saliva are destroyed

How common is celiac disease?

Celiac disease affects people in all parts of the world. Originally thought to be a rare childhood syndrome, celiac disease is now known to be a common genetic disorder. More than two million people in the United States have the disease, or about one in 133 people.[1] Among people who have a first-degree relative—a parent, sibling, or child—diagnosed with celiac disease, as many as one in 22 people may have the disease.[2]

Celiac disease is also more common among people with other genetic disorders including Down syndrome and Turner syndrome, a condition that affects girls' development.

How is celiac disease diagnosed?

Recognizing celiac disease can be difficult because some of its symptoms are similar to those of other diseases. Celiac disease can be confused with irritable bowel syndrome, iron-deficiency anemia caused by menstrual blood loss, inflammatory bowel disease, diverticulitis, intestinal infections, and chronic fatigue syndrome. As a result, celiac disease has long been underdiagnosed or misdiagnosed. As doctors become more aware of the many varied symptoms of the disease and reliable blood tests become more available, diagnosis rates are increasing.

Blood Tests: People with celiac disease have higher than normal levels of certain autoantibodies—proteins that react against the body's own cells or tissues—in their blood. To diagnose celiac disease, doctors will test blood for high levels of anti-tissue transglutaminase antibodies (tTGA) or anti-endomysium antibodies (EMA). If test results are negative but celiac disease is still suspected, additional blood tests may be needed.

Before being tested, one should continue to eat a diet that includes foods with gluten, such as breads and pastas. If a person stops eating foods with gluten before being tested, the results may be negative for celiac disease even if the disease is present.

Intestinal Biopsy: If blood tests and symptoms suggest celiac disease, a biopsy of the small intestine is performed to confirm the diagnosis. During the biopsy, the doctor removes tiny pieces of tissue from the small intestine to check for damage to the villi. To obtain the tissue sample, the doctor eases a long, thin tube called an endoscope through the patient's mouth and stomach into the small intestine. The doctor then takes the samples using instruments passed through the endoscope.

Dermatitis Herpetiformis: Dermatitis herpetiformis (DH) is an intensely itchy, blistering skin rash that affects 15 to 25 percent of people with celiac disease.[3] The rash usually occurs on the elbows, knees, and buttocks. Most people with DH have no digestive symptoms of celiac disease.

DH is diagnosed through blood tests and a skin biopsy. If the antibody tests are positive and the skin biopsy has the typical findings of DH, patients do not need to have an intestinal biopsy. Both the skin disease and the intestinal disease respond to a gluten-free diet and recur if gluten is added back into the diet. The rash symptoms can be controlled with antibiotics such as dapsone. Because dapsone does not treat the intestinal condition, people with DH must maintain a gluten-free diet.

Screening: Screening for celiac disease means testing for the presence of autoantibodies in the blood in people without symptoms. Americans are not routinely screened for celiac disease. However, because celiac disease is hereditary, family members of a person with the disease may wish to be tested. Four to 12 percent of an affected person's first-degree relatives will also have the disease.[4]

How is celiac disease treated?

The only treatment for celiac disease is a gluten-free diet. Doctors may ask a newly diagnosed person to work with a dietitian on a gluten-free diet plan. A dietitian is a health care professional who specializes in food and nutrition. Someone with celiac disease can learn from a dietitian how to read ingredient lists and identify foods that contain gluten in order to make informed decisions at the grocery store and when eating out.

For most people, following this diet will stop symptoms, heal existing intestinal damage, and prevent further damage. Improvement begins within days of starting the diet. The small intestine usually heals in three to six months in children but may take several years in adults. A healed intestine means a person now has villi that can absorb nutrients from food into the bloodstream.

To stay well, people with celiac disease must avoid gluten for the rest of their lives. Eating even a small amount of gluten can damage the small intestine. The damage will occur in anyone with the disease, including people without noticeable symptoms. Depending on a person's age at diagnosis, some problems will not improve, such as short stature and dental enamel defects.

Some people with celiac disease show no improvement on the gluten-free diet. The most common reason for poor response to the diet is that small amounts of gluten are still being consumed. Hidden sources of gluten include additives such as modified food starch, preservatives, and stabilizers made with wheat. And because many corn and rice products are produced in factories that also manufacture wheat products, they can be contaminated with wheat gluten.

Rarely, the intestinal injury will continue despite a strictly gluten-free diet. People with this condition, known as refractory celiac disease, have severely damaged intestines that cannot heal. Because their intestines are not absorbing enough nutrients, they may need to receive nutrients directly into their bloodstream through a vein, or intravenously. Researchers are evaluating drug treatments for refractory celiac disease.

The Gluten-Free Diet

A gluten-free diet means not eating foods that contain wheat, rye, and barley. The foods and products made from these grains should also be avoided. In other words, a person with celiac disease should not eat most grain, pasta, cereal, and many processed foods.

Despite these restrictions, people with celiac disease can eat a well-balanced diet with a variety of foods. They can use potato, rice, soy, amaranth, quinoa, buckwheat, or bean flour instead of wheat flour. They can buy gluten-free bread, pasta, and other products from stores that carry organic foods, or order products from special food companies. Gluten-free products are increasingly available from mainstream stores.

"Plain" meat, fish, rice, fruits, and vegetables do not contain gluten, so people with celiac disease can freely eat these foods. In the past, people with celiac disease were advised not to eat oats. New evidence suggests that most people can safely eat small amounts of oats, as long as the oats are not contaminated with wheat gluten during processing. People with celiac disease should work closely with their health care team when deciding whether to include oats in their diet. Examples of other foods that are safe to eat and those that are not are provided in Table 28.1.

The gluten-free diet requires a completely new approach to eating. Newly diagnosed people and their families may find support groups helpful as they learn to adjust to a new way of life. People with celiac disease must be cautious about what they buy for lunch at school or work, what they purchase at the grocery store, what they eat at restaurants or parties, and what they grab for a snack. Eating out can be a challenge. When in doubt about a menu item, a person with celiac disease should ask the waiter or chef about ingredients and preparation or if a gluten-free menu is available.

Gluten is also used in some medications. People with celiac disease should ask a pharmacist if prescribed medications contain wheat. Because gluten is sometimes used as an additive in unexpected products—such as lipstick and play dough—reading product labels is important. If the ingredients are not listed on the label, the manufacturer should provide a list upon request. With practice, screening for gluten becomes second nature.

New Food Labeling

The Food Allergen Labeling and Consumer Protection Act (FALCPA), which took effect on January 1, 2006, requires food labels to clearly identify wheat and other common food allergens in the list of ingredients. FALCPA also requires the U.S. Food and Drug Administration to develop and finalize rules for the use of the term "gluten free" on product labels.

Points To Remember

- People with celiac disease cannot tolerate gluten, a protein in wheat, rye, and barley.

- Untreated celiac disease damages the small intestine and interferes with nutrient absorption.

- Without treatment, people with celiac disease can develop complications such as osteoporosis, anemia, and cancer.

- A person with celiac disease may or may not have symptoms.

- Diagnosis involves blood tests and, in most cases, a biopsy of the small intestine.

- Since celiac disease is hereditary, family members of a person with celiac disease may wish to be tested.

Table 28.1. The Gluten-free Diet: Some Examples. In 2006, the American Dietetic Association updated its recommendations for a gluten-free diet. The following chart is based on the 2006 recommendations. This list is not complete, so people with celiac disease should discuss gluten-free food choices with a dietitian or physician who specializes in celiac disease. People with celiac disease should always read food ingredient lists carefully to make sure the food does not contain gluten.

Allowed Foods

amaranth	Job's tears	sago
arrowroot	legumes	seeds
buckwheat	millet	sorghum
cassava	nuts	soy
corn	potatoes	tapioca
flax	quinoa	teff
Indian rice grass	rice	wild rice
		yucca

Foods To Avoid

wheat: including einkorn, emmer, spelt, kamut, wheat starch, wheat bran, wheat germ, cracked wheat, hydrolyzed wheat protein	barley
	rye
	triticale (a cross between wheat and rye)

Other Wheat Products

bromated flour	graham flour	self-rising flour
durum flour	phosphated flour	semolina
enriched flour	plain flour	white flour
farina		

Processed Foods That May Contain Wheat, Barley, Or Rye*

bouillon cubes	communion wafers	sauces
brown rice syrup	French fries	seasoned tortilla chips
candy	gravy	self-basting turkey
chips/potato chips	imitation fish	soups
cold cuts, hot dogs, salami, sausage	matzo	soy sauce
	rice mixes	vegetables in sauce

* Most of these foods can be found gluten-free. When in doubt, check with the food manufacturer.

Source: Thompson T. *Celiac Disease Nutrition Guide, 2nd ed.* Chicago: American Dietetic Association; 2006. © American Dietetic Association. Adapted with permission. For a complete copy of the Celiac Disease Nutrition Guide, please visit www.eatright.org.

- Celiac disease is treated by eliminating all gluten from the diet. The gluten-free diet is a lifetime requirement.

- A dietitian can teach a person with celiac disease about food selection, label reading, and other strategies to help manage the disease.

Notes

1. Fasano A, Berti I, Gerarduzzi T, et al. Prevalence of celiac disease in at-risk and not-at-risk groups in the United States. *Archives of Internal Medicine*. 2003;163(3):268–292.

2. Ibid.

3. Rodrigo L. Celiac disease. *World Journal of Gastroenterology*. 2006;12(41):6585–6593.

4. Ibid.

Chapter 29

Histamine Intolerance

Overview

"True" allergic reactions involve histamine, but histamine intolerance is different. Histamine intolerance refers to a reaction to foods that have high levels of naturally occurring histamine; in contrast, during a normal allergic reaction, the body itself produces high levels of histamine in response to a food it perceives as an invader. People with histamine intolerance often have low levels of either of two enzymes—diamine oxidase (DAO) and histamine-N-methyltransferase (HNMT)—that bind to and metabolize histamine. In these people, histamine can build up over time and cause symptoms throughout the body.

What Histamine Is

Histamine is one of a group of nitrogen-containing compounds called amines. (Other common amines include amphetamines and pseudoephedrine.) Histamine is bioactive, which means that in the body, it has biological effects. It binds to special receptors in tissues throughout the body, thereby causing a variety of skin, gastrointestinal, nervous system and cardiac symptoms.

Symptoms

The most common symptoms of histamine intolerance are migraine headaches, gastrointestinal symptoms (such as diarrhea), flushing, hives, eczema, and allergic rhinitis.

Histamine intolerance can also cause more severe symptoms. It can trigger asthma attacks or anaphylactic shock, can cause arrhythmia, and may be associated with serious chronic conditions like Crohn disease.

High-Histamine Foods

Most foods that are high in histamine are highly processed or fermented: wine, aged cheese, yeast-containing foods, and sauerkraut. Spinach and tomatoes are also high in histamine. In addition, while citrus fruits are not themselves considered high in histamine, they can release histamine in the body that is bound to mast cells. Therefore, people on a strict histamine-free diet are generally advised to avoid citrus.

Histamine And Alcohol

[Ed. Note: Teens should not drink alcohol. The following facts are provided for general information purposes.] "Red wine migraines" are often histamine intolerance headaches, and red wine is indeed high in histamine. But all alcoholic beverages can be problematic for people with histamine intolerance because alcohol can make DAO, one of the enzymes that metabolizes histamine in the body, less effective. Alcohol is therefore not allowed on a histamine-free diet.

Diagnosing Histamine Intolerance

Recurring symptoms after eating high-histamine foods may lead doctors to suspect a histamine intolerance; a food log may be useful in this stage of diagnosis. Histamine intolerance differs from IgE-mediated food allergies in that concentrations of histamine in the body can build up over time. This can make diagnosing a histamine intolerance challenging, especially since traditional allergy tests like prick tests and RAST tests can't be used to diagnose non-IgE mediated allergies. Histamine intolerance can be diagnosed by a trial of a histamine-free diet followed by a double-blind food challenge.

Living With And Treating Histamine Intolerance

Maintaining a strict histamine-free diet is the key to relief from histamine intolerance symptoms. Your doctor will discuss which foods you should avoid, but in general, fermented and aged foods and certain high-histamine vegetables are most likely to cause problems.

You should also let your doctor know about any medications, prescription or non-prescription, you're taking. Some medications can affect the action of DAO and HNMT.

If you are on such a medication, your doctor may want to adjust your dosage, switch you to a similar medication that doesn't inhibit these enzymes, or, if possible, have you go off the medicines entirely.

While a histamine-free diet is the only long-term treatment for histamine intolerance, there are a couple other treatments that may be useful. Benadryl (an antihistamine) may be useful in case you accidentally eat histamine-containing food or have to take a drug that can block DAO activity.

There are also supplements that some doctors recommend for people with histamine intolerance. They include high doses of vitamin C and vitamin B6 (which can stimulate the activity of DAO in the body) and capsules of DAO to supplement the body's natural supply. However, these treatments are, at this time, recommended for use alongside a histamine-free diet and not to allow people with histamine intolerance to eat foods containing histamine.

Sources

Maintz, Laura, et al.. "Evidence for a Reduced Histamine Degradation Capacity in a Subgroup of Patients with Atopic Eczema." *Journal of Allergy and Clinical Immunology*. May 2006, 117(5): 1106-12.

Maintz, Laura and Natalija Novak. "Histamine and Histamine Intolerance." *American Journal of Clinical Nutrition*. May 2007, 85(5): 1185-96. 8 June 2008.

Chapter 30

Sulfite Sensitivity

- **Note:** This information was produced by the Australasian Society of Clinical Immunology and Allergy (ASCIA). ASCIA is an Australasian Society and as such any ASCIA articles may include region-specific information.

- **Note:** This information uses spelling according to the Australian Therapeutic Goods Administration (TGA) approved terminology for medicines (1999) in which the terms sulfur, sulfite, sulfate, and sulfonamide replace sulphur, sulphite, sulphate and sulphonamide.

Sulfites are preservatives used in some drinks, foods, and occasionally medication. Sulfites can cause allergy like reactions (intolerances), most commonly asthma symptoms in those with underlying asthma, sometimes allergic rhinitis (hay fever) like reactions, occasionally urticaria (hives) and very rarely, anaphylaxis (severe allergic reaction). Wheezing is the most common reaction.

Sulfites Are Preservatives

Sulfites have been used since Roman times to preserve food flavor and color, inhibit bacterial growth, reduce spoilage, stop fresh food from spotting and turning brown, and help preserve medication and increase shelf life.

How Do They Work?

Sulfites release sulfur dioxide, which is the active component that helps preserve food and medication.

About This Chapter: "Sulfite Allergy," © Australasian Society of Clinical Immunology and Allergy, 2010. All rights reserved. Reprinted with permission. For additional information, visit www.allergy.org.au.

Asthma Is The Most Common Adverse Effect

The most common adverse reactions, including wheezing, chest tightness, and coughing are estimated to affect 5–10% of people with asthma. Symptoms are more likely when asthma is poorly controlled. However, adverse reactions to sulfites can also occur when there is no preceding history of asthma. Reactions can be mild through to potentially life threatening.

Anaphylaxis Is Much Less Common

Anaphylaxis has been described, but is very rare. Symptoms include flushing, fast heartbeat, wheezing, hives, dizziness, stomach upset and diarrhoea, collapse, tingling, or difficulty swallowing.

Sensitivity To Sulfites Is A Different Condition From Sulfonamide Antibiotic Allergy

Some patients will have allergic reactions to sulfonamide molecule-containing medication or sulfonamide antibiotics. This is a very different condition from sulfite sensitivity and is covered in a separate article: Sulfonamide antibiotic allergy (available online at http://www.allergy.org.au/patients/medication-allergy/sulfonamide-antibiotic-allergy).

The Mechanism By Which Reactions Occur Is Unclear

- Sulfur dioxide gas (SO2) is an irritant, and so reflex contraction of the airways from inhaling sulfur dioxide gas is one possible explanation. This mechanism may explain the rapid onset of symptoms when drinking liquids like beer or wine, when SO2 gas is inhaled during the swallowing process. [Ed. Note: Irrespective of their sensitivity to sulfites, teens should not drink alcohol.]

- Some people with asthma who react to sulfites have a partial deficiency of the enzyme sulfite oxidase which helps to break down sulphur dioxide.

- Some people (but not many) have positive skin allergy tests to sulfites indicating true (IgE-mediated) allergy.

Diagnosis Of Suspected Sulfite Sensitivity

Most people with sulfite sensitivity do not have positive allergy tests and there is currently no reliable blood or skin allergy test to test for sulfite intolerances.

At times, it may be important to undertake a deliberate food challenge with sulfites in a graded fashion under medical supervision to confirm or exclude sensitivity.

Information on food intolerances is available on the ASCIA website: Food intolerances (http://www.allergy.org.au/patients/food-other-adverse-reactions/food-intolerance).

Sulfites Are Present In Many Foods

Sulfites have a useful role to play in helping preserve many foods and beverages. The addition of sulfites to some foods like beer and wine is permitted in most countries. In many countries, it is illegal to add sulfites to foods like fresh salads or fruit salads, or to meats like mincemeat or sausage meat. Unfortunately, these can be added from time to time illegally. The following is a list of the most common sources of accidental exposure to sulfites.

- **Drinks:** Cordials, some fruit juices, beer and wine, some soft drinks, instant tea.
- **Other Liquids:** Commercial preparations of lemon and lime juice, vinegar, grape juice.
- **Commercial Foods:** Dry potatoes, some gravies and sauces and fruit toppings, maraschino cherries, pickled onions, maple syrup, jams, jellies, some biscuits and bread or pie or pizza dough
- **Fruit:** Dried apricots, and sometimes grapes will be transported with sachets of the sulfite containing preservative. (Dried sultanas do not normally contain sulfites).
- **Salads And Fruit Salads:** Sometimes restaurant salads and fruit salads will have sulfites added to preserve their color.
- **Crustaceans:** Sulphur powder is sometimes added over the top of crustaceans to stop them discoloring.
- **Meat:** Sulfites are sometimes added illegally to mincemeat or sausage meat.
- **Other Foods:** Gelatin, coconut.

The Presence Of Sulfites Can Be Recognized On Labelled Food

By Australian law, the presence of sulfites must be indicated on the label by code numbers 220 to 228, or the word "sulfite": 220—sulphur dioxide; 221—sodium sulfite; 222—sodium bisulfite; 223—sodium metabisulfite; 224—potassium metabisulfite; 226—calcium sulfite; 227—calcium and bisulfite; and 228—potassium bisulfite. [Ed. Note: U.S. law also requires that the presence of sulfites be indicated on food labels (except in cases of trace amounts below 10 ppm).]

Low Or No Sulfite Wines And Beers

[Ed. Note: These details are for general information purposes only. Irrespective of their sensitivity to sulfites, teens should not drink alcohol.] Sulfites are generally found at higher levels in the cask wine than bottled wine, and are at much higher concentrations in white wine than red wine, which is preserved by natural tannins. Some wine makers in Australia produce wines that state that they do not add sulfites into the wine. Some brewers produce beer and state that they do not add sulfites. There are various technical reasons related to wine making and brewing, which may mean that very low levels of sulfites are still present, even when not deliberately added.

Sulfites Are Also Used In Some Medications

- **Topical:** Some eye drops and creams

- **Oral Medication:** At the time of writing, no adverse reactions to sulfites have occurred from swallowed medication that might have been contaminated with sulfites.

- **Injectable Medication:** Adrenaline (epinephrine), isoprenaline, phenylephrine, dexamethasone and some other injectable corticosteroids, dopamine, local anaesthetics/dental anaesthetics containing adrenaline and aminoglycoside antibiotics are the most common potential sources of exposure. It should be noted that even in patients with serious sulfite sensitivity, the benefit of adrenaline is considered to outweigh any theoretical risk from sulfites in an emergency.

Management Of Sulfite Sensitivity

- **Time:** There is no evidence that sulfite sensitivity reduces with time.

- **Avoidance:** This is the mainstay of management. Commercial test strips to test food for the presence of sulfites are available in some other countries, but are not 100% reliable; these are not available in Australia at this time.

- **Switching Off The Sensitivity:** There is no proven way of desensitization or immunotherapy to reduce the severity of sulfite sensitivity.

- **Emergency Action Plan:** Those with relatively mild reactions like mild wheezing should carry their asthma puffers when eating away from home. Those with more serious reactions are managed along the same lines as anyone else with anaphylaxis, with provision of an ASCIA action plan for anaphylaxis, and training in the use of an adrenaline autoinjector (EpiPen or Anapen).

Part Four
Other Common Allergy Triggers

Chapter 31

Pollen Allergies

Each spring, summer, and fall, tiny pollen grains are released from trees, weeds, and grasses. These grains hitch rides on currents of air. Although the job of pollen is to fertilize plants, many grains never reach their targets. Instead, pollen can enter your eyes, nose, and throat and trigger pollen allergy.

Many people know pollen allergy as hay fever, but health experts usually refer to it as "seasonal allergic rhinitis." This simply means an allergy to pollen that makes your nose run during certain seasons.

Of all the things that can cause an allergy, pollen is one of the most common. To a great extent, people can avoid many of the foods, medicines, or animals that cause allergies. But, short of staying indoors with the windows closed when the pollen count is high—and even that may not help—people have no easy way to avoid breathing in pollen that floats in the air.

What is an allergy?

An allergy is a specific reaction of your body's immune system to a normally harmless substance. People who have allergies often are sensitive to more than one substance. Symptoms of pollen allergy include any of the following: Runny nose, sneezing, itchy eyes, congestion of the nose, or red and watery eyes.

What is pollen?

Plants produce round pollen grains. Individual grains are too tiny to see with the naked eye, but some can form large, visible clusters. For fertilization to take place and seeds to form

About This Chapter: From "Pollen Allergy," National Institute of Allergy and Infectious Diseases (www.niaid.nih .gov), October 2011.

in some plants, pollen must be moved from the flower of one plant to that of another of the same species—for example, from one oak tree to another oak tree—by a process called cross-pollination. Insects do this job for certain flowering plants, while other plants, such as ragweed, rely on wind to transport their pollen grains.

Which types of pollen cause allergies?

Most of the pollen that causes allergic reactions comes from plants that don't have showy flowers, such as trees, weeds, and grasses. These plants make small, light, and dry pollen grains that are made to be carried by wind.

Because airborne pollen can drift for many miles, removing an offending plant may not help. Amazingly, scientists have collected samples of ragweed pollen 400 miles out at sea and two miles high in the air. In addition, most allergy-causing pollen comes from plants that produce it in huge quantities. For example, a single ragweed plant can generate a million grains of pollen every day.

The components of a pollen grain are the main factors that determine whether that pollen is likely to cause allergic rhinitis. For example, pine tree pollen is produced in large amounts by a common tree, but it is not a major cause of pollen allergy because the components of pine pollen are less likely to cause an allergic reaction.

Some grasses that produce pollen include timothy grass, Kentucky bluegrass, Johnson grass, Bermuda grass, redtop grass, orchard grass, and sweet vernal grass. Some trees that produce pollen include oak, ash, elm, hickory, pecan, box elder and mountain elder.

Among North American plants, weeds produce the largest amounts of allergenic pollen. Ragweed is the major culprit, but other important sources of weed pollen come from sagebrush, redroot pigweed, lamb's quarters, Russian thistle (tumbleweed), and English plantain. Some species of grasses and trees also produce highly allergenic pollen.

Although some people may think they are allergic to colorful or scented flowers like roses, it's not usually the case. Only florists, gardeners, and others who have close contact with flowers over a long period of time are likely to be sensitive to pollen from these plants. In fact, most people have little contact with the large, heavy, and waxy pollen grains of flowering plants because this type of pollen is not carried by wind, but by insects such as butterflies and bees.

When do plants make pollen?

One of the obvious features of pollen allergy is its seasonal nature—people have symptoms only when the pollen grains to which they are allergic are in the air. Each plant pollinates more or less at the same time from year to year. Exactly when a plant starts to pollinate seems to depend on the relative length of night and day—and therefore on geographical location—rather than on the weather. But weather conditions during pollination can affect the amount of pollen produced and carried by the wind in a specific year. For example, in the Northern Hemisphere, areas farther north experience a later start to the pollinating period and the pollen allergy season.

What is a pollen count?

A pollen count, often reported by local weather broadcasts or allergy websites each year, is a measure of how much pollen is in the air. This count represents the concentration of all the pollen (or of one particular type, like ragweed) in the air in a certain area at a specific time. It is reported as grains of pollen per cubic meter of air collected over 24 hours.

Pollen counts tend to be the highest early in the morning on warm, dry, breezy days and the lowest during chilly, wet periods. Although the pollen count changes, it is useful as a general guide for when it may be wise for you to stay indoors and avoid contact with that pollen.

Preventing Ragweed Pollen Allergy Symptoms

Ragweed and other weeds such as curly dock, lambs quarters, pigweed, plantain, sheep sorrel, and sagebrush are some of the most prolific producers of pollen allergens.

Although the ragweed pollen season runs from August to November, ragweed pollen levels usually peak in mid-September in many areas in the country.

In addition, pollen counts are highest between 5:00–10:00 a.m. and on dry, hot and windy days.

Preventive Strategies

- Avoid the outdoors between 5:00–10:00 a.m. Save outside activities for late afternoon or after a heavy rain, when pollen levels are lower.

- Keep windows in your home and car closed to lower exposure to pollen. To keep cool, use air conditioners and avoid using window and attic fans.

- Be aware that pollen can also be transported indoors on people and pets.

- Dry your clothes in an automatic dryer rather than hanging them outside. Otherwise pollen can collect on clothing and be carried indoors.

Source: Excerpted from "Pollen," National Institute of Environmental Health Sciences (www.niehs.nih.gov), April 21, 2011.

How is pollen allergy diagnosed?

Skin Test: A doctor with expertise in allergic diseases, known as an allergist, or other healthcare professional will use a skin prick test to find out whether you have antibodies that react to a specific allergen. These antibodies, produced by the immune system, attach to mast cells in your skin. When the allergen binds to its antibody like a lock and key, the mast cells release histamine and other chemicals that cause allergy symptoms. A skin test is simple and relatively safe, and the results are ready in minutes.

With a skin prick test, your healthcare professional uses a needle to place a tiny amount of pollen extract (liquid substance) just below the surface of the skin on your lower arm or back. If you are allergic, there will be swelling or redness at the test site. Although such a reaction shows that you produce antibodies to a specific allergen, you might not have the respiratory and eye symptoms (runny nose, sneezing, itchy eyes) of an allergic reaction.

Blood Tests: Instead of the skin test, your healthcare professional can take a blood sample to measure the levels of pollen-specific antibodies your body produces.

As with skin testing, positive blood tests don't necessarily mean that you have pollen allergy.

What medicines are used to treat pollen allergy?

Because it is nearly impossible to avoid contact with pollen, you might be able to control your symptoms with medicines. You can buy some allergy medicines without a prescription.

Preventing Grass Pollen Allergy Symptoms

As with tree pollen, grass pollen is regional as well as seasonal. In addition, grass pollen levels can be affected by temperature, time of day and rain. Of the 1,200 species of grass that grow in North America, only a small percentage of these cause allergies. The following are the most common grasses that can cause allergies: Bermuda grass, Johnson grass, Kentucky bluegrass, Orchard grass, Sweet vernal grass, and Timothy grass.

Preventive Strategies

- If you have a grass lawn, have someone else do the mowing. If you must mow the lawn yourself, wear a mask.
- Keep grass cut short.
- Choose ground covers that don't produce much pollen, such as Irish moss, bunch, and dichondra.

Source: Excerpted from "Pollen," National Institute of Environmental Health Sciences (www.niehs.nih.gov), April 21, 2011.

Preventing Tree Pollen Allergy Symptoms

Trees are the earliest pollen producers, releasing their pollen as early as January in the Southern states and as late as May or June in the Northern states. Trees can aggravate your allergy whether or not they are on your property, since trees release large amounts of pollen that can be distributed miles away from the original source.

Of the 50,000 different kinds of trees, less than 100 have been shown to cause allergies. Most allergies are specific to one type of tree such as catalpa, elm, hickory, olive, pecan, sycamore, or walnut or to the male cultivar of certain trees. The female of these species are totally pollen-free: ash, box elder, cottonwood, date palm, maple (red), maple (silver), Phoenix palm, poplar, and willow. Some people, though, do show cross-reactivity among trees in the alder, beech, birch, and oak family, and the juniper and cedar family.

Preventive Strategies

In addition to following the suggestions given for avoiding ragweed pollen, consider this tip: If you buy trees for your yard, look for species that do not aggravate allergies—such as crape myrtle, dogwood, fig, fir, palm, pear, plum, redbud, and redwood trees or the female cultivars of ash, box elder, cottonwood, maple, palm, poplar or willow trees.

Source: Excerpted from "Pollen," National Institute of Environmental Health Sciences (www.niehs.nih.gov), April 21, 2011.

Most over-the-counter medicines are antihistamines. These medicines are often helpful in people who have mild disease. If these medicines don't give you relief or they cause unwanted side effects, your healthcare professional may write a prescription for a more powerful medicine. For example, you may be prescribed a topical nasal steroid to take with an antihistamine. Some people with seasonal allergic rhinitis develop complications, including asthma and sinusitis. If these complications develop, it's important to see a healthcare professional.

Types of medicines available to treat pollen allergy symptoms include antihistamines, topical nasal steroids, cromolyn sodium, and decongestants.

Antihistamines: Antihistamines have proven useful in relieving sneezing and itching in the nose and eyes and in reducing swelling and drainage in the nose because of pollen allergy.

Many people who take some types of antihistamines, available over the counter or by prescription, have some unwelcome side effects, such as drowsiness and loss of alertness and coordination. When children have such reactions, adults may interpret those reactions as behavior problems.

Effective antihistamines that cause fewer of these side effects are available over the counter or by prescription.

Topical Nasal Steroids: Topical nasal steroids are anti-inflammatory medicines that inhibit the allergic reaction. The combination of antihistamines and nasal steroids is a very effective way to treat pollen allergy, especially if your reaction to pollen is moderate or severe.

You should not confuse topical nasal steroids with anabolic steroids, which athletes sometimes use to improve their performance. The chemicals in nasal steroids are different from those in anabolic steroids.

Although topical nasal steroids can have side effects, they are safe when used at the recommended doses and for the recommended times.

Cromolyn Sodium: Cromolyn sodium is a nasal spray that helps prevent allergic rhinitis from starting in some people. When used as a nasal spray, it can safely inhibit the release of chemicals that cause allergy symptoms. It has few side effects when used as directed and significantly helps some people manage their allergies.

Decongestants: Decongestants can help shrink your nasal passages. This, in turn, can help relieve congestion, swelling, and general discomfort in the sinus areas caused by nasal allergies. Your healthcare professional may recommend using oral or nasal decongestants to reduce congestion, along with an antihistamine to control your symptoms.

You shouldn't use over-the-counter or prescription decongestant nose drops and sprays for more than a few days. When you use them for longer periods, these medicines can lead to even more congestion and swelling inside your nose and sinuses.

Allergy Shots: Currently, a series of allergy shots, called allergen immunotherapy, is the only available treatment that can provide a long-lasting benefit against allergies, even after the treatment is stopped. Allergy shots are given as subcutaneous (under the skin) injections. They contain increasing concentrations of the pollen allergen(s) to which you are sensitive. These shots reduce the level of antibodies to pollen in your blood and cause your body to make another protective antibody called IgG. Because these shots may have significant side effects, people need to stay in the healthcare professional's office for a period of time after receiving the shots.

Health experts recommend that people who benefit from allergy shots continue receiving them for three years and then consider stopping them with the guidance of an allergy specialist. Although many people are able to stop the injections with good results lasting for several years, others do get worse after the shots are stopped.

As researchers improve allergy shots, they promise to become an even more effective treatment.

Chapter 32

Pet Allergies

Who gets pet allergies?

Six out of 10 people in the United States come in contact with cats or dogs. The total pet population is more than 100 million, or about four pets for every 10 people.

Allergies to pets with fur or feathers are common, especially among people who have other allergies or asthma. From 15 percent to 30 percent of people with allergies have allergic reactions to cats and dogs.

People with dog allergies may be allergic to all dogs or to only some breeds. Cat allergies are about twice as common as dog allergies.

What causes a pet allergy?

The job of immune system cells is to find foreign substances such as viruses and bacteria and get rid of them. Normally, this response protects us from dangerous diseases. People with pet allergies have supersensitive immune systems that react to harmless proteins in the pet's dander (dead skin that is shed), saliva, or urine. These proteins are called allergens.

Dogs and cats secrete fluids and shed dander that contain the allergens. They collect on fur and other surfaces. The allergens will not lose their strength for a long time, sometimes for several months. They appear to be sticky and adhere to walls, clothing, and other surfaces.

Pet hair is not an allergen. It can collect dander, though. It also harbors other allergens like dust and pollen.

About This Chapter: "Pet Allergies," reprinted with permission from the Asthma and Allergy Foundation of America (www.aafa.org), © 2005. Reviewed by David A. Cooke, MD, FACP, September 2012.

Cat and dog allergens are everywhere. Pet dander is even in homes never occupied by these animals because it is carried on people's clothing. The allergens get in the air with petting, grooming, or stirring the air where the allergens have settled. Once airborne, the particles can stay suspended in the air for long periods of time.

What are the symptoms?

Reactions to cat and dog allergens that land on the membranes that line eyes and nose include swelling and itching of the membranes, stuffy nose, and inflamed eyes. A pet scratch or lick can cause the skin area to become red.

If allergen levels are low or sensitivity is minor, symptoms may not appear until after several days of contact with the pet.

Many airborne particles are small enough to get into the lungs. When inhaled, the allergens combine with antibodies. This can cause severe breathing problems—coughing, wheezing, and shortness of breath—in highly sensitive people within 15 to 30 minutes. Sometimes highly sensitive people also get an intense rash on the face, neck, and upper chest.

For about 20 percent to 30 percent of people with asthma, cat contact can trigger a severe asthma attack. Cat allergies also can lead to chronic asthma.

The Truth About Pet And Animal Allergies

Many people think animal allergies are caused by the fur or feathers of their pet. In fact, allergies are actually aggravated by other substances:

- Proteins secreted by oil glands and shed as dander

- Proteins in saliva (which stick to fur when animals lick themselves)

- Aerosolized urine from rodents and guinea pigs

Keep in mind that you can sneeze with and without your pet being present. Although an animal may be out of sight, their allergens are not. This is because pet allergens are carried on very small particles. As a result pet allergens can remain circulating in the air and remain on carpets and furniture for weeks and months after a pet is gone. Allergens may also be present in public buildings, schools, etc. where there are no pets present.

Source: Excerpted from "Pets and Animals," National Institute of Environmental Health Sciences (www.niehs.nih.gov), April 21, 2011.

How is a pet allergy diagnosed?

If a pet allergy is suspected, the doctor may diagnose it by taking a medical history and testing the blood of the patient. Some people are so attached to their pets that they will deny the pets could cause their symptoms. In these cases, the patient is removed from the animal's environment to see if symptoms go away. It does not help to remove the dog or cat. Allergens still in the area can cause symptoms months after the animal is gone.

To diagnose cat-induced asthma, the patient must have both of the following:

• Asthma symptoms when exposed to cat or cat allergen

• An allergic reaction to a skin test or to a blood test called RAST (radioallergosorbent test). To make sure the diagnosis is correct, the doctor will watch what happens when a cat is added then removed from the patient's environment several times.

What is the best treatment?

The best treatment is to avoid contact with cats or dogs or their dander. Keep the pets out of the house, and avoid visiting people with pets. Avoiding cats and dogs may give you enough relief that you will not need medication.

Keeping the pet outdoors will help, but will not rid the house of pet allergens. Another option is to have pets that do not have fur or feathers. Fish, snakes, or turtles are some choices.

What if I want to keep my pet?

To test the effect of household pets on your quality of life, remove them from your home for at least two months and clean thoroughly every week. After two months, if you still want pets, bring a pet into the house. Measure the change in your symptoms, then decide if the change in your symptoms is worth keeping the pet.

If you decide to keep a pet, bar it from the bedroom. You spend from one-third to one-half of your time there. Keep the bedroom door closed and clean the bedroom aggressively:

• Because animal allergens are sticky, you must remove the animal's favorite furniture, remove wall-to-wall carpet, and scrub the walls and woodwork. Keep surfaces throughout the home clean and uncluttered. Bare floors and walls are best.

• If you must have carpet, select ones with a low pile and steam clean them frequently. Better yet, use throw rugs that can be washed in hot water.

- Wear a dust mask to vacuum. Vacuum cleaners stir up allergens that have settled on carpet and make allergies worse. Use a vacuum with a HEPA (high efficiency particulate air) filter if possible.

- Forced-air heating and air-conditioning can spread allergens through the house. Cover bedroom vents with dense filtering material like cheesecloth.

- Adding an air cleaner with a HEPA filter to central heating and air conditioning can help remove pet allergens from the air. The air cleaner should be used at least four hours per day. Another type of air cleaner that has an electrostatic filter will remove particles the size of animal allergens from the air. No air cleaner or filter will remove allergens stuck to surfaces, though.

- Washing the pet every week may reduce airborne allergens, but is of questionable value in reducing a person's symptoms.

- Have someone without a pet allergy brush the pet outside to remove dander as well as clean the litter box or cage.

Chapter 33

Allergies And Other Health Effects Of Mold

Introduction To Molds

Molds produce tiny spores to reproduce. Mold spores waft through the indoor and outdoor air continually. When mold spores land on a damp spot indoors, they may begin growing and digesting whatever they are growing on in order to survive. There are molds that can grow on wood, paper, carpet, and foods. When excessive moisture or water accumulates indoors, mold growth will often occur, particularly if the moisture problem remains undiscovered or un-addressed. There is no practical way to eliminate all mold and mold spores in the indoor environment; the way to control indoor mold growth is to control moisture.

Molds In The Environment

Molds live in the soil, on plants, and on dead or decaying matter. Outdoors, molds play a key role in the breakdown of leaves, wood, and other plant debris. Molds belong to the kingdom *Fungi*, and unlike plants, they lack chlorophyll and must survive by digesting plant materials, using plant and other organic materials for food. Without molds, our environment would be overwhelmed with large amounts of dead plant matter.

Molds produce tiny spores to reproduce, just as some plants produce seeds. These mold spores can be found in both indoor and outdoor air, and settled on indoor and outdoor surfaces. When mold spores land on a damp spot, they may begin growing and digesting whatever they are growing on in order to survive. Molds gradually destroy the things they grow on.

About This Chapter: This chapter includes excerpts from "Mold Resources" and "Mold Remediation in Schools and Commercial Buildings: Appendix B—Introduction to Molds," U.S. Environmental Protection Agency (www .epa.gov), November 10, 2011.

Moisture control is the key to mold control. Molds need both food and water to survive; since molds can digest most things, water is the factor that limits mold growth. Molds will often grow in damp or wet areas indoors. Common sites for indoor mold growth include bathroom tile, basement walls, areas around windows where moisture condenses, and near leaky water fountains or sinks. Common sources or causes of water or moisture problems include roof leaks, deferred maintenance, condensation associated with high humidity or cold spots in the building, localized flooding due to plumbing failures or heavy rains, slow leaks in plumbing fixtures, and malfunction or poor design of humidification systems. Uncontrolled humidity can also be a source of moisture leading to mold growth, particularly in hot, humid climates.

Health Effects And Symptoms Associated With Mold Exposure

When moisture problems occur and mold growth results, building occupants may begin to report odors and a variety of health problems, such as headaches, breathing difficulties, skin irritation, allergic reactions, and aggravation of asthma symptoms; all of these symptoms could potentially be associated with mold exposure.

All molds have the potential to cause health effects. Molds produce allergens, irritants, and in some cases, toxins that may cause reactions in humans. The types and severity of symptoms depend, in part, on the types of mold present, the extent of an individual's exposure, the ages of the individuals, and their existing sensitivities or allergies. Specific reactions to mold growth can include the following:

Allergic Reactions: Inhaling or touching mold or mold spores may cause allergic reactions in sensitive individuals. Allergic reactions to mold are common—these reactions can be immediate or delayed. Allergic responses include hay fever-type symptoms, such as sneezing, runny nose, red eyes, and skin rash (dermatitis). Mold spores and fragments can produce allergic reactions in sensitive individuals regardless of whether the mold is dead or alive. Repeated or single exposure to mold or mold spores may cause previously non-sensitive individuals to become sensitive. Repeated exposure has the potential to increase sensitivity.

Asthma: Molds can trigger asthma attacks in persons who are allergic (sensitized) to molds. The irritants produced by molds may also worsen asthma in non-allergic (non-sensitized) people.

Hypersensitivity Pneumonitis: Hypersensitivity pneumonitis may develop following either short-term (acute) or long-term (chronic) exposure to molds. The disease resembles bacterial pneumonia and is uncommon.

Irritant Effects: Mold exposure can cause irritation of the eyes, skin, nose, throat, and lungs, and sometimes can create a burning sensation in these areas.

Opportunistic Infections: People with weakened immune systems (that is, immune-compromised or immune-suppressed individuals) may be more vulnerable to infections by molds (as well as more vulnerable than healthy persons to mold toxins). *Aspergillus fumigatus*, for example, has been known to infect the lungs of immune-compromised individuals. These individuals inhale the mold spores which then start growing in their lungs. *Trichoderma* has also been known to infect immune-compromised children.

Healthy individuals are usually not vulnerable to opportunistic infections from airborne mold exposure. However, molds can cause common skin diseases, such as athlete's foot, as well as other infections such as yeast infections.

Mold Toxins (Mycotoxins)

Molds can produce toxic substances called mycotoxins. Some mycotoxins cling to the surface of mold spores; others may be found within spores. More than 200 mycotoxins have been identified from common molds, and many more remain to be identified. Some of the molds that are known to produce mycotoxins are commonly found in moisture-damaged buildings. Exposure pathways for mycotoxins can include inhalation, ingestion, or skin contact. Although some mycotoxins are well known to affect humans and have been shown to be responsible for human health effects, for many mycotoxins, little information is available.

Aflatoxin B_1 is perhaps the most well known and studied mycotoxin. It can be produced by the molds *Aspergillus flavus* and *Aspergillus parasiticus* and is one of the most potent carcinogens known. Ingestion of aflatoxin B_1 can cause liver cancer. There is also some evidence that inhalation of aflatoxin B_1 can cause lung cancer. Aflatoxin B_1 has been found on contaminated grains, peanuts, and other human and animal foodstuffs.

Much of the information on the human health effects of inhalation exposure to mycotoxins comes from studies done in the workplace and some case studies or case reports.

Many symptoms and human health effects attributed to inhalation of mycotoxins have been reported including: mucous membrane irritation, skin rash, nausea, immune system suppression, acute or chronic liver damage, acute or chronic central nervous system damage, endocrine effects, and cancer and a wide range of health effects has been reported following ingestion of moldy foods including liver damage, nervous system damage, and immunological effects. More studies are needed to get a clear picture of the health effects related to most mycotoxins. However, it is clearly prudent to avoid exposure to molds and mycotoxins.

Microbial Volatile Organic Compounds

Some compounds produced by molds are volatile and are released directly into the air. These are known as microbial volatile organic compounds (mVOCs). Because these compounds often have strong and/or unpleasant odors, they can be the source of odors associated with molds. Exposure to mVOCs from molds has been linked to symptoms such as headaches, nasal irritation, dizziness, fatigue, and nausea. Research on mVOCs is still in the early phase.

Glucans Or Fungal Cell Wall Components

Glucans are small pieces of the cell walls of molds which may cause inflammatory lung and airway reactions. These glucans can affect the immune system when inhaled. Exposure to very high levels of glucans or dust mixtures including glucans may cause a flu-like illness known as organic dust toxic syndrome (ODTS). This illness has been primarily noted in agricultural and manufacturing settings.

Spores

Mold spores are microscopic and are naturally present in both indoor and outdoor air. Molds reproduce by means of spores. Some molds have spores that are easily disturbed and waft into the air and settle repeatedly with each disturbance. Other molds have sticky spores that will cling to surfaces and are dislodged by brushing against them or by other direct contact. Spores may remain able to grow for years after they are produced. In addition, whether or not the spores are alive, the allergens in and on them may remain allergenic for years.

Basic Mold Cleanup

The key to mold control is moisture control. It is important to dry water damaged areas and items within 24–48 hours to prevent mold growth. If mold is a problem in your home, clean up the mold and get rid of the excess water or moisture. Fix leaky plumbing or other sources of water. Wash mold off hard surfaces with detergent and water, and dry completely. Absorbent materials (such as ceiling tiles and carpet) that become moldy may have to be replaced.

Homes And Molds

Water in your home can come from many sources. Water can enter your home by leaking or by seeping through basement floors. Showers or even cooking can add moisture to the air in your home. The amount of moisture that the air in your home can hold depends on the

Ten Things You Should Know About Mold

1. Potential health effects and symptoms associated with mold exposures include allergic reactions, asthma, and other respiratory complaints.

2. There is no practical way to eliminate all mold and mold spores in the indoor environment; the way to control indoor mold growth is to control moisture.

3. If mold is a problem in your home or school, the mold must be cleaned up and the sources of moisture must be eliminated.

4. Fixing the source of the water problem or leak will prevent mold growth.

5. Reduce indoor humidity (to 30–60%) to decrease mold growth by venting bathrooms, dryers, and other moisture-generating sources to the outside; using air conditioners and de-humidifiers; increasing ventilation; and using exhaust fans whenever cooking, dishwashing, and cleaning.

6. Clean and dry any damp or wet building materials and furnishings within 24–48 hours to prevent mold growth.

7. Clean mold off hard surfaces with water and detergent, and dry completely. Absorbent materials such as ceiling tiles, that are moldy, may need to be replaced.

8. Prevent condensation: Reduce the potential for condensation on cold surfaces (such as windows, piping, exterior walls, roof, or floors) by adding insulation.

9. In areas where there is a perpetual moisture problem, do not install carpeting (that is, by drinking fountains, by classroom sinks, or on concrete floors with leaks or frequent condensation).

10. Molds can be found almost anywhere; they can grow on virtually any substance, providing moisture is present. There are molds that can grow on wood, paper, carpet, and foods.

Source: "Mold Resources," EPA, November 10, 2011.

temperature of the air. As the temperature goes down, the air is able to hold less moisture. This is why, in cold weather, moisture condenses on cold surfaces (for example, drops of water form on the inside of a window). This moisture can encourage biological pollutants to grow.

There are many ways to control moisture in your home. If necessary, talk to your parents about these issues:

- Fix leaks and seepage. If water is entering the house from the outside, options range from simple landscaping to extensive excavation and waterproofing. (The ground should slope away from the house.) Water in the basement can result from the lack of gutters or a water flow toward the house. Water leaks in pipes or around tubs and sinks can provide a place for biological pollutants to grow.

- Put a plastic cover over dirt in crawlspaces to prevent moisture from coming in from the ground. Be sure crawlspaces are well-ventilated.

- Use exhaust fans in bathrooms and kitchens to remove moisture to the outside (not into the attic). Vent your clothes dryer to the outside.

- Turn off certain appliances (such as humidifiers or kerosene heaters) if you notice moisture on windows and other surfaces.

- Use dehumidifiers and air conditioners, especially in hot, humid climates, to reduce moisture in the air, but be sure that the appliances themselves don't become sources of biological pollutants.

- Raise the temperature of cold surfaces where moisture condenses. Use insulation or storm windows. (A storm window installed on the inside works better than one installed on the outside.) Open doors between rooms (especially doors to closets which may be colder than the rooms) to increase circulation. Circulation carries heat to the cold surfaces. Increase air circulation by using fans and by moving furniture from wall corners to promote air and heat circulation. Be sure that your house has a source of fresh air and can expel excessive moisture from the home.

- Pay special attention to carpet on concrete floors. Carpet can absorb moisture and serve as a place for biological pollutants to grow. Use area rugs which can be taken up and washed often. In certain climates, if carpet is to be installed over a concrete floor, it may be necessary to use a vapor barrier (plastic sheeting) over the concrete and cover that with sub-flooring (insulation covered with plywood) to prevent a moisture problem.

- Moisture problems and their solutions differ from one climate to another. The Northeast is cold and wet; the Southwest is hot and dry; the South is hot and wet; and the Western Mountain states are cold and dry. All of these regions can have moisture problems. For example, evaporative coolers used in the Southwest can encourage the growth of biological pollutants. In other hot regions, the use of air conditioners which cool the air too quickly may prevent the air conditioners from running long enough to remove excess moisture from the air. The types of construction and weatherization for the different climates can lead to different problems and solutions.

Moisture On Windows

The humidistat in your house is set too high if excessive moisture collects on windows and other cold surfaces. Excess humidity for a prolonged time can damage walls especially when outdoor air temperatures are very low. Excess moisture condenses on window glass because the glass is cold. Other sources of excess moisture besides overuse of a humidifier may be long showers, running water for other uses, boiling or steaming in cooking, plants, and drying clothes indoors. A tight, energy-efficient house holds more moisture inside; you may need to run a kitchen or bath ventilating fan sometimes, or open a window briefly. Storm windows and caulking around windows keep the interior glass warmer and reduce condensation of moisture there.

Air Ducts

If there is substantial visible mold growth inside hard surface (for example, sheet metal) ducts or on other components of your heating and cooling system your parents may want to consider having them cleaned. There are several important points to understand concerning mold detection in heating and cooling systems:

- Many sections of your heating and cooling system may not be accessible for a visible inspection, so your parents should ask the service provider to show them any mold they say exists.

- Although a substance may look like mold, a positive determination of whether it is mold or not can be made only by an expert and may require laboratory analysis for final confirmation. For about $50, some microbiology laboratories can tell you whether a sample sent to them on a clear strip of sticky household tape is mold or simply a substance that resembles it.

- If your house has insulated air ducts and the insulation gets wet or moldy it cannot be effectively cleaned and should be removed and replaced.

- If the conditions causing the mold growth in the first place are not corrected, mold growth will recur.

Schools And Mold And Indoor Air Quality

Moisture problems in school buildings can be caused by a variety of conditions, including roof and plumbing leaks, condensation, and excess humidity. Some moisture problems in schools have been linked to changes in building construction practices during the past twenty to thirty years. These changes have resulted in more tightly sealed buildings that may not allow moisture to escape easily. Moisture problems in schools are also associated with delayed maintenance or insufficient maintenance, due to budget and other constraints. Temporary structures in schools, such as trailers and portable classrooms, have frequently been associated with moisture and mold problems.

Reducing Mold Growth In Schools

Talk to your school administration if you believe any of these steps are necessary:

- Reduce indoor humidity
  - Vent showers and other moisture-generating sources to the outside.
  - Control humidity levels and dampness by using air conditioners and de-humidifiers.
  - Provide adequate ventilation to maintain indoor humidity levels between 30–60%.
  - Use exhaust fans whenever cooking, dishwashing, and cleaning in food service areas.
  - Inspect the building for signs of mold, moisture, leaks, or spills

- Check for moldy odor
  - Look for water stains or discoloration on the ceiling, walls, floors, and window sills.
  - Look around and under sinks for standing water, water stains, or mold.
  - Inspect bathrooms for standing water, water stains, or mold.
  - Do not let water stand in air conditioning or refrigerator drip pans.

- Respond promptly to signs of problems
  - Clean and dry any damp or wet building materials and furnishings within 24–48 hours of occurrence to prevent mold growth.
  - Fix the source of the water problem or leak to prevent mold growth.
  - Clean mold off hard surfaces with water and detergent, and dry completely.
  - Absorbent materials such as ceiling tiles, that are moldy, may need to be replaced.
  - Check the mechanical room and roof for unsanitary conditions, leaks, or spills.

- Prevent moisture condensation
  - Reduce the potential for condensation on cold surfaces (that is, windows, piping, exterior walls, roof, or floors) by adding insulation.

- Floor and carpet cleaning
  - Remove spots and stains immediately, using the flooring manufacturer's recommended techniques.
  - Use care to prevent excess moisture or cleaning residue accumulation and ensure that cleaned areas are dried quickly.
  - In areas where there is a perpetual moisture problem, do not install carpeting (that is, by drinking fountains, by classroom sinks, or on concrete floors with leaks or frequent condensation).

Chapter 34

House Dust Allergy

Many people recognize allergy symptoms such as a runny or stuffy nose, itchy, watery eyes, and sneezing (allergic rhinoconjunctivitis) from dust exposure related to common household chores such as vacuuming, sweeping, and dusting. House dust exposure can also trigger asthma symptoms such as wheezing, coughing, chest tightness and shortness of breath.

Dust Allergy Diagnosis

If you think you may have an allergy to any of the components of house dust, consult a board certified allergist-immunologist. To pinpoint the cause of your symptoms, the allergist will ask detailed questions about your work and home environments, family medical history, frequency and severity of symptoms, exposure to pets and a variety of other questions. Sometimes the history will reveal obvious triggers, like someone who develops symptoms every time they are around a certain animal. More often though, the history may suggest triggers, but it may not be obvious in identifying the exact ones.

Sometimes the medical history may not suggest any triggers, yet allergy may be the cause. In this case, your allergist finds out what you are allergic to by doing skin tests. Skin tests involve either pricking the skin (prick tests) or injecting into the skin (intradermal tests) with different allergens and observing for a reaction. A positive reaction (a raised welt with redness around it) may indicate that you are allergic to that allergen. Occasionally, your allergist may order a blood test in addition to the skin test to confirm the diagnosis of allergy. The blood tests are generally less sensitive than skin testing.

Dust Allergy Treatment

Once your allergy triggers have been identified, steps should be taken to avoid them. Research has confirmed that targeted avoidance (environmental control aimed at relevant triggers) can be as effective as medications in reducing symptoms. The usual case requires targeted avoidance, medications prescribed by your allergist, and in many cases, specific allergen immunotherapy (allergy shots) to bring the problems under control.

Dust Mite Allergy

Dust mites (sometimes called bed mites) are the most common cause of allergy from house dust. They belong to the family of eight-legged creatures called arachnids that also includes spiders, chiggers, and ticks. Dust mites are hardy creatures that live and multiply easily in warm, humid places. They prefer temperatures at or above 70 degrees Fahrenheit with a relative humidity of 75 percent to 80 percent. They die when the humidity falls below 40 percent to 50 percent. They are not usually found in dry climates.

High levels of exposure to dust mite are an important factor in the development of asthma in children. People who are allergic to dust mites react to proteins within the bodies and feces of the mites. These particles are found mostly in pillows, mattresses, carpeting, and upholstered furniture. They float into the air when anyone vacuums, walks on a carpet, or disturbs bedding, but settle out of the air soon after the disturbance is over.

Dust mite-allergic people who inhale these particles frequently experience allergy symptoms. There may be many as 19,000 dust mites in one gram of dust, but usually between 100 to 500 mites live in each gram. (A gram is about the weight of a paper clip.) Each mite produces about 10 to 20 waste particles per day and lives for 30 days. Egg-laying females can add 25 to 30 new mites to the population during their lifetime.

Mites eat particles of skin and dander, so they thrive in places where there are people and animals. Dust mites don't bite, cannot spread diseases, and usually do not live on people. They are harmful only to people who become allergic to them. While usual household insecticides have no effect on dust mites, there are ways to reduce exposure to dust mites in the home.

Tips For Reducing House Dust Allergens

1. Measure the indoor humidity and keep it below 55 percent. Do not use vaporizers or humidifiers. You may need a dehumidifier. Use vent fans in bathrooms and when cooking to remove moisture. Repair all water leaks. (Dust mite, cockroach, and mold allergy.)

Excellent references regarding mold prevention and remediation can be found at http://www.epa.gov/mold and http://www.nyc.gov/html/doh/html/epi/moldrpt1.shtml

2. Remove wall-to-wall carpets from the bedroom if possible. Use a central vacuum or a vacuum with a HEPA (high-efficiency particulate air) filter regularly. If you are allergic, wear a N95 filter mask while dusting, sweeping, or vacuuming. Remember, it takes over two hours for the dust to settle back down, so if possible clean when the allergic patient is away and don't clean the bedroom at night. (Mold, animal, and house dust mite allergies.)

Why does house dust cause allergic reactions?

House dust is a mixture of many substances. Its content may vary from home to home, but the most common allergy triggers are:

- Dust mites
- Cockroaches
- Fungi (mold)
- Animals

Any of these allergens can cause a response in the immune system which results in the production of a special antibody (immunoglobulin E or IgE). IgE brings about an allergic inflammatory response. Exposure to only small amounts of the offending allergen can cause allergy symptoms.

3. Keep pets out of the bedroom at ALL times. Consider using a HEPA Air Cleaner in the bedroom. It is best to remove the animal from the home. (Animal allergy.)

4. Encase mattresses and pillows with "mite-proof" covers. Wash all bed linens regularly using hot water. (Dust mites allergy.)

5. Do not leave out uncovered food at night. Dispose of food wastes (including fast food wraps) in a tightly sealed garbage can. Use roach traps. Schedule regular professional pest control utilizing integrated pest management (IPM) methods. (Cockroach, mouse, and mold allergy.)

6. Install a high efficiency media filter with a MERV (minimum efficiency reporting value) rating of 11 or 12 in the furnace and air-conditioning unit. Leave the fan on to create a "whole house" air filter that removes particulates. Change the filter at least every three months (with the change of the seasons) to keep the air cleaner year round. Have your heating and air-conditioning units inspected and serviced every six months. (Animal, mold, and house dust mites allergies.)

7. Your board-certified allergist is the best resource for effective help with these issues. Many expensive, unproven products are of no benefit.

Is Dust Allergy A Sign Of A Dirty House?

No. A dirty house can make a house dust allergy problem worse, however. Normal housekeeping may not be enough to get rid of house dust allergies. This is because many of the substances in dust cannot be removed by normal cleaning procedures. Vigorous cleaning methods can actually put more dust into the air making symptoms worse. Even if the house is very clean, some people are so allergic to dust that even minimal exposures may trigger their symptoms.

Chapter 35

Cockroach Allergy

What is cockroach allergy?

When most people think of allergy triggers, they often focus on plant pollens, dust, animals, and stinging insects. In fact, cockroaches also can trigger allergies and asthma.

Cockroach allergy was first reported in 1943, when skin rashes appeared immediately after the insects crawled over patients' skin. Skin tests first confirmed patients had cockroach allergy in 1959.

In the 1970s, studies made it clear that patients with cockroach allergies develop acute asthma attacks. The attacks occur after inhaling cockroach allergens and last for hours. Asthma has steadily increased over the past 30 years. It is the most common chronic disease of childhood. Now we know that the frequent hospital admissions of inner-city children with asthma often is directly related to their contact with cockroach allergens—the substances that cause allergies. From 23 percent to 60 percent of urban residents with asthma are sensitive to the cockroach allergen.

The increase in asthma is not fully understood. Experts think one reason for the increase among children is that they play indoors more than in past years and thus have increased contact with the allergen. This is especially true in the inner cities where they stay inside because of safety concerns.

What causes the allergic reaction?

The job of immune system cells is to find foreign substances such as viruses and bacteria and get rid of them. Normally, this response protects us from dangerous diseases. People with

About This Chapter: "Cockroach Allergy," reprinted with permission from the Asthma and Allergy Foundation of America (www.aafa.org). © 2011.

allergies have supersensitive immune systems that react when they inhale, swallow, or touch certain harmless substances such as pollen or cockroaches. These substances are the allergens.

Cockroach allergen is believed to derive from feces, saliva, and the bodies of these insects. Cockroaches live all over the world, from tropical areas to the coldest spots on earth. Studies show that 78 percent to 98 percent of urban homes have cockroaches. Each home has from 900 to 330,000 of the insects.

Private homes also harbor them, especially if the homes are well insulated. When one roach is seen in the basement or kitchen, it is safe to assume that at least 800 roaches are hidden under the kitchen sink, in closets, and the like. They are carried in with groceries, furniture, and luggage used on trips. Once they are in the home, they are hard to get rid of.

The amount of roach allergen in house dust or air can be measured. In dwellings where the amount is high, exposure is high and the rate of hospitalization for asthma goes up. Allergen particles are large and settle rapidly on surfaces. They become airborne when the air is stirred by people moving around or by children at play.

Who develops cockroach allergy?

People with chronic severe bronchial asthma are most likely to have cockroach allergy. Also likely to have it are people with a chronic stuffy nose, skin rash, constant sinus infection, repeat ear infection, and asthma.

Cockroach allergy is a problem among people who live in inner-cities or in the South and are of low socioeconomic status. In one study of inner-city children, 37 percent were allergic to cockroaches, 35 percent to dust mites, and 23 percent to cats. Those who were allergic to cockroaches and were exposed to the insects were hospitalized for asthma 3.3 times more often than other children. This was true even when compared with those who were allergic to dust mites or cats.

Cockroach allergy is more common among poor African Americans. Experts believe that this is not because of racial differences; rather, it is because of the disproportionate number of African Americans living in the inner cities.

What are its symptoms?

Symptoms vary. They may be a mildly itchy skin, scratchy throat, or itchy eyes and nose. Or the allergy symptoms can become stronger, including severe, persistent asthma in some people. Asthma symptoms often are a problem all year, not just in some seasons. This can make it hard to determine that a cockroach allergy is the cause of the asthma.

Cockroaches And Asthma

- Cockroaches are one of the most common and allergenic of indoor pests.
- Recent studies have found a strong association between the presence of cockroaches and increases in the severity of asthma symptoms in individuals who are sensitive to cockroach allergens.
- These pests are common even in the cleanest of crowded urban areas and older dwellings. They are found in all types of neighborhoods.
- The proteins found in cockroach saliva are particularly allergenic but the body and droppings of cockroaches also contain allergenic proteins.

Source: Excerpted from "Cockroaches," National Institute of Environmental Health Sciences (www.niehs.nih.gov), April 21, 2011.

How is cockroach allergy diagnosed?

The National Heart, Lung, and Blood Institute recommends that all patients with persistent asthma be tested for allergic response to cockroach as well as to the other chief allergens, dust mites, cats, dogs, and mold.

Diagnosis can be made only by skin tests. The doctor scratches or pricks the skin with cockroach extract. Redness, an itchy rash, or swelling at the site suggests you are allergic to the insect.

Cockroaches should be suspected, though, when allergy symptoms—stuffy nose, inflamed eyes or ears, skin rash, or bronchial asthma—persist year round.

How can I manage cockroach allergy?

- If you have cockroach allergy, avoid contact with roaches and their droppings.
- The first step is to rid your home of the roaches. Because they resist many control measures, it is best to call in pest control experts.
- For ongoing control, use poison baits, boric acid, and traps. Don't use chemical agents. They can irritate allergies and asthma.
- Do not leave food and garbage uncovered.
- To manage nasal and sinus symptoms, use antihistamines, decongestants, and anti-inflammatory medications. Your doctor will also prescribe anti-inflammatory medications and bronchodilators if you have asthma.
- If you keep having serious allergic symptoms, see an allergist about "allergy injections" with the cockroach extract. They can reduce symptoms over time.

Chapter 36

Sting Allergies

Overview

Although less common than pollen allergy, insect venom allergy is anything but trivial—it can be life-threatening. The primary offenders are most often insects that sting rather than those that bite. These insects are members of the order of *Hymenoptera* of the class *Insecta*. Stinging insects of concern are found in three families:

- Vespids (*Vespidae*): Including yellow jackets, hornets, and wasps.

- Bees (*Apidae*): Honeybees are the most frequent offenders with bumblebees causing significantly fewer reactions. Sweatbees infrequently cause allergic reactions.

- Ants (*Formicidae*): Including fire ants and harvester ants. Although painful, harvester ant stings are a less common cause of anaphylaxis. Imported fire ant stings are known to cause systemic (whole body) allergic reactions in their habitat in the southeastern U.S. and along the Gulf Coast. They characteristically bite to attach themselves to their victim and then sting multiple times in a semicircular pattern with a sterile pustule forming after several hours at each sting site.

There have been isolated case reports of systemic allergic reactions to bites from deer flies, kissing bugs, bed bugs, and mosquitoes, but such reactions are rare. More common are large local reactions to these bites that, although unpleasant, are not life threatening.

About This Chapter: "Insect Sting Allergy," June 2012. Copyright © National Jewish Health (www.njhealth.org). All rights reserved. Used by permission. Although some of the text in this chapter addresses parents, the information is still beneficial for teens.

Symptoms

Insect sting reactions can be classified as immediate or delayed based upon their timing. Reactions can also be toxic or allergic. A toxic reaction is due to compounds in the venom itself acting on cells and tissues of the body. A true allergic response is a result of the immune system making specific allergic antibodies (IgE) to components of the insect venom, leading—with exposure—to the generation and release of a variety of chemicals such as histamine that act on surrounding tissue to cause the symptoms associated with allergic reaction.

Immediate Reactions

Immediate reactions are those reactions occurring within minutes to hours of a sting and can be further divided into local, large local, anaphylactic, and toxic reactions. Immediate local reactions are often considered the "normal reaction." Signs and symptoms of immediate localized reactions are limited to the area of the sting site. Local reactions can occur in individuals who are not insect allergic.

Signs and symptoms may consist of:

- pain
- redness
- swelling
- mild itching that may last for several hours

Delayed Reactions

Reactions occurring more than four hours after a sting are classified as delayed reactions. There have been isolated reports of serum sickness-like syndromes occurring about a week after a sting. Other unusual reactions that have been reported in association with insect stings include Guillain-Barré syndrome, glomerulonephritis, myocarditis, vasculitis and encephalitis. Signs and symptoms may include:

- hives
- fever
- general discomfort
- joint pain
- pain or partial paralysis of extremities (hands, arms, feet, and legs)
- kidney pain

- chest pain (angina)
- swelling
- headache, dizziness, loss of consciousness

Large Local Reactions

Large local reactions are characterized by redness and swelling that extends from the sting site over a large surrounding area. These reactions often peak within 48 to 72 hours and last up to 10 days. They may be accompanied by fatigue, low-grade fever, mild nausea, and discomfort and are often misdiagnosed as cellulitis.

Anaphylaxis

Anaphylaxis is the most severe insect sting reaction. This reaction, involving multiple organ systems at the same time, most often begins within minutes of the sting although it can occasionally begin an hour or so later. If an anaphylactic reaction is suspected, give injectable epinephrine and an antihistamine (if available) and call 911 immediately. Signs and symptoms may consist of:

- flushing, itching
- hives
- sneezing, runny nose
- nausea, vomiting, diarrhea
- abdominal cramping
- heart irregularities
- swelling in the throat
- severe trouble breathing
- drop in blood pressure (hypotension)
- loss of consciousness
- shock

Toxic Reactions

In the event of a sting from a poisonous spider or insect; or multiple, simultaneous stings from otherwise non-poisonous insects (as might be the case when a nest is disturbed, or when Africanized honeybees are involved); a toxic reaction may result. Toxic reactions are not caused by an allergic response, but rather by the effects of venom that acts as a poison. Local and toxic reactions can be seen in individuals who are not insect sting allergic, although some patients who experience toxic reactions can become allergic to insect venom later. Symptoms of a toxic reaction vary depending on the toxicity of the venom of the insect or spider, the amount of venom injected, and the individual's tolerance for that particular venom. Signs and symptoms may consist of:

- rapid swelling at the site of the sting

- headache

- weakness

- lightheadedness

- drowsiness

- fever

- diarrhea

- muscle spasms

- fainting (syncope)

- seizures

Usually, symptoms lessen or go away within 48 hours. Hives and shortness of breath may occur in an allergic reaction, but not in a toxic reaction. Though it is possible to have both a toxic reaction and an allergic reaction at the same time, this rarely occurs. A toxic reaction can be life-threatening and may lead to heart problems, shock, and death.

If a toxic reaction is suspected, call 911, or seek professional medical attention immediately.

Diagnosis

The first step in making the diagnosis of insect venom sensitivity consists of taking a careful history and attempting to identify the responsible insect. Nesting and behavior patterns and a description of the insect and the sting may aid identification. For example, honeybees, because their stinger is barbed, usually lose their stinging apparatus, leaving it stuck in the victim at the site of the sting. Thus, stinging is a fatal event for a honeybee. However, this alone is not diagnostic of a honeybee sting because vespids can also lose their stingers about eight percent of the time.

Unfortunately, accurate identification of the insect based on the history alone is not always possible. People with histories suggestive of significant sting sensitivity should be referred to an allergist. The usual procedure is to skin test with the five commercially available venoms: honey bee, paper wasp, yellow jacket, yellow hornet, and white-faced hornet. When appropriate whole-body extracts for imported fire ant, harvester ant, and several biting insects are also available for testing. If the history is very suggestive of a generalized reaction and skin tests are negative, they should be repeated as well as obtaining blood tests for specific venoms (RAST [radioallergosorbent test]).

Treatment

Venom allergy shots (immunotherapy) are highly effective in preventing subsequent sting reactions. After reaching maintenance doses of immunotherapy, 95 percent of venom-treated patients are able to tolerate single stings, and sting reactions that occur are generally milder. Adult patients who have a positive venom skin test generally are considered candidates for specific-venom immunotherapy. Children with skin symptoms alone have only a 10 percent risk of systemic reactions and aren't considered candidates for skin testing or immunotherapy. Nonetheless, children with more severe or life-threatening reactions are candidates for venom immunotherapy.

Treatment of local reactions in people without a history of insect sting sensitivity include aspirin for pain and ice to reduce swelling.

For those with a history of large local reactions, taking an oral antihistamine (preferably non-sedating) and, in some cases, taking a single dose of oral steroids soon after the sting is recommended.

Wear a medical alert bracelet or necklace stating that you (or your child) are allergic to insect stings.

Be familiar with the potential symptoms of allergic reactions to insect stings. Your family should also be familiar with this information. Ask your healthcare provider to give you a written action plan. If an epinephrine injection device is prescribed, learn when and how to use it. Make sure that all caretakers understand the action plan and how to give the epinephrine and any other medication prescribed for treatment of reactions.

Carry an emergency pack at all times. The emergency pack should contain each of the medications needed to treat a sting reaction, such as an epinephrine injection device and an antihistamine in the form of syrup or chewable tablet. If you or your child has asthma, a rescue inhaler should also be kept in the emergency pack. An action plan card indicating the actions to take and the importance of calling 911 or going to the closest medical facility once the medication is given is also helpful.

Reduce Insect Exposure

Knowing how to lessen the risk of being stung is an important part of learning how to care for yourself or someone else with insect sting allergy. For a child, make sure that all caretakers also are taught how to respond when avoidance strategies fail and a sting occurs. This means being prepared to treat insect sting reactions in a variety of settings including at home, school, day care, friend's houses and all other sites where the child spends time.

- Wear protective clothing while outside to decrease exposed skin. Wear long pants when hiking or mowing the grass and wear gloves while gardening.

- Wear white or light colored clothing. Dark clothing and clothing with flowery designs are more likely to attract insects.

- Wear shoes rather than bare feet or sandals.

- Use unscented deodorant and rinse off perspiration after vigorous exercise. Insects are attracted to the scent of deodorants and perspiration.

- Avoid the use of strong smelling perfume, cologne, hair oil, hair spray, or lotions because insects may be attracted by their fragrance.

- Cover food and drinks at outdoor events as much as possible. Outside garbage should remain covered. The smell of food attracts insects.

- Use insect repellents and keep insecticide available.

- Do not knowingly approach or disturb the nests of stinging insects.

Insect Sting Allergy: Frequently Asked Questions

Question: Are there ways I can protect myself from insect stings while outdoors?

Answer: Wear protective clothing while outside to decrease exposed skin. For example, wear long pants when hiking or mowing the grass, gloves while gardening, and shoes or sandals rather than running around in bare feet.

Question: Is any color of clothing better?

Answer: Wear white or light colored clothing; dark clothing and clothing with flowery designs are more likely to attract insects.

Question: Can I protect myself if I exercise outdoors?

Answer: Use unscented deodorant and rinse off perspiration after vigorous exercise. Insects are attracted to the scent of deodorants and perspiration. Avoid any strong smelling perfume, cologne, hair oil, hair spray, or lotions because insects may be attracted by the smell. Use insect repellants and keep insecticide available.

Question: How can I protect myself from insect stings during a picnic?

Answer: Cover food and drinks at outdoor events as much as possible. The smell of food is a strong attraction for insects. Don't forget to cover garbage, as well.

Question: I've had severe reactions to insect stings in the past. What should I do to protect myself and let others know about my condition?

Answer: Wear a medical alert bracelet or necklace stating that you are allergic to insect stings. The person with insect allergies should always carry an emergency pack. Talk with your healthcare provider about exactly what to have in the emergency pack, but generally it should contain each of the medications needed to treat a sting reaction, such as an oral antihistamine—syrup or chewable tablet—and an epinephrine injection device (EpiPen). If you have asthma, also keep a rescue inhaler and spacer in the pack. Ask your healthcare provider about potential symptoms of allergic reactions to insect stings. It also can be helpful to carry a small action plan card listing the actions to take and the importance of calling 911 or going to the closest medical facility once the medication is given. Review how to take all the medications that are prescribed in your action plan. If an epinephrine injection device is prescribed, review when it should be used and demonstrate the correct technique for your healthcare provider. Talk with family about how they can help you follow your action plan.

Chapter 37

Medication And Drug Allergies

Overview

Allergies to medications/drugs are complicated because they can be caused by many different medications, resulting in a wide variety of signs and symptoms that may affect various organs or parts of the body. Furthermore, some drugs can cause adverse effects with symptoms that closely resemble those of an allergic reaction. The difference is that true drug allergy is caused by a hypersensitive immune system that creates IgE and other antibodies and/or cytotoxic immune cells in response to an otherwise harmless substance in the medication.

One characteristic of all drug allergies is that similar symptoms will occur every time soon after the offending medicine is taken. Penicillin and other antibiotics are the medicines that most commonly cause allergic reactions. Women appear to have an increased risk for adverse drug reactions.

Symptoms

The signs and symptoms of medication/drug allergy can involve the skin, lungs, gastrointestinal tract (digestive system), and rarely other organs. Occasionally, allergic-like reactions to drugs may take several days to develop and may include other symptoms such as fever, joint aches, and rashes. Such reactions may not be due to an IgE antibody but due to other types of immune reactions, although the term "allergic reaction" is commonly used to refer these conditions.

About This Chapter: "Medication/Drug Allergy," November 2011. Copyright © National Jewish Health (www .njhealth.org). All rights reserved. Used by permission.

Symptoms after drug ingestion can also result from conditions other than drug allergy. Often drugs elicit a side effect, which is the result of a direct action of the drug (pharmacological or non-pharmacological) but not due to an immune/allergic reaction. Sometimes the symptoms are caused by the illness for which the drug was taken. Occasionally, symptoms are caused by drug interactions when a patient is taking multiple medications at the same time.

Medication/drug allergy symptoms include:

- **Skin Symptoms:** Include itching, flushing, and hives or other forms of rash.

- **Gastrointestinal (Digestive System) Symptoms:** Include tingling and burning of the mouth and throat, swelling, nausea, vomiting, abdominal pain, and diarrhea.

- **Respiratory Symptoms:** Include nasal congestion, runny nose, sneezing, throat swelling, wheezing and/or difficulty breathing.

- **Life-Threatening Anaphylactic Reactions:** These may cause a person to lose consciousness and stop breathing. Call 911 immediately if you suspect anaphylaxis.

Diagnosis And Treatment

Every medication/drug allergy diagnosis should begin with a detailed medical history and physical examination. The doctor will ask lots of questions about the nature of the reaction, where and when it occurs, etc. Since the drug allergy may be genetic, expect some questions about other family members who may be allergic.

Depending upon the findings of the initial evaluation, the following tests may be necessary:

- Allergy skin testing may be performed to check for presence of allergic antibodies to selected drug allergens.

- Blood testing is occasionally indicated.

- A drug challenge to the suspected drug is sometimes necessary to confirm the diagnosis. If indicated, drug challenges are coordinated with safety as the highest priority.

The best way to treat drug allergy is to avoid the medication, since there is no cure for allergy. Antihistamines and steroids can be used to alleviate symptoms, but once a drug allergy is determined, the medication should be avoided.

Reduce Drug Exposure

The best way to treat drug allergy is to avoid the medication. Here are a few tips to help prevent an allergic reaction to drugs:

- Memorize trade and generic names of the medications that cause a reaction and check labeling on products you buy.

- Make sure you tell all caregivers about your allergy.

- Wear a med-alert bracelet or necklace describing your allergy just in case you ever need emergency care.

- If your doctor prescribes an injectable epinephrine pen for anaphylactic reactions, remember to carry it with you.

"Treat Through" Medication Allergies

In very rare cases, it may be required to "treat through" a medication allergy in which the drug may be required despite the reaction. This can be dangerous and is only used as a last resort and in a hospital setting.

Patients may be pre-treated with steroids or antihistamines in such cases. Drug desensitization can be performed in a hospital setting where the patient is given gradually increasing doses of the medication either by mouth or by I.V. under constant monitoring until he or she can tolerate a full dose.

It is very important to remember that desensitization works only for that particular course of the medicine, so if it is discontinued, the person once again becomes allergic and needs to be desensitized each time the medicine is administered.

Chapter 38

Latex Allergy

Overview

Latex—a natural rubber made from the sap of the *Hevea brasiliensis* tree—is used to manufacture many items, including bicycle and wheelchair tires, toys, some balloons, examining gloves, household gloves, surgical tubing, rubber bands, and condoms. The major exposure of concern is to the powder from latex gloves, because the latex proteins adhere to the powder and become airborne when these gloves are put on, taken off, or snapped.

A person allergic to latex is actually allergic to one or more proteins (allergens) found in the sap from the rubber tree. Interestingly, these proteins—or ones very similar—can be found in banana, kiwi, avocado, potato, strawberries, peaches, and chestnuts. Both latex and these foods are plant-derived, and contain chitinase I, a pan allergen responsible for the latex-fruit syndrome. Therefore, people who are allergic to latex may have cross-reactions to these foods. Interestingly, the chitinase I allergen is destroyed by heating, so many people can eat the cooked food but not the raw form.

In addition, raw latex is mixed with a variety of different chemicals that allow the latex proteins to polymerize, or take shape, into long chains that can then be manipulated to form solid objects. Some of these chemicals can cause contact dermatitis, an allergic skin reaction that appears as mild to severe itchy, red bumps or rashes on the skin directly exposed to the rubber product, typically the hands. However, these chemicals do not cause specific IgE type symptoms such as asthma, hives, or hayfever.

About This Chapter: "Latex Allergy," January 2012, Copyright © National Jewish Health (www.njhealth.org). All rights Reserved. Used by permission.

Symptoms

Latex allergy can present a wide range of symptoms, including:

- hives (contact urticaria);
- itchy, watery eyes (conjunctivitis);
- sneezing, runny nose (rhinitis);
- wheezing, shortness of breath, chest tightness (asthma symptoms); and
- in severe cases, systemic anaphylaxis including critical asthma symptoms, throat swelling, fall in blood pressure, loss of consciousness, and, very rarely, death.

Risk Factors

Genetics and the environment both play a role in developing a latex allergy. There are groups of people who are more likely to develop a latex allergy than others.

High Exposure To Latex

Since the amount of exposure to latex is a key factor in developing a latex allergy, healthcare workers and patients (especially children) who undergo multiple surgeries are at risk. Children with spina bifida are the most likely group to develop a latex allergy, in part because their exposures are more likely to be mucosal, for example, through latex catheters and tubing.

Genetic Links To Allergies

There is a genetic link to allergies. Therefore, people are at an increased risk for developing an allergy to latex if they have other allergic conditions such as these:

- Allergy-induced asthma
- Eczema (atopic dermatitis)
- Hives (chronic urticaria)
- Food allergies

People who have experienced a reaction after eating banana, kiwi, avocado, potato, strawberries, peaches, or chestnuts may also have increased risk for latex allergy.

Treatment

The best way to treat latex allergy is to avoid latex. There is no cure for allergy, and continued exposure to latex may make the condition worse.

Antihistamines may be used to control some symptoms, but they also may help mask allergic reactions to small amounts of latex in the environment.

Latex is a very complex biological compound, and the specific proteins within latex that cause allergic reactions have not been fully identified and characterized and may vary from person to person. Therefore, there is no standardized extract, so immunotherapy (allergy shots) is not currently a treatment option.

Reduce Latex Exposure

Environmental control—decreasing or eliminating exposure to the latex allergen—is the best way to reduce symptoms in those already latex allergic, and prevent the allergy from developing in other exposed patients and health care workers. Evidence shows that allergy and asthma symptoms may improve over time if the recommended environmental control changes are made. Environmental control measures to consider for allergy to latex include:

- Generally, the most important latex exposure to avoid is powder from powdered latex gloves. Solid objects containing latex, such as rubber bands, blood pressure tubing, bicycle tires, and the like, are not a hazard for asthma or hay fever symptoms because they do not emit latex particles.

- A latex-safe environment is one where latex allergic patients and staff do not use any latex-containing items, and co-workers and other patients do not use powdered latex gloves, but instead use non-powdered latex, or, preferably, non-latex gloves. Both latex-allergic and non-allergic patients and staff are protected against allergic reactions in this environment.

What is latex?

Latex is a milky fluid that comes from the tropical rubber tree. Hundreds of everyday products contain latex. Repeated exposure to a protein in natural latex can make you more likely to develop a latex allergy. If your immune system detects the protein, a reaction can start in minutes. You could get a rash, asthma and in rare cases shock from latex exposure.

Latex products are all around you. Some common ones are gloves, condoms, balloons, rubber bands, shoe soles, and pacifiers. If you are allergic to latex, it is a good idea to learn which products contain it. That way, you can reduce your exposure.

The most common reactions are to gloves and condoms. Latex-free alternatives exist for both.

SOURCE: From "Latex Allergy," U.S. National Library of Medicine (www.nlm.nih.gov), February 9, 2012.

- Healthcare workers allergic to latex should wear alternative products such as nitrile examining gloves instead of latex, and they should ask their coworkers to wear nitrile gloves, or at least a non-powdered latex glove. If this is not possible, seek reassignment to an area where powdered latex gloves are not used.

- Non-healthcare professionals allergic to latex should communicate their allergic conditions to medical staff when undergoing a checkup or medical procedure. This is especially important in the case of surgery. You could even bring your own non-latex gloves to any medical appointment in case your caregiver doesn't have any.

- Check labeling on products you buy. "Hypoallergenic" does not necessarily mean "no latex."

- Wear a med-alert bracelet or necklace describing your allergy, in case you ever need emergency care.

- Carry an injectable epinephrine pen in case of an anaphylactic reaction, although these are very rare.

Chapter 39

Nickel Allergy

Nickel allergy is one of the most common causes of contact allergic dermatitis. In affected individuals, dermatitis (eczema) develops in places where nickel-containing metal is touching the skin. The most common sites are the earlobes (from earrings), the wrists (from a watch strap) and the lower abdomen (from a jeans stud); the affected areas become intensely itchy and may become red and blistered (acute dermatitis) or dry, thickened, and pigmented (chronic dermatitis).

Who Is Affected By Nickel Allergy?

Contact allergic dermatitis to nickel may develop at any age. Once this nickel allergy has occurred, it persists for many years, often life-long.

Nickel allergy is more common in women, probably because they are more likely to have pierced ears than men, although this is changing. The degree of allergy varies. Some people develop dermatitis (also called eczema) from even brief contact with nickel-containing items, while others break out only after many years of skin contact with nickel.

Can It Affect Areas That Are Not In Contact With Metal?

Some people develop intermittent or persistent eczema on their hands and feet. It is usually a blistering type of eczema, known as pompholyx. Sometimes it is due to contact with metal items containing nickel, but often there is no obvious reason for it.

About This Chapter: "Nickel Allergy," reprinted with permission from DermNet NZ, the web site of the New Zealand Dermatological Society. Visit www.dermnetnz.org for patient information about skin diseases, conditions, and treatment. © December 22, 2010 New Zealand Dermatological Society. All rights reserved.

It has been suggested that in some, dyshidrotic hand dermatitis is due to nickel in the diet. Unfortunately it is not possible to avoid ingesting nickel, as it is present in most foodstuffs. A low-nickel diet is only rarely helpful.

Diagnosis

Nickel allergy is diagnosed by the clinical history and by special allergy tests, patch tests.

Subjects are specifically tested to nickel sulphate-hexahydrate. The chemical formula for this is $NiO4S.6H2O$.

Treatment

- **Compresses:** Dry up blisters with diluted vinegar compresses.
- **Topical Steroids:** Apply topical steroid to the dermatitis as directed.
- **Antibiotics:** Antibiotic creams or pills may be necessary for secondary infection. Usually a penicillin antibiotic such as flucloxacillin is chosen.
- **Emollients:** Apply soothing emollient creams frequently to relieve itch and dry skin.

Unfortunately, desensitization with injections or pills is not possible.

Low Nickel Diet

Foods Allowed

- Meat, poultry, fish, eggs, milk, yogurt, cheese, quark, butter, margarine
- Cereals, bread, flour, rice, pasta
- Small servings of wholemeal flour, wholegrain cereals, wheat bran and wheat germ
- Most vegetables
- Small servings of beetroot, cabbage, cauliflower, leeks, parsnips, potatoes, spinach
- Fruit, raw and stewed
- Tea, coffee, soft drinks, cordials, beer, wine

Foods To Avoid

- Canned spaghetti and baked beans
- Green beans, broccoli, peas including split peas, canned vegetables
- Canned fruit, dried fruit, nuts
- Cocoa, drinking chocolate, chocolate

Avoid Nickel

It is essential to avoid contact with nickel-containing metals.

Test Your Metal Items

Test your metal items to see if they contain nickel. Obtain a nickel-testing kit from your dermatologist or pharmacist. The kit consists of two small bottles of clear fluid; one contains dimethylglyoxime and the other ammonium hydroxide. When mixed together in the presence of nickel, a pink color results.

Apply a drop from each bottle on to the metal item to be tested—first try it on a 10-cent coin. Use a cotton bud to rub gently—observe the color on the bud. If it remains clear, the item has no free nickel and will not cause dermatitis. If it is pink it contains nickel and may cause problems if the metal touches your skin. The chemicals will not harm your jewelry.

Jewelry

Necklaces, necklace-clips, earrings, bracelets, watch-straps, and rings may contain nickel. "Hypoallergenic," solid gold (12 carat or more), and silver jewelry should be safe. Nine carat gold and white gold both contain nickel. Plastic covers for earring studs can be obtained. Coating the stud with nail varnish is not recommended.

Clothing

Metal zips, bra hooks, suspender clips, hair-pins, buttons, studs, spectacle frames, etcetera, are likely to contain nickel. Use substitutes made of plastic, coated, or painted metal or some other material.

Personal Articles

Consider mobile phones, lipstick holders, powder compacts, handbag catches, cigarette lighters, razors, keys, key rings, pocket knives, and pens as potential causes of dermatitis.

Metal Items In The Home

Cupboard handles, kitchen utensils, cutlery, toaster, metal teapots, scissors, needles, pins, thimbles, vacuum cleaners, torches [flashlights], bath plugs... may all contain nickel. Choose tools with plastic handles. Stainless steel does not usually cause dermatitis unless it is nickel-plated.

Money

Silver coins are composed of cupronickel. Cashiers with nickel allergy may develop hand dermatitis from this source. Wear gloves to handle money or pay with a credit card or check.

Metal At Work

Nickel dermatitis may be aggravated by contact with paper clips, typewriter keys, instruments, and metal fragments from a lathe or chain saw.

Chapter 40

Hair Dye Allergy

What Is Paraphenylenediamine And Where Is It Found?

Paraphenylenediamine (PPD) is a chemical substance that is widely used as a permanent hair dye. It may also been found in textile or fur dyes, dark colored cosmetics, temporary tattoos, photographic developer and lithography plates, photocopying and printing inks, black rubber, oils, greases, and gasoline.

The use of PPD as a hair dye is popular because it is a permanent dye that gives a natural look. Hair can also be shampooed without becoming discolored and perming to achieve waves or curls can be done without difficulty. PPD hair dyes usually come packaged as two bottles, one containing the PPD dye preparation and the other containing the developer or oxidizer. PPD is a colorless substance that requires oxygen for it to become colored. It is this intermediate, partially oxidized state that may cause allergy in sensitive individuals. Fully oxidized PPD is not a sensitizer thus individuals with PPD allergy can wear wigs or fur coats dyed with PPD safely.

What Are The Reactions To PPD Allergy?

Reaction caused by the use of hair dye in mild cases usually only involves dermatitis to the upper eyelids or the rims of the ears. In more severe cases, there may be marked reddening and swelling of the scalp and the face. The eyelids may completely close and the allergic contact dermatitis reaction may become widespread.

About This Chapter: "Allergy to Paraphenylenediamine," reprinted with permission from DermNet NZ, the web site of the New Zealand Dermatological Society. Visit www.dermnetnz.org for patient information about skin diseases, conditions, and treatment. © September 25, 2011 New Zealand Dermatological Society. All rights reserved.

Severe allergy to PPD can result in contact urticaria and rarely, anaphylaxis.

People working with PPD such as hairdressers and film developers may develop dermatitis on their hands; patch testing usually reveals hypersensitivity to PPD. Occupational allergy to PPD has been found in a milk tester whom through laboratory work was in frequent contact with PPD solution. Dermatitis on the hands and occasional spreading to the arms and upper chest occurred.

Am I Allergic To PPD?

Most hair color preparations, particularly those containing PPD, carry a warning on the packaging to the effect that a patch test should be done prior to use of the dye. There are basically two patch testing methods available to test for allergic sensitivity to PPD.

Alternative Names For Paraphenylenediamine

- PPD or PPDA
- Phenylenediamine base
- p-Phenylenediamine
- 4-Phenylenediamine
- 1,4-Phenylenediamine
- 4-Benzenediamine
- 1,4-Benzenediamine
- para-Diaminobenzene (p-Diaminobenzene)
- para-Aminoaniline (p-Aminoaniline)
- Orsin
- Rodol
- Ursol

Further Information

- **Formula:** 4-Phenylenediamine base—$C_6H_8N_2$
- **CAS Number:** 106–50–3
- **Cross Reactions:** Azo and aniline dyes; Benzocaine; Procaine; Para-aminobenzoic acid (PABA); Para-aminosalicylic acid; Sulfonamides; Carbutamide; Hydrochlorothiazide
- **Appearance:** White to slightly red solid crystals that darken on exposure to air.
- **Sensitizer:** Intermediate, partially oxidized PPD
- **Patch Test:** 2% PPD in petrolatum

Patch Test Method 1: Uncovered

- Routine technique used by consumers for testing hair dye sensitivity.

- Instructions for testing should be included with every package of hair dye preparation.

- Essentially the test involves applying a 25-cent sized spot of solution (dye and developer mixed together) to either the neck (behind the ear) or the inner bend of the elbow. Allow to dry and leave uncovered for 48–72 hours. If no irritation or rash occurs during this time then the test is negative and one can assume that the risk of developing a rash will be much less when the dye is applied to the whole head.

- Any immediate signs of irritation or rash are more likely to be an irritant contact dermatitis (nonallergic).

- A 1+ to 2+ reaction (scale measuring PPD sensitivity) to PPD hair dye usually indicates that dermatitis will develop if the mixture is used.

Patch Test Method 2: Covered

- Diagnostic test used to determine PPD sensitivity.

- Patch testing using 2% PPD in petrolatum.

- A +/- reaction (scale measuring PPD sensitivity) to this patch test method usually means that these individuals can use PPD hair dyes without difficulty.

- A 1+ to 3+ reaction indicates allergic dermatitis will most likely occur with use of hair dyes thus preventing their use.

- Positive reaction from both methods provides confirmation that PPD is the cause of dermatitis and PPD containing products should be avoided.

Treatment Of PPD Dermatitis

In acute severe cases of PPD hair dye dermatitis, wash the hair and scalp thoroughly with a mild soap or soapless shampoo to remove the excess dye. Apply a 2% hydrogen peroxide solution or compresses of potassium permanganate in a 1:5000 dilution to completely oxidize the PPD. To soothe, soften the crust and alleviate the tight feeling of the scalp, a wet dressing of cold olive oil and lime may be used. Further treatment with a topical application of an emulsion of water and water-miscible corticosteroid cream, or oral corticosteroids may be indicated.

Management of PPD dermatitis on other parts of the body may be treated as for any acute dermatitis/eczema; this may include treatment with topical corticosteroids and emollients.

What Should I Do To Avoid PPD Allergy?

If you have an allergy to PPD and have your hair dyed, you should avoid the use of all oxidation type hair dyes. These are usually recognized by coming in a two-bottle preparation. Inform your hairdresser that you are allergic to PPD. Semi-permanent hair dyes may be a suitable alternative but approximately 10% of individuals who are allergic to PPD also react to these; patch testing to confirm sensitivity should be performed prior to their use. Metallic hair dyes and vegetable rinse hair dyes may be used but these do not provide permanent coloring. Some newer permanent and semipermanent hair dyes use para-toluenediamine sulfate (PTDS) instead of PPD. This is likely to be tolerated by about 50% of people who are allergic to PPD. Patch testing is recommended prior to use.

In cases of occupational exposure, avoid contact with PPD by wearing suitable protective garments such as gloves and protective sleeves.

Alert your doctor or dentist to the fact that you have an allergy to PPD, this is particularly important if you a receiving treatment which may require the use of a local anesthetic.

Allergy to PPD may make you sensitive to other related compounds. As a precaution you should avoid using products containing any of these substances.

Related Substances To PPD Which May Also Cause An Allergic Reaction

- **Azo Dyes:** Used in semi-permanent and temporary hair dyes, ballpoint pen inks, gasoline and diesel oil, and as coloring agent in foods and medications.

- **Benzocaine And Procaine:** These are local anaesthetics used by doctors and dentists.

- **Sulfonamides, Sulfones, Sulfa Drugs:** PPD allergy may make you sensitive to the use of these drugs also, discuss with your doctor before changing or stopping your medication.

- **Para-Aminobenzoic Acid (PABA):** This is used in sunscreens and creams that are readily available in over-the-counter preparations. You should only used sunscreens that are labeled 'PABA-free'. Ask your pharmacist for suitable alternatives.

- **Para-Aminosalicylic Acid:** Used for tuberculosis.

Your dermatologist may have further specific advice, particularly if you are highly sensitive to PPD.

Chapter 41

Fragrance Allergy

There are more than 5000 different fragrances that are in use today. In any one product the number of fragrances used can be many. Fortunately only a small number of fragrances are actually common sensitizers and cause allergy in sensitive individuals.

What Is Fragrance Mix And Where Is It Found?

Fragrance mix is a mixture of eight individual fragrances that is used to screen for fragrance allergy. The eight listed are the most common allergy-causing fragrances that are used across many products for their fragrant and flavoring properties.

Components of Fragrance Mix

Cinnamic Alcohol

- Odor of hyacinth
- Ester in natural fragrances such as Balsam of Peru, storax, cinnamon leaves, hyacinth oil, and propolis
- Used/found in:
  - Fragrance in perfumes, cosmetics, deodorants, paper, laundry detergent products, toilet soap, personal hygiene products
  - Flavoring in beverages (cola, bitters, Vermouth), chewing gums, toothpaste, and mouthwash

Cinnamic Aldehyde

- Warm spicy odor with a taste of cinnamon
- Constituent of cinnamon oil

Eugenol

- Powerful spicy odor of clove with a pungent taste
- Found in oils of clove and cinnamon leaf
- Also found in roses, carnations, hyacinths, and violets
- Used/found in:
  - Fragrance in perfume, cosmetics, colognes, toilet waters, hair cosmetics, aftershave, personal hygiene products
  - Flavoring in toothpaste, mouthwash, and food flavorings
  - Used in dental cement and packing agents thus giving the characteristic odor of dental surgeries
  - Inherent insecticidal and fungicidal properties—used to preserve meats and other foods
  - Pharmaceutical creams and lotions for its antiseptic properties

Isoeugenol

- Odor of clove weaker than that of eugenol
- Constituent of nutmeg oil and ylang ylang oil
- Isomerization of eugenol

Geraniol

- Sweet floral odor of rose
- Constitutes a large portion of rose and palmarosa oil, geranium oil, lavender oil, jasmine oil and citronella oil
- Present in over 250 essential oils
- Used/found in:
  - Most widely used fragrance in perfumes, colognes, facial make-up, and skin care products

Alpha Amyl Cinnamic Alcohol

- Intense odor of jasmine
- Synthetic essential oil
- Used/found in:
  - Found in perfumes, soaps, cosmetics, and toothpaste

Hydroxycitronellal

- Sweet fresh odor of lily of the valley
- Synthetic floral fragrance
- Used/found in:
  - Found in perfumes, soaps, cosmetics, eye cream, aftershaves
  - Also used in insecticides and antiseptics

Oak Moss Absolute

- Earthy, woody, masculine odor
- Essential oil produced by solvent extraction of tree lichen
- Used/found in:
  - Commonly used in colognes, aftershaves, and scented products for men

Fragrances may also be found in the workplace. Paints, cutting fluids, and metal working fluids may contain fragrances to mask offending odors. Fragrances may also be circulated through air conditioning.

What Are The Reactions To Fragrance Mix Allergy?

Typical allergic contact dermatitis reactions may occur in individuals allergic to fragrance mix or any other chemically related substances. The rash is characteristically located on the face, hands, and arms. There may be intense swelling and redness of the affected area within a few hours or the rash may appear after a day or two of the product being used. Sometimes symptoms may only be redness, dryness, and itching.

Oral exposure may cause sore mouth (tongue) and rash of the lips or angles of the mouth. Flare-ups of dermatitis in fragrance-sensitive individuals may occur if they use or consume products containing fragrance allergens.

Am I Allergic To Fragrances?

Sensitivity to a perfume, cream, or lotion is usually the first indicator of an allergy to fragrance. Patch testing using fragrance mix and Balsam of Peru detects approximately 75% of fragrance allergy cases. A positive patch to fragrance mix indicates that you are allergic to one or more fragrance chemicals. An estimated 1–2% of the general population is allergic to fragrance.

Self-testing a product for fragrance allergy is possible but should be done only after first talking with your doctor. This should be done only with products that are designed to stay on the skin such as cosmetics and lotions. Apply a small amount (50 cent sized area) of the product to a small tender area of skin such as the bend of your arm or neck for several days in a row. Examine the area each day and if no reaction occurs, it is unlikely you are allergic to it. However, it may still not be suitable for you as it can still cause an irritant reaction. Products such as shampoos, conditioners, soaps, and cleansers should not be tested in this way as they frequently cause an irritant dermatitis, which is not allergic, if they are covered or overused on tender areas.

Treatment Of Dermatitis Caused By Fragrance Allergy

Once the dermatitis appears on the skin, treatment is as for any acute dermatitis/eczema, that is, topical corticosteroids, emollients, treatment of any secondary bacterial infection (*Staphylococcus aureus*), etc.

What Should I Do To Avoid Fragrance Allergy?

If you have a fragrance allergy the best way to avoid any problems is by avoiding all products that contain fragrances of any sort. Unfortunately, fragrance allergy is usually life-long and gets worse with continued exposure.

There are more than 5000 different fragrances that are in use today. In any one product the number of fragrances used can be many. Fortunately only a small number of fragrances are actually common sensitizers and cause allergy in sensitive individuals.

Often products are only labeled as containing fragrance and do not identify the individual chemicals used to make up the fragrance. You should avoid all products that are labeled with any of the following names. These include other names for fragrances, individual fragrance allergens and other related substances that you may also be allergic to.

Other Names For Fragrances

- Perfumes
- Toilet water
- Colognes
- Masking perfumes
- Unscented perfumes
- Aroma chemicals
- Essential oils

Individual Fragrance Allergens

- Amyl cinnamic alcohol
- Anisyl alcohol
- Benzyl alcohol
- Benzyl salicylate
- Cinnamic alcohol
- Cinnamic aldehyde
- Coumarin
- Eugenol
- Geraniol
- Hydroxycitronellal
- Isoeugenol
- Musk ambrette
- Oak moss absolute
- Sandalwood oil
- Wood tars

Other Potential Allergens

- Balsam of Peru
- Cassia oil
- Cinnamon
- Cloves
- Citronella candles
- Ethylene brassylate

Be wary of products that are labelled "fragrance free" or "unscented" as these terms may not necessarily mean they do not contain fragrance chemicals, they just imply the product has no perceptible odor. These products may possibly contain a masking fragrance that is used to cover up the odor of other ingredients.

Note that clothes washed in scented laundry detergent can be a problem with prolonged skin contact of the garment in the presence of moisture and heat. It would be best to use fragrance-free laundry detergent.

Alert your doctor or dentist to the fact that you have an allergy to fragrance mix. If you are highly sensitive, your doctor may also recommend a special diet that eliminates foods to which these allergens or related allergens are added as flavoring.

Your dermatologist may have further specific advice, particularly if you are highly sensitive to fragrance mix.

Reference

Book: *Fisher's Contact Dermatitis*. Ed Rietschel RL, Fowler JF. Lippincott Williams & Wilkins, 2001.

Further Information

- Compound; Cinnamic alcohol; Formula: $C_9H_{10}O$; Chemical Abstracts Service (CAS) number: 104-54-1
- Compound: Cinnamic aldehyde; Formula: C_9H_8O; CAS number: 104-55-2
- Compound: Alpha amyl cinnamic aldehyde: Formula $C_{14}H_{18}O$; CAS number: 122-40-7
- Compound: Eugenol; Formula: $C_{10}H_{12}O_2$; CAS number: 97-53-0
- Compound: Isoeugenol; Formula: $C_{10}H_{22}N_2$; CAS number: 97-54-1
- Compound: Hydroxycitronellal; Formula: $C_{10}H_{18}O_2$; CAS number: 107-75-5
- Compound: Geraniol; Formula: $C_{10}H_{18}O$; CAS number: 106-24-1
- Compound: Oak moss absolute

Cross Reactions

- Balsam of Peru
- Cassia oil
- Cinnamon
- Cloves
- Citronella candles
- Ethylene brassylate
- Tiger balm

Sensitizer

- Cinnamic alcohol, cinnamic aldehyde, alpha amyl cinnamic aldehyde, eugenol, isoeugenol, hydroxycitronellal, geraniol, oak moss absolute

Patch Test

- Fragrance mix 8%

Chapter 42

Lanolin Allergy

What Are Wool Alcohols?

Wool alcohols are the principle component of lanolin in which allergens are found. Lanolin is a natural product obtained from the fleece of sheep. Sebum is extracted from the wool, cleaned, and refined to produce anhydrous lanolin. This comprises three parts, wool alcohols, fatty alcohols, and fatty acids. Currently the wool alcohols are considered the main sensitizers in lanolin but whether they are the sole sensitizers, needs further investigation. Nowadays there is also chemically modified lanolin that may be less sensitizing than natural lanolin.

Wool alcohols, wool fat, anhydrous lanolin, lanolin alcohol, wool wax, and wool grease are just some of the terms used interchangeably with lanolin. In this article we will use wool alcohols, as it is this fraction of lanolin that is the main cause of contact allergies.

What Products Contain Wool Alcohols?

Lanolin is a good emulsifier; this means it binds well with water thus it is particularly useful in the manufacture of pharmaceutical and cosmetic formulations. Wool alcohols are found in many pharmaceutical preparations, cosmetics, and toiletries. They also have some industrial uses.

About This Chapter: "Allergy to Wool Alcohols," reprinted with permission from DermNet NZ, the web site of the New Zealand Dermatological Society. Visit www.dermnetnz.org for patient information about skin diseases, conditions, and treatment. © June 15, 2009 New Zealand Dermatological Society. All rights reserved.

Pharmaceuticals

- Steroid-containing creams/ointments
- Hemorrhoidal preparations
- Medicated shampoos
- Veterinary products
- Liniments

Cosmetics And Toiletries

- Hand creams
- Moisturizers
- Protective creams
- Self-tanners
- Sunscreens
- Glossy lipsticks
- Makeup removers
- Foundations, powders
- Eye makeup
- Hairspray
- Shaving creams
- Baby oils, diaper lotions

Industrial

- Printing ink
- Furniture and shoe polishers
- Textile finishers
- Lubricants, cutting fluids
- Paper
- Leather

What Are The Reactions Of Allergy To Wool Alcohols?

Typical allergic contact dermatitis reactions may occur in individuals allergic to wool alcohols. The rash is characteristically located on the face, hands, and arms. There may be intense swelling and redness of the affected area within a few hours or the rash may appear after a day or two of the product being used.

Am I Allergic To Wool Alcohols?

Patch testing using 30% wool alcohol in petrolatum is what is routinely used to test for sensitivity to wool alcohols. Although wool alcohols are the main sensitizers in lanolin they may not always be the cause of the sensitivity and patch testing with natural lanolin from several sources is also recommended.

The development of chemically modified lanolin may help to reduce the incidence of skin reactions to natural lanolin. However, there have been cases where patients have shown marked sensitivity to modified lanolin, yet not to natural lanolin. Dermatitis caused by modified lanolin may be missed if patch testing is confined to testing with wool alcohols and natural lanolin only.

Since lanolin is a natural product, its constituents vary depending on its source. Therefore an individual may be allergic to some lanolin-containing products but not to others. Self-testing a product for allergy to lanolin-containing products is possible but should be done only after first talking with your doctor. This should be done only with products that are designed to stay on the skin such as cosmetics and lotions. Apply a small amount (50 cent sized area) of the product to a small tender area of skin such as the bend of your arm or neck daily for five to seven days. Examine the area each day and if no reaction occurs, it is unlikely you are allergic to it, although it may still act as an irritant. Products such as soaps, polishers, and waxes should not be tested in this way.

Alternative Names For Wool Alcohol

Wool alcohol is also known by several other names. These include:

- Adeps lanae anhydrous
- Aloholes lanae
- Amerchol
- Anhydrous lanolin
- Lanolin
- Wool fat
- Wool grease
- Wool wax

Avoid all of these. At work, request a material safety data sheet to help identify potential sources of exposure.

Further Information

- **Cross Reactions:** Cetyl or stearyl alcohols (Eucerin, Aquaphor)
- **Sensitizer:** Wool alcohol is the main sensitizer in lanolin
- **Patch Test:** Wool alcohol 30% in petrolatum

Management Of Dermatitis Caused By Wool Alcohol Allergy

Once the dermatitis appears on the skin, the first thing to do is to remove the source. In most instances this would entail stopping the use of all products that contain lanolin.

Standard treatment with emollients and topical steroids must not contain lanolin.

What Should I Do To Avoid Wool Alcohol Allergy?

If you have wool alcohol allergy the best way to avoid any problems is by avoiding all products that contain wool alcohols. Check all product labels for the list of ingredients and do not use if they contain wool alcohols or any of the other names for wool alcohols. If you are unsure, ask your pharmacist for advice and a suitable alternative.

Alert your doctor to the fact that you have an allergy to wool alcohols. This is particularly important as some topical medications that your doctor may want to prescribe to you contain wool alcohols.

Your dermatologist may have further specific advice, particularly if you are highly sensitive to wool alcohols.

Chapter 43

Formaldehyde Allergy

What Is Formaldehyde And Where Is It Found?

Formaldehyde is a chemical that is used widely across many products in our environment. It would be difficult to list all the possible sources of formaldehyde; the list below shows some of the more common sources of formaldehyde exposure.

Sources Of Formaldehyde

- Fabrics treated with formaldehyde resins and in which some free formaldehyde remains. Formaldehyde resins provide the unique qualities of the following fabrics:

  - Permanent press

  - Anti-cling, anti-static, anti-wrinkle, and anti-shrink finishes

  - Chlorine-resistant finishes

  - Stiffening on lightweight nylon knits

  - Waterproof finishes

  - Perspiration proof finishes

  - Moth proof and mildew resistant finishes

  - Suede and chamois

- Cosmetics and toiletries including fingernail polishers and hardeners, antiperspirants, makeup, bubble bath, bath oils, shampoos, creams, mouthwashes, and deodorants. In many cases formaldehyde is used as a preservative.

- Household cleansers, disinfectants, and polishes

- Paper products—formaldehyde is used to improve the water resistance, grease resistance, shrink resistance, and other characteristics of paper

- Building materials—urea-formaldehyde glue or adhesive is used in pressed wood products such as particle board, plywood, and medium-density fiberboard (MDF)

- Medications including wart remedies, anhidrotics, medicated creams, orthopaedic casts, and root canal preparation disinfectant

- Paints, primers, and paint-stripping agents

- Embalming fluid and as a preservative for laboratory specimens

- Formaldehyde is released in the smoke from burning wood, coal, charcoal, cigarettes, natural gas, and kerosene.

What Are The Reactions To Formaldehyde Allergy?

Reactions to formaldehyde depend on the type of exposure that has occurred. Formaldehyde is not only a sensitizer but also a potent primary irritant. Exposure to formaldehyde gas may cause burning sensations in the eye, nose and throat, skin rashes, tightness of the chest and wheezing, fatigue, and headaches. These symptoms may be a result of a primary irritant effect or an allergic sensitization to formaldehyde.

Frequent or prolonged exposure may cause hypersensitivity, leading to the development of allergic contact dermatitis. This may occur through skin contact with formaldehyde containing products or with clothing made from fabrics containing formaldehyde. Dermatitis caused by clothing tends to affect parts of the body where there is greatest friction between the skin and fabric, for example "trouser dermatitis" is usually apparent on the inner thighs, gluteal folds, and backs of the knees. Sweating may also be a factor in causing the allergic dermatitis as sweat or sebum appears to leach free formaldehyde from formaldehyde resins. Individuals sensitive to formaldehyde are not necessarily hypersensitive to formaldehyde resins. Clothing dermatitis appears to affect women more than men.

In individuals who are highly sensitive, contact with minute amounts of formaldehyde or being in a room where a bottle of formaldehyde may have been open previously thus leaving residual gas, can cause dermatitis.

Am I Allergic To Formaldehyde?

Formaldehyde allergy is diagnosed from the clinical history and by performing special allergy tests (patch tests).

Patch testing of formalin (40% solution of formaldehyde gas) is performed using a 2% aqueous solution of formalin. Some investigators have stated that 75% of positive patch tests have no clinical significance and only 20% of these can be related with actual instances of formaldehyde dermatitis.

The diagnosis of clothing dermatitis due to free formaldehyde can only be confirmed if the following standard criteria are fulfilled. In some cases, clothing dermatitis may not be a problem, even if the suspected fabric tests positive for free formaldehyde and an individual has a positive patch test reaction to 2% formalin.

Patch testing of products for formaldehyde resins is performed using 10% urea formaldehyde in petrolatum, 10% melamine formaldehyde in petrolatum, and 1% other formaldehyde resins in petrolatum or isopropyl alcohol.

Self-testing a product for formaldehyde is possible but should be done only after first talking with your doctor. This should be done only with products that are designed to stay on the skin such as cosmetics and lotions. Apply a small amount of the product to a small tender area of skin such as the bend of your arm or neck. Examine the area each day for several days and if no reaction occurs, the product is most probably suitable for you to use.

Treatment Of Contact Dermatitis Due To Formaldehyde Exposure

If you are diagnosed with formaldehyde allergy then if at all possible avoid exposure to formaldehyde containing products, otherwise take means to reduce potential exposure.

Formaldehyde Clothing Dermatitis: Criteria To Fulfill

- Suspected fabric shows the presence of free formaldehyde.
- Patient shows a positive patch test reaction to 2% formalin.
- Formaldehyde resin impregnated fabric show a positive patch test reaction—the piece of fabric tested should have been worn and subjected to sweat, sebum, and friction.
- Wearing the fabric causes a clinical allergic contact dermatitis.

Once the dermatitis appears on the skin, treatment is as for any acute dermatitis/eczema, that is topical corticosteroids, emollients, treatment of any secondary bacterial infection (*Staphylococcus aureus*), etcetera.

What Should I Do To Avoid Formaldehyde Allergy?

It is difficult to avoid all exposure to formaldehyde because it is normally present at low levels (usually <0.03 ppm) in both indoor and outdoor air. For most people low-level exposure (up to 0.1 ppm) does not cause any problems. Methods to avoid or minimize exposure are described below.

Methods To Avoid Or Minimize Exposure To High Levels Of Formaldehyde

- Wear clothing made of 100% cotton, polyester, nylon or acrylic; these fabrics generally contain less formaldehyde and are usually well tolerated by sensitive individuals.

  - Avoid all clothing made with fabrics that have been treated with formaldehyde.

- In general, machine wash all new clothing and bedding in hot, soapy water several times before use.

- Purchase furniture made of pressed wood products only if the surfaces and edges are laminated or coated.

- Occupational exposure can be reduced by identifying potential sources of exposure (material safety data sheets should be available to employees) and taking precautions to minimize exposure by wearing suitable protective garments.

- To reduce the formaldehyde content in the air, increase ventilation by opening doors and windows and/or installing exhaust fans in closed areas.

- Read product labels and avoid not only formaldehyde itself but also formaldehyde-releasing preservatives. Some of these are known by the following names:
  - Quaternium-15
  - 2-bromo-2nitropropane-1,3-diol
  - imidazolidinyl urea
  - diazolidinyl urea

Alternative Names For Formaldehyde

Formaldehyde is also known by several other names. These include:

- Formalin
- Methanal
- Methyl aldehyde
- Methylene oxide
- Morbicid acid
- Oxymethylene

Avoid all of these. At work, request a material safety data sheet to help identify potential sources of exposure.

Further Information

- Formula: CH_2O
- CAS Number: 50-00-0
- Cross Reactions: Possibly glutaraldehyde
- Appearance: Clear, colorless liquid
- Sensitizer: Free formaldehyde, formaldehyde resins
- Patch Test: 2% aqueous solution of formalin (40% solution of formaldehyde gas); 10% urea formaldehyde in petrolatum; 10% melamine formaldehyde in petrolatum; 1% other formaldehyde resins in petrolatum or isopropyl alcohol.

Sources Of Exposure To Formaldehyde

- Anhidrotics and antiperspirants
- Building materials—pressed wood products such as particleboard, plywood, and MDF
- Canned ice
- Cellulose esters
- Clothing made from fabrics finished with formaldehyde resins
- Coatings—melamine, urea, sulfonamide, phenol resins
- Cosmetics and toiletries
- Disinfectants and cleaning agents
- Embalming fluid and fixatives
- Fabric and textiles
- Glues, pastes
- Medications
- Mildew preventative in fruits and vegetables
- Paints and primers
- Paper products
- Phenolic resins and urea plastics found in buttons, footwear, and jewelry
- Photographic plates
- Polishes
- Preservatives
- Printing/etching materials
- Rubber cements

- Smoke

- Tanning agents

- Toxoids and vaccines

References

Book: *Fisher's Contact Dermatitis.* Ed Rietschel RL, Fowler JF. Lippincott Williams & Wilkins, 2001

Reich HC, Warshaw EM. Allergic contact dermatitis from formaldehyde textile resins. *Dermatitis.* 2010 Apr;21(2):65-76.

Part Five
Managing Allergies In Daily Life

Chapter 44

Learning To Avoid Allergy Triggers

Allergens are organic substances that trigger over reactions of the immune system in people who have a hereditary tendency toward allergies (including allergic asthma). The most common allergens are the proteins in plant pollens, mold spores, dust mite droppings, animal dander, cockroaches, and latex. Foods generally do not trigger asthma alone, although respiratory symptoms may be part of a food allergy reaction that can also include hives, swelling, eczema, diarrhea, vomiting, and loss of consciousness.

How Can You Control Allergens?

Identify your allergens. Each individual can be allergic to a different allergen or group of allergens. Allergy tests can identify the ones that are a problem for you, along with a physical examination and careful medical history discussed with your doctor.

Learn how to control triggers both at home and away from home using the information below.

Dust Mites

Dust mites are microscopic bugs related to ticks and spiders. They eat dead skin that people shed every day and prefer warm humid environments. Dust mites live mostly in mattresses, pillows, carpets, bedding, stuffed toys, and fabric-covered furniture. Dust mite droppings are the most allergenic part.

About This Chapter: "Controlling Asthma Triggers," reviewed July 2012 by Frank J. Twarog, M.D., Ph.D. Reprinted with permission from the Asthma and Allergy Foundation of American, New England Chapter. All rights reserved. For additional information, visit www.asthmaandallergies.org.

How Can You Avoid Dust Mites?

- Wash sheets, blankets and comforters once a week in hot water and dry in a clothes dryer. This applies to bedding at day care as well as at home.

- Use allergy-proof mattress and pillow encasings (or pillows that can be washed and tumble-dried weekly).

- Keep the humidity low, between 30% and 50%.

- Avoid stuffed animals except for ones that can be thoroughly washed in hot water and tumble-dried.

- Avoid dust collectors. Store books and toys in enclosed book cases or toy chests. Do not use drapes and fabric hangings, other than light curtains that can be washed regularly in hot water.

- If rugs or carpets must be used, vacuum frequently (every day or two) with a vacuum that has a HEPA (high-efficiency particulate air) filter or uses double-layer dust bags.

Pets/Animal Dander

Through allergy tests and discussions with your doctor, determine the pets to which you are allergic. Some people, for instance, may be allergic to cats, but not to dogs, birds, mice, rats, or guinea pigs. Others may be allergic to all or several of them. All pets can cause allergies, no matter what size, what breed, or how long their hair is, or whether they shed. The asthma trigger (the sticky dander) is found in the animal's skin flakes, saliva, and urine (which dries, floats through the air, and attaches to everything from floors to ceilings, clothing, and furniture). Dander can stay around for months after a pet has gone.

How Can You Avoid Animal Dander?

- The best method of avoidance is to find a new home for any pet causing allergies in your family or child care setting.

- The next best method of control is to keep the pet outdoors and wash it frequently.

- Avoid feather-stuffed furnishings, pillows, and toys.

- Animal dander left by a previous pet is very difficult to remove without thorough cleaning.

Mold And Mildew

Indoor mold and mildew spores grow in damp and humid places such as bathrooms, kitchens, and basements. They can also be found in old books. The best way to control mold is to control moisture and humidity.

How Can You Avoid Mold?

- Any damp surface where molds can grow—refrigerator drip pans, shower stalls and curtains, damp areas under sinks, and around toilets—should be cleaned weekly with a weak bleach solution.

- Use exhaust fans or open windows in kitchens, bathrooms, and basements when showering, cooking, cleaning, or using the dishwasher.

- Fix leaky plumbing or other sources of moisture.

- Check periodically for leaks and areas of standing water.

- Absorbent moldy materials, such as ceiling tiles or carpets, may need to be replaced.

- Never lay carpeting on concrete floors or in damp areas like basements or bathrooms. It is almost impossible to keep these carpets dry.

- Maintain low indoor humidity, ideally between 30% and 50%, as measured by a humidity gauge (hygrometer) that can be purchased at a hardware store. If you use a dehumidifier (to take moisture out of the air), be sure to empty and clean the machine regularly.

- Do not use a humidifier (which puts moisture into the air).

- Keep air conditioner filters clean and dry.

- Vent clothes dryers to the outside.

Pests (Cockroaches, Mice, Or Rats)

- Do not leave food or garbage out. Quickly clean up all food crumbs or spilled liquids.

- Store food in airtight containers.

- Throw away piles of paper where pests hide.

- Plug up cracks and holes in walls, floors and ceilings, where rats and roaches can get in.

- Try using poison baits, boric acid (for cockroaches), or traps before using pesticidal sprays.

- If these steps are not enough, limit any spraying to infested areas, carefully follow instructions on the label, make sure there is plenty of fresh air when you spray, and keep the person with asthma out of the room.

Latex

- In some people latex can trigger an asthmatic reaction. They need to avoid exposure to latex (such as latex gloves and balloons).

Outdoor Plant Pollens And Mold Spores

Outdoor allergens can follow you home and become indoor allergens.

- Identify, through testing, which pollens affect you. Learn when they are in season (for example, in New England, tree and grass pollens come in the spring; ragweed grows from mid-August to the first frost; molds grow on wet piles of leaves and compost).

- During your pollen season, or moldy times, keep windows closed and use a clean air conditioner instead for air circulation.

- Wash hair and shower nightly to remove pollens brought in from the outside. Wash pollens off clothes. Don't hang laundry outside to dry.

- Check pollen counts to see if it may be a bad time for you.

Irritants: Smoke And Fumes

Irritants aggravate the inflammation in the airways that is characteristic of asthma. Below is a list of common irritants, and ways to avoid or control them:

- Smoke from cigarettes, wood fires, and charcoal grills:

  - These irritants should be avoided. Tobacco smoke is the most preventable trigger of asthma. Smoking is dangerous to everyone—the person smoking and those who breathe in secondhand smoke. Don't smoke and don't allow smoking in your home, car, or child care setting. Children of mothers who smoke are twice as likely to develop asthma.

- Fumes and odors from household cleaners, paint, perfumes, cosmetics, and gasoline:

  - Whenever possible, choose products without fumes, labeled "fragrance-free."

  - Instead of spraying products into the air, use them to wet a cloth for cleaning. Use a plain cloth dampened with water alone, whenever possible.

  - Avoid newly painted areas and construction areas until they are dry and free of odors and dust.

  - Use a face mask to avoid breathing in fumes that can't be avoided.

- Fumes and air pollution from outside:
  - Avoid having cars, trucks, or buses idle where fumes can be drawn in through air intake vents or open windows.
  - Stay indoors as much as possible on high ozone days.
  - Support efforts to retrofit or eliminate diesel buses.

Infections

Respiratory infections and colds can trigger asthma. Try to control the spread of infections through frequent hand-washing and wiping frequently touched surfaces (such as faucets) with a mild bleach solution rather than disinfectant sprays. People with respiratory conditions are generally advised to get flu shots, unless they are allergic to eggs. Ask your doctor how to adjust your medications to deal with infections.

General Maintenance Issues

- Use a vacuum cleaner with a high efficiency (HEPA) filter or double-layer dust bags. (Other vacuums blow tiny dust particles back into the air.)
- Dust often, with a damp cloth, to avoid stirring up the dust.
- If you have a forced air system, use a HEPA or electrostatic filter for your furnace. Clean or replace furnace filters often. You can also cover duct vents with filters.
- Air cleaning machines can remove smoke and odors, but not heavier particles that do not stay airborne. It is important to try to avoid the things that produce airborne triggers.

Other Triggers

- Cold air, humidity, and sudden weather changes:
  - Plan outdoor activities to avoid your triggers when possible.
  - Use a mask or scarf over your nose and mouth to avoid cold air.
- Exercise and activities that make you breathe harder or take in cold air quickly, if your asthma is not under control (such as laughing, yelling, and crying):
  - Learn warm-up activities that warm the air you breathe in.
  - Exercise is important for general health and fitness.
  - Pre-medication before exercise helps people with exercise-induced asthma.

Chapter 45

Your Rights Regarding Allergy Medication At School

Take Two: Always Carry Two Epinephrine Auto-Injectors At School

Kelsey never leaves home without it—her auto-injectable epinephrine, that is. In fact she always has two. You see, Kelsey is allergic to peanuts and while she does everything she can to avoid being exposed to them, she knows that accidents happen, especially now that she's an active teenager. And she knows that if an accidental exposure does occur, she could develop the life-threatening allergic reaction called anaphylaxis.

Some common allergies that are prone to anaphylaxis include peanut, tree nut, shellfish, and insect sting. Not everyone who is allergic to one or more of these will develop anaphylaxis— but it's happened to Kelsey before, so she's always watchful.

Every person—and every episode—is different, however. It's important to understand that an anaphylactic reaction can progress quickly and turn deadly with little warning. That's why doctors recommend that at-risk patients carry auto-injectable epinephrine with them at all times and use it at the first sign of symptoms.

Symptoms include the following:

- Hives (red, itchy bumps on your skin)

- Lip, tongue, and throat swelling

About This Chapter: This chapter includes text from "Take Two: Always Carry Two Epinephrine Auto-Injectors at School" and "Medications at School," both © 2012 Allergy and Asthma Network Mothers of Asthmatics (AANMA). Reprinted with permission. Information about state laws was current at the time of publication, but readers should check the AANMA website (www.aanma.org) for the most up to date facts.

- Nausea, vomiting, diarrhea, cramping

- Shortness of breath, wheezing, coughing

- Drop in blood pressure

- Loss of consciousness

Thanks to the Allergy and Asthma Network Mothers of Asthmatics (AANMA)'s Breathe: It's the Law campaign (sponsored by Dey Pharma, LP, now Mylan Specialty) and tireless efforts from volunteers across the country, laws have been passed in 49 states guaranteeing students like Kelsey the right to keep their auto-injectable epinephrine close at hand at school and school-sponsored events. It's lifesaving legislation. To get involved, contact AANMA through their website (www.aanma.org).

What Is "Breathe: It's The Law"?

Breathe: It's the Law is a campaign to make sure students in every state can carry and self-administer their life-saving asthma and anaphylaxis medications. AANMA and supporters pushed for years to make sure all 50 states had laws protecting students' rights to carry and

Epinephrine Tips

- Epinephrine is very efficient at stopping anaphylaxis when it is used right away; most anaphylaxis-related fatalities occur when treatment is delayed.

- As many as 25 percent of people who have an anaphylactic reaction will have a second wave of symptoms, so keep two doses of epinephrine with you at all times and get to a hospital as quickly as possible after using your first dose.

- Store your auto-injectors as close to room temperature as possible, since extremely hot or cold temperatures may make the epinephrine ineffective or cause the injector to malfunction. If you're outside on a cold day, keep it close to your body to keep it warm.

- Auto-injectable epinephrine is one of those medicines you hope you never have to use. But as such, it's easy to forget about it and let it get out of date. Check yours today and renew it if necessary.

- At the pharmacy, make sure the device you're given is the one your physician prescribed and that you know how to use it.

Source: From "Take Two: Always Carry Two Epinephrine Auto-Injectors at School," © 2012 Allergy and Asthma Network Mothers of Asthmatics (AANMA).

Medications At School

In 2002, Allergy and Asthma Network Mothers of Asthmatics (AANMA) held an Asthma Awareness Day Capitol Hill field hearing about the plight of school children whose asthma medications were locked in the clinic instead of by their side at all times as prescribed by their physicians. Tragically, each school year there were reports of students who did not receive medication in time. They died. The same was true of students with anaphylaxis and their access to prescribed auto-injectable epinephrine.

As a result of those hearings, members of Congress joined with AANMA and advocates across the country to pass the Asthmatic Schoolchildren's Treatment and Health Management Act of 2004 (first introduced in the House of Representatives in 2003 as HR2023). Signed into law in October 2004, this groundbreaking legislation gave funding preference to states that protect student's rights to carry and self-administer asthma and anaphylaxis medications at school.

Today, all 50 states have laws protecting students' rights to carry and use prescribed asthma medications; 49 have similar laws regarding anaphylaxis medications.

Source: From "Medications at School," © 2012 Allergy and Asthma Network Mothers of Asthmatics (AANMA).

---

use asthma and anaphylaxis medications at school. It wasn't easy, but the last state passed its asthma-medication law in 2010. Now that Rhode Island passed legislation in May 2012, New York is the last state that still needs an anaphylaxis law.

Why is it important?

Every school year students die because they were unable to get to their asthma or anaphylaxis medications on time. The medications were locked in a nurse's cabinet or stowed away in a place too far to get to when the student needed them. Minutes count when asthma or anaphylaxis strikes. Students need to carry these medications on them, know when and how to use them—and then do it.

How can I help get these laws passed in the remaining state?

Contact AANMA's Director of Patient Advocacy, through the AANMA website (www .aanma.org) or 800-878-4403. They will help you contact your local legislators and send you a sample letter you can send to them urging them to pass this legislation.

I live in a state that has passed these laws—how can I make sure my school knows about the laws and allows students to carry and use their medications?

Visit your school and hand them this chapter or ask them to read the facts at www.aanma.org/advocacy/meds-at-school. Bring copies for the principal and school nurse, and a few extra for other teachers. When they visit www.aanma.org/advocacy/meds-at-school and click on their state, they can read exactly what the law is.

The Breathe: It's the Law campaign was sponsored by Dey Pharma, LP, now Mylan Specialty.

Chapter 46

Using Cosmetics Safely

Eye Cosmetic Safety

Eye cosmetics are intended to make eyes more attractive, or in some cases to cleanse the eye area. One thing they shouldn't do is cause harm. Most are safe when used properly. However, there are some things to be careful about when using these products, such as the risk of infection, the risk of injury from the applicator, and the use of unapproved color additives. The following information provides an introduction to some safety concerns and legal issues related to eye cosmetics.

Keep It Clean

Eye cosmetics are usually safe when you buy them, but misusing them can allow dangerous bacteria or fungi to grow in them. Then, when applied to the eye area, a cosmetic can cause an infection. In rare cases, women have been temporarily or permanently blinded by an infection from an eye cosmetic. See the Safety Checklist below for tips on keeping your eye cosmetics clean and protecting against infections. Occasionally, contamination can be a problem for some eye cosmetics even when they are new.

Don't Share! Don't Swap!

Don't share or swap eye cosmetics—not even with your best friend. Another person's germs may be hazardous to you. The risk of contamination may be even greater with "testers" at retail

About This Chapter: This chapter includes excerpts from the following documents produced by the U.S. Food and Drug Administration (www.fda.gov): "Eye Cosmetic Safety," April 15, 2011; "Color Additives and Cosmetics," December 22, 2011; and "Bad Reaction to Cosmetics? Tell FDA," August 9, 2012.

stores, where a number of people are using the same sample product. If you feel you must sample cosmetics at a store, make sure they are applied with single-use applicators, such as clean cotton swabs.

Hold Still!

It may seem like efficient use of your time to apply makeup in the car or on the bus, but resist that temptation, even if you're not in the driver's seat. If you hit a bump, come to a sudden stop, or are hit by another vehicle, you risk injuring your eye (scratching your cornea, for example) with a mascara wand or other applicator. Even a slight scratch can result in a serious infection.

What's In It?

As with any cosmetic product sold on a retail basis to consumers, eye cosmetics are required to have an ingredient declaration on the label, according to regulations implemented under the Fair Packaging and Labeling Act, or FPLA—an important consumer protection law. If you wish to avoid certain ingredients or compare the ingredients in different brands, you can check the ingredient declaration.

If a cosmetic sold on a retail basis to consumers does not have an ingredient declaration, it is considered misbranded and is illegal in interstate commerce. Very small packages in tightly compartmented display racks may have copies of the ingredient declaration available on tear-off sheets accompanying the display. If neither the package nor the display rack provides the ingredient declaration, you aren't getting the information you're entitled to. Don't hesitate to ask the store manager or the manufacturer why not.

What's That Shade You're Wearing?

In the United States, the use of color additives is strictly regulated (see "Color Additives And Cosmetics" below). A number of color additives approved for cosmetic use in general are not approved for use in the area of the eye.

Keep Away From Kohl—And Keep Kohl Away From Kids

One color additive of particular concern is kohl. Also known as al-kahl, kajal, or surma, kohl is used in some parts of the world to enhance the appearance of the eyes, but is unapproved for cosmetic use in the United States. Kohl consists of salts of heavy metals, such as antimony and lead. It may be tempting to think that because kohl has been used traditionally as an eye cosmetic in some parts of the world, it must be safe. However, there have been reports linking the use of kohl to lead poisoning in children.

Some eye cosmetics may be labeled with the word "kohl" only to indicate the shade, not because they contain true kohl. If the product is properly labeled, you can check to see whether the color additives declared on the label are in U.S. Food and Drug Administration's (FDA's) list of color additives approved for use in cosmetics, then make sure they are listed as approved for use in the area of the eye.

Dying To Dye Your Eyelashes?

Permanent eyelash and eyebrow tints and dyes have been known to cause serious eye injuries, including blindness. There are no color additives approved by FDA for permanent dyeing or tinting of eyelashes and eyebrows.

Thinking Of False Eyelashes Or Extensions?

FDA considers false eyelashes, eyelash extensions, and their adhesives to be cosmetic products, and as such they must adhere to the safety and labeling requirements for cosmetics. False eyelashes and eyelash extensions require adhesives to hold them in place. Remember that the eyelids are delicate, and an allergic reaction, irritation, or other injury in the eye area can be particularly troublesome. Check the ingredients before using these adhesives.

Bad Reaction?

If you have a bad reaction to eye cosmetics, first contact your healthcare provider. FDA also encourages consumers to report any adverse reactions to cosmetics. (See "Bad Reaction to Cosmetics? Tell FDA" below.)

Safety Checklist

If you use eye cosmetics, FDA urges you to follow these safety tips:

- If any eye cosmetic causes irritation, stop using it immediately. If irritation persists, see a doctor.

- Avoid using eye cosmetics if you have an eye infection or the skin around the eye is inflamed. Wait until the area is healed. Discard any eye cosmetics you were using when you got the infection.

- Be aware that there are bacteria on your hands that, if placed in the eye, could cause infections. Wash your hands before applying eye cosmetics.

- Make sure that any instrument you place in the eye area is clean.

- Don't share your cosmetics. Another person's bacteria may be hazardous to you.

- Don't allow cosmetics to become covered with dust or contaminated with dirt or soil. Keep containers clean.

- Don't use old containers of eye cosmetics. Manufacturers usually recommend discarding mascara two to four months after purchase.

- Discard dried-up mascara. Don't add saliva or water to moisten it. The bacteria from your mouth may grow in the mascara and cause infection. Adding water may introduce bacteria and will dilute the preservative that is intended to protect against microbial growth.

- Don't store cosmetics at temperatures above 85 degrees F. Cosmetics held for long periods in hot cars, for example, are more susceptible to deterioration of the preservative.

- When applying or removing eye cosmetics, be careful not to scratch the eyeball or other sensitive area. Never apply or remove eye cosmetics in a moving vehicle.

- Don't use any cosmetics near your eyes unless they are intended specifically for that use. For instance, don't use a lip liner as an eye liner. You may be exposing your eyes to contamination from your mouth, or to color additives that are not approved for use in the area of the eye.

- Avoid color additives that are not approved for use in the area of the eye, such as "permanent" eyelash tints and kohl. Be especially careful to keep kohl away from children, since reports have linked it to lead poisoning.

Some More Eye Cosmetic Safety Tips

- The Food and Drug Administration (FDA) regulates all cosmetics marketed in the United States, including mascara, eye shadows, eye liner, concealers, and eyebrow pencils.
- Keep everything clean. Dangerous bacteria or fungi can grow in some cosmetic products, as well as their containers. Cleanliness can help prevent eye infections.
- Always wash your hands before applying eye cosmetics, and be sure that any instrument you place near your eyes is clean. Be especially careful not to contaminate cosmetics by introducing microorganisms. For example, don't lay an eyelash wand on a countertop where it can pick up bacteria. Keep containers clean, since these may also be a source of contamination.
- Don't use eye cosmetics that cause irritation. Stop using a product immediately if irritation occurs. See a doctor if irritation persists.

Source: Excerpted from "Use Eye Cosmetics Safely," U.S. Food and Drug Administration (www.fda.gov), August 9, 2012.

Color Additives And Cosmetics

Color additives are subject to a strict system of approval under U.S. law.

Some Basic Requirements

If a product (except coal-tar hair dyes) contains a color additive, by law it must adhere to these requirements:

- **Approval:** All color additives used in cosmetics (or any other FDA-regulated product) must be approved by FDA. There must be a regulation specifically addressing a substance's use as a color additive, specifications, and restrictions.

- **Certification:** In addition to approval, a number of color additives must be batch certified by FDA if they are to be used in cosmetics (or any other FDA-regulated product) marketed in the U.S.

- **Identity And Specifications:** All color additives must meet the requirements for identity and specifications stated in the Code of Federal Regulations (CFR).

- **Use And Restrictions:** Color additives may be used only for the intended uses stated in the regulations that pertain to them. The regulations also specify other restrictions for certain colors, such as the maximum permissible concentration in the finished product.

How Are Color Additives Categorized?

Approved color additives fall into two main categories: those subject to certification (sometimes called "certifiable") and those exempt from certification. In addition, the regulations refer to other classifications, such as straight colors and lakes.

Colors Subject To Certification: These color additives are derived primarily from petroleum and are sometimes known as "coal-tar dyes" or "synthetic-organic" colors. Except in the case of coal-tar hair dyes, these colors must not be used unless FDA has certified that the batch in question has passed analysis of its composition and purity in FDA's own labs.

These certified colors generally have three-part names. The names include a prefix "FD&C," "D&C," or "External D&C"; a color; and a number. An example is "FD&C Yellow No. 5." Certified colors also may be identified in cosmetic ingredient declarations by color and number alone, without a prefix (such as "Yellow 5").

Colors Exempt From Certification: These color additives are obtained primarily from mineral, plant, or animal sources. They are not subject to batch certification requirements.

However, they still are considered artificial colors, and when used in cosmetics or other FDA-regulated products, they must comply with the identity, specifications, uses, restrictions, and labeling requirements stated in the regulations.

Straight Color: "Straight color" refers to any color additive listed as such in FDA regulations (in 21 CFR 73, 74, and 81 [21 CFR 70.3(j)]). A lake is a straight color. Because lakes are not soluble in water, they often are used when it is important to keep a color from "bleeding," as in lipstick. In some cases, special restrictions apply to their use.

Regulations That Restrict Intended Use

Eye-Area Use: Manufacturers may not use a color additive in the area of the eye unless the regulation for that additive specifically permits such use. Although there are color additives approved for use in products such as mascara and eyebrow pencils, none is approved for dyeing the eyebrows or eyelashes.

Externally Applied Cosmetics: This term does not apply to the lips or any body surface covered by mucous membrane. For instance, if a color additive is approved for use in externally applied cosmetics, it may not be used it in products such as lipsticks unless the regulation specifically permits this use.

Injection: No color additive may be used in injections unless its listing in the regulations specifically provides for such use. This includes injection into the skin for tattooing or permanent makeup. The fact that a color additive is listed for any other use does not mean that it may be used for injections.

Special Effects And Novelty Use

No matter how exotic or novel the color additive or its intended use, it is subject to the same regulations as the more everyday colors and products. The following items are a sampling of some out-of-the-ordinary color additives. This list is not exhaustive. Rather, it is intended to show how the regulations apply to such colors:

Color-Changing Pigments: Colors that change in response to such factors as change in pH or exposure to oxygen or temperature are subject to the same regulations as all other color additives.

Composite Pigments: Color additives used in combination to achieve variable effects, such as those found in pearlescent products, are subject to the same regulations as all other color additives. Some color additives, when used in combination, may form new pigments, which may not be approved for the intended use. An example is a "holographic" glitter, consisting of aluminum, an approved color additive, bonded to an etched plastic film.

Halloween Makeup: These products are considered cosmetics and are therefore subject to the same regulations as other cosmetics, including the same restrictions on color additives.

Tattoo Pigments: No color additives are approved for injection into the skin, as in tattoos and permanent makeup.

Theatrical Makeup: Like Halloween makeup, these products are considered cosmetics and are therefore subject to the same regulations as other cosmetics, including the same restrictions on color additives.

Bad Reaction To Cosmetics?

You break out in a head-to-toe rash after applying a sunless tanning lotion. Your skin is red and blotchy after getting your face painted at the school carnival. Your scalp is burned after using a hair relaxer. If you've had a negative reaction to a beauty, personal hygiene, or makeup product, the Food and Drug Administration (FDA) wants to hear from you.

From morning until night—styling hair for school to showering before bed—Americans depend upon personal care products. Most are safe, but some cause problems, and that's when FDA gets involved.

"Even though these products are widely used, most don't require FDA approval before they're sold in stores, salons, and at makeup counters," says Linda Katz, M.D., director of the agency's Office of Cosmetics and Colors. "So, consumers are one of FDA's most important resources when it comes to identifying problems."

What are "hypoallergenic" cosmetics?

Hypoallergenic cosmetics are products that manufacturers claim produce fewer allergic reactions than other cosmetic products. Consumers with hypersensitive skin, and even those with "normal" skin, may be led to believe that these products will be gentler to their skin than non-hypoallergenic cosmetics.

There are no federal standards or definitions that govern the use of the term "hypoallergenic." The term means whatever a particular company wants it to mean. Manufacturers of cosmetics labeled as hypoallergenic are not required to submit substantiation of their hypoallergenicity claims to the U.S. Food and Drug Administration (FDA).

The term "hypoallergenic" may have considerable market value in promoting cosmetic products to consumers on a retail basis, but dermatologists say it has very little meaning.

Source: "Cosmetics Q&A: Hypoallergenic," U.S. Food and Drug Administration (www.fda.gov), May 2, 5012.

The federal Food, Drug, and Cosmetic Act defines "cosmetics" as products that are intended to be applied to the body "for cleansing, beautifying, promoting attractiveness, or altering the appearance." But the legal definition includes items that most Americans might not ordinarily think of as cosmetics, including these: Face and body cleansers; Deodorants; Moisturizers and other skin lotions and creams; Baby lotions and oils; Hair care products, dyes, conditioners, straighteners, perms; Makeup; Hair removal creams; Nail polishes; Shaving products; Perfumes and colognes; Face paints and temporary tattoos; and Permanent tattoos and permanent makeup.

What To Report

Katz says consumers should contact FDA if they experience a rash, hair loss, infection, or other problem—even if they didn't follow product directions. FDA also wants to know if a product has a bad smell or unusual color—which could signal contamination—or if the item's label is incomplete or inaccurate. If you have any concerns about a cosmetic, contact MedWatch, FDA's problem-reporting program, on the web (http://www.fda.gov/Safety/MedWatch) or by phone at 800-332-1088; or contact the consumer complaint coordinator in your area.

When you contact FDA, include the following information in your report: The name and contact information for the person who had the reaction; The age, gender, and ethnicity of the product's user; The name of the product and manufacturer; A description of the reaction—and treatment, if any; The healthcare provider's name and contact information, if medical attention was provided; When and where the product was purchased.

And be sure to give the age, gender, and ethnicity of the person who had the reaction, says FDA scientist Wendy Good, Ph.D. Good, who analyzes reports about problems with cosmetics. That information is important because it can help scientists spot trends.

When a consumer report is received, FDA enters the information into a database of negative reactions. Experts then look for reports related to the same product or similar ones. FDA scientists will use the information to determine if the product has a history of problems and represents a public health concern that needs to be addressed.

If you file a consumer report, your identity will remain confidential.

"Cosmetics are usually safe, but when they aren't, consumer reporting is essential so FDA can take action when appropriate," Katz says. Those actions could—depending upon the product and the problem—range from issuing a consumer safety advisory to taking legal action.

Chapter 47

Use Caution With Face Painting And Tattoos

Novelty Makeup

Painting your face can be a big part of the fun on Halloween and lots of other special occasions. Most of the time people do this without a problem, but not always. Here are some pointers to help keep your fun from leaving you with a rash, swollen eyelids, or other grief.

Painting Your Face: Special Effects Without After Effects

Decorating your face with face paint or other makeup lets you see better than you can if you're wearing a mask. A mask can make it hard to see where you're going and watch out for cars. But make sure your painted-on designs don't cause problems of their own.

- Follow all directions carefully.

- Don't decorate your face with things that aren't intended for your skin.

- If your face paint has a very bad smell, this could be a sign that it is contaminated. Throw it away and use another one.

- Like soap, some things are OK on your skin, but not in your eyes. Some face paint or other makeup may say on the label that it is not for use near the eyes. Believe this, even if the label has a picture of people wearing it near their eyes. Be careful to keep makeup from getting into your eyes.

- Even products intended for use near your eyes can sometimes irritate your skin if you use too much.

About This Chapter: This chapter includes excerpts from documents produced by the U.S. Food and Drug Administration (www.fda.gov): "Novelty Makeup," June 27, 2011; "Temporary Tattoos, Henna/Mehndi, and Black Henna," July 2, 2012; and "Tattoos and Permanent Make-up," October 5, 2009.

- If you're decorating your skin with something you've never used before, you might try a dab of it on your arm for a couple of days to check for an allergic reaction before you put it on your face. This is an especially smart thing to do if you tend to have allergies.

Color Additives: A Little Detective Work Won't Hurt

A big part of Halloween makeup is color. But this is your skin we're talking about. Think about what you're putting on it. You might not want to put the same coloring on your skin that a car company uses in its paint.

Luckily, you don't have to. The law says that color additives have to be approved by the U.S. Food and Drug Administration (FDA) for use in cosmetics, including color additives in face paints and other cosmetics that may be used around Halloween time. It also includes theatrical makeup.

Plus, FDA has to decide how they may be used, based on safety information. A color that's OK on your tough fingernails or your hair may not be OK on your skin. Colors that are OK for most of your skin may not be OK near your eyes.

How do you know which ones are OK to use, and where? Do some detective work and check two places:

1. The list of ingredients on the label. Look for the names of the colors. THEN...

2. Check the Summary of Color Additives on FDA's website (http://www.fda.gov/ForIndustry/ ColorAdditives/ColorAdditiveInventories/ucm115641.htm). There's a section especially on colors for cosmetics. If there's a color in your makeup that isn't on this list, the company that made it is not obeying the law. Don't use it. Even if it's on the list, check to see if it has FDA's OK for use near the eyes. If it doesn't, keep it away from your eyes.

For That Ghoulish Glow

There are two kinds of "glow" effects you might get from Halloween-type makeup. Ready for some ten-dollar words? There are "fluorescent" (say "floor-ESS-ent") and "luminescent" (say "loo-min-ESS-ent") colors. Here's the difference:

Fluorescent Colors: These are the make-you-blink colors sometimes called "neon" or "day-glow." There are eight fluorescent colors approved for cosmetics, and like other colors, there are limits on how they may be used. None of them are allowed for use near the eyes. (Check the Summary of Color Additives again.) These are their names: D&C Orange No. 5, No. 10, and No. 11; D&C Red No. 21, No. 22, No. 27 and No. 28; and D&C Yellow No. 7.

Luminescent Colors: These colors glow in the dark. In August 2000, FDA approved luminescent zinc sulfide for limited cosmetic use. It's the only luminescent color approved for cosmetic use, and it's not for every day and not for near your eyes. You can recognize it by its whitish-yellowish-greenish glow.

When The Party's Over

Don't go to bed with your makeup on. Wearing it too long might irritate your skin, and bits of makeup can flake off or smear and get into your eyes, not to mention mess up your pillow and annoy your parents.

How you take the stuff off is as important as how you put it on. Remove it the way the label says. If it says to remove it with cold cream, use cold cream. If it says to remove it with soap and water, use soap and water. If it says to remove it with eye makeup remover, use eye makeup remover. You get the picture. The same goes for removing glue, like the stuff that holds on fake beards.

And remember, the skin around your eyes is delicate. Remove makeup gently.

But Just In Case

What if you followed all these steps and still had a bad reaction? In March 2005 and May 2009, some face paint products were recalled from the market because they caused problems such as a skin rash, irritation, itching, or minor swelling where the paints were applied. If you have a reaction that seems to be caused by face paints, your parents may want to call a doctor, and they can call FDA, too. We like to keep track of reactions to cosmetics so we know if there are problem products on the market. To report a bad reaction to face paint, novelty makeup, or any other cosmetic product, see "Bad Reaction to Cosmetics?" at the end of the preceding chapter, or you can look for the document "Your Guide to Reporting Problems to FDA" available online at http://www.fda.gov/ForConsumers/ConsumerUpdates/ucm095859.htm.

Temporary Tattoos, Henna/Mehndi, And "Black Henna"

FDA has received reports of adverse reactions to some temporary skin-staining products. The following information is intended to respond to questions about the safety and legality of such products.

Decal-Type Temporary Tattoos: Temporary tattoos, such as those applied to the skin with a moistened wad of cotton, fade several days after application. Under the law, color additives used in them must be approved by FDA for use on the skin.

FDA has received reports of allergic reactions to some decal-type temporary tattoos. An import alert [a regulatory process that enables FDA to keep potentially dangerous imported goods out of the U.S. marketplace] is in effect for several foreign-made temporary tattoos. The temporary tattoos subject to the import alert are not allowed into the United States because they contain colors not permitted for use in cosmetics applied to the skin or they don't have the required ingredient declaration on the label.

Henna, Or Mehndi, And Black Henna: Henna, a coloring made from a plant, is approved only for use as a hair dye. It is not approved for direct application to the skin, as in the body-decorating process known as mehndi. This unapproved use of a color additive makes these products adulterated and therefore illegal. An import alert is in effect for henna intended for use on the skin.

Because henna typically produces a brown, orange-brown, or reddish-brown tint, other ingredients must be added to produce other colors, such as those marketed as "black henna" and "blue henna." Even brown shades of products marketed as henna may contain other ingredients intended to make them darker or make the stain last longer on the skin.

So-called "black henna" may contain the coal tar color p-phenylenediamine, also known as PPD, which is only permitted for use as a hair dye. In some cases, the so-called black henna consists only of hair dye, which the artist mixes straight from the package and applies to the customer's skin.

PPD and some other hair dye ingredients may cause reactions in some individuals. That's the reason hair dyes have a caution statement and instructions to do a patch test on a small area of the skin before using them.

FDA has received reports of injuries to the skin from products marketed as henna and products marketed as "black henna."

Finding Out What's In A Temporary Tattoo Or Henna/Mehndi Product

Cosmetics, including temporary skin-staining products that are sold on a retail basis to consumers must have their ingredients listed on the label. Without such an ingredient declaration, they are considered misbranded and are illegal in interstate commerce. FDA requires the ingredient declaration under the authority of the Fair Packaging and Labeling Act (FPLA).

Because the FPLA does not apply to cosmetic samples and products used exclusively by professionals—for example, for application at a salon, or a booth at a fair or boardwalk—the requirement for an ingredient declaration does not apply to these products.

Tattoos And Permanent Make-Up

Before getting a tattoo or permanent make-up, here is what you should know. A tattoo is a mark or design on the skin. A permanent tattoo is meant to last forever. It is made with a needle and colored ink. The needle puts the ink into the skin. Some of these colors are also used in printing or painting cars and have not been tested for safety. In fact, no colors are approved by FDA for injecting into the skin. Allergic reactions have been reported from individuals who have received either temporary or permanent tattoos.

Types Of Tattoos

There are many different kinds of tattoos. For example:

- **Permanent Tattoos:** A needle is used to insert colored ink into the skin.

- **Permanent Make-Up:** This is a permanent tattoo that looks like make-up, such as eyebrow pencil, lip liner, eyeliner or blush.

- **Henna (Mehndi) Tattoos:** A natural plant dye called henna, or mehndi, is used to stain the skin. This kind of tattoo does not use needles. The color lasts two to three weeks. Henna is only approved by FDA for use as a hair dye. It is not approved for use on the skin.

- **Sticker-Type Temporary Tattoos:** The tattoo design is on a piece of coated paper. It is put on the skin with water or may be rubbed off onto the skin. Temporary tattoos last only a few days. They must contain only colors permitted for use in cosmetics applied to the skin.

Why Would Someone Want A Tattoo Or Permanent Make-Up?

- They want to restore a natural look to the face or breast, especially after surgery.

- They have trouble putting on make-up as a result of a medical condition.

How To Report A Bad Reaction To A Temporary Tattoo, Tattoo, Or Other Cosmetic

If you have concerns about temporary tattoos, tattoo ink, or any other cosmetic, you can contact MedWatch, the U.S. Food and Drug Administration's problem-reporting program, through the website at http://www.fda.gov/Safety/MedWatch, by phone at 800-332-1088, or contact the consumer complaint coordinator in your area.

Source: FDA, 2009–2012.

- They have lost their eyebrows.
- They find it appealing.
- Cultural or societal influences.

What Are The Risks?

- Infection—dirty needles can pass infections from one person to another person. These can be serious like hepatitis and HIV.
- You might be allergic to something used in your tattoo. This is rare, but can cause serious problems. In one case, involving one manufacturer, more than 150 reports of bad reactions to certain shades of permanent make-up inks were reported to FDA. Some women were permanently disfigured. The company recalled many of its inks.
- Lumps or bumps may form around the tattoo color.
- People may have swelling or burning in the tattoo when they have magnetic resonance imaging (MRI). This happens rarely and does not last very long.

What If I Don't Like My Tattoo?

- You may not like your tattoo even if it was done well. Not liking the tattoo is a common reason for having one removed.
- If you decide you want to get rid of a tattoo, it usually takes many treatments and costs a lot of money.
- Scars may form when getting or removing a tattoo.

Remember ... Think very carefully before getting a tattoo. Most tattoos are permanent. Removing tattoos and permanent make-up can be hard and can cost a lot of money. Sometimes, it cannot be done. It often means surgery and scarring.

How Can I Get Rid Of A Tattoo?

Tattoo removal should be done by a doctor or clinic and not by a tattoo parlor. There are several ways to try to remove a tattoo, and they don't always work. It can cost a lot of money and you may need a lot of treatment. Talk to your doctor or other health care provider to learn the best way to remove your tattoo.

Chapter 48

Nail Care Product Safety

There are many nail products on the market. It is important to know how to use them safely. As with any cosmetic product, follow the labeled directions carefully and pay careful attention to any warning statements. The following information will answer commonly asked questions about some nail products and ingredients.

How Nail Products Are Regulated

Nail products for both home and salon use are regulated by the Food and Drug Administration. Under the Federal Food, Drug, and Cosmetic Act (FD&C Act), these products are cosmetics.

By law, nail products sold in the United States must be free of poisonous or deleterious (harmful) substances that might injure users when used as labeled or under the usual or customary conditions of use. Many nail products contain potentially harmful ingredients, but are allowed on the market because they are safe when used as directed. For example, some nail ingredients are harmful only when ingested, which is not their intended use.

The labels of all cosmetics, whether marketed to consumers or salons, must include a warning statement whenever necessary or appropriate to prevent a health hazard that may occur with use of the product. Cosmetics sold on a retail basis to consumers also must bear an ingredient declaration, with the names of the ingredients listed in descending order of predominance. The requirement for an ingredient declaration does not apply, for example, to products used at professional establishments or samples distributed free of charge. However,

About This Chapter: Excerpted from "Nail Care Products," U.S. Food and Drug Administration (www.fda.gov), April 22, 2011.

the requirement does apply if these products are also sold at retail, even if they are labeled "For professional use only."

Nail Product Ingredient Safety

Infections and allergic reactions can occur with some nail products. As mentioned previously, some ingredients in nail products may be harmful if ingested. Some can easily catch fire if exposed to the flame of the pilot light of a stove, a lit cigarette, or other heat source, such as the heating element of a curling iron. Nail products also can be dangerous if they get in the eyes. Consumers should read labels of nail products carefully and heed any warnings.

Some Common Nail Product Ingredients

Acetonitrile In Artificial Nail Removers

Artificial nail removers consist primarily of acetonitrile. Child-resistant packaging is required for all household glue removers in liquid form containing more than 500 milligrams of acetonitrile in a single container. The Consumer Product Safety Commission (CPSC) enforces this requirement under authority of the Poison Prevention Packaging Act. However, the fact that a product is in "child-resistant" packaging does not mean that a child could not open it.

Like any cosmetic product that may be hazardous if misused, it is important for these artificial nail removers to carry an appropriate warning on the label, along with directions for safe use.

Formaldehyde In Nail Hardeners

Nail hardeners that contain formaldehyde may cause an irritation or allergic reaction to those sensitized to this compound. There is also some evidence that certain individuals may become allergic to toluene sulfonamide–formaldehyde resin, a common ingredient in nail preparations.

In 1984, the Cosmetic Ingredient Review (CIR) Expert Panel reported that available toxicological data and other information were insufficient to conclude that cosmetics containing formaldehyde in excess of 0.2% are safe. However, the CIR was referring to cosmetic products applied to the skin, not nail products. The concentration of formaldehyde needed for nail hardening is higher than 0.2%, but formaldehyde is less likely to cause skin sensitization when shields are used to keep the hardener away from the skin. If you are allergic to formaldehyde, have previously experienced an allergic reaction to nail preparations or for any other reason wish to avoid this ingredient, be sure to read the product ingredient statement on the label to determine if formaldehyde and toluene sulfonamide-formaldehyde resin are present.

Methacrylate Monomers In Artificial Nails ("Acrylics")

Artificial nails are composed primarily of acrylic polymers and are made by reacting together acrylic monomers, such as ethyl methacrylate monomer, with acrylic polymers, such as polymethylmethacrylate. When the reaction is completed, traces of the monomer are likely to remain in the polymer. For example, traces of methacrylate monomers remain after artificial nails are formed. The polymers themselves are typically quite safe, but traces of the reactive monomers could result in an adverse reaction, such as redness, swelling, and pain in the nail bed, among people who have become sensitive (allergic) to methacrylates.

Ethyl methacrylate monomer is commonly used today in acrylic nails, although methyl methacrylate monomer may still be found in some artificial nail products. In the early 1970s, FDA received a number of complaints of injury associated with the use of artificial nails containing methyl methacrylate monomer. Among these injuries were reports of fingernail damage and deformity, as well as contact dermatitis. Unlike methyl methacrylate monomer, methyl methacrylate polymers were not associated with these injuries. Based on its investigations of the injuries and discussions with medical experts in the field of dermatology, the agency chose to remove from the market products containing 100 percent methyl methacrylate monomer through court proceedings, which resulted in a preliminary injunction against one firm as well as several seizure actions and voluntary recalls. No regulation specifically prohibits the use of methyl methacrylate monomer in cosmetic products.

The CIR Expert Panel determined in 2002 that ethyl methacrylate is safe as used when application is accompanied by directions to avoid skin contact because of its sensitizing potential (that is, the possibility that a person might develop an allergy to this material).

Methacrylic Acid In Nail Primers

Despite the similar names, methacrylic acid is different from methacrylate monomers. It also is used differently and raises different safety concerns. Methacrylic acid (MAA) has been used in nail primers to help acrylic nails adhere to the nail surfaces. In response to cases of poisoning and injury, the CPSC issued a regulation requiring child-resistant packaging for household products containing MAA. A number of serious injuries have occurred to children who ingested such products or spilled them, receiving burns to their skin.

311

Nail primers that contain MAA are most commonly distributed through wholesale suppliers to nail salons and retail beauty supply stores, and they usually are labeled "For Professional Use Only." However, some of these retail stores sell to both professionals and consumers.

The CPSC regulation, established in accordance with the Poison Prevention Packaging Act, requires child- resistant packaging for liquid household products containing more than five percent MAA, weight to volume, in a single retail package. That means that it applies, for example, to a product containing more than 5 grams of MAA per 100 milliliters.

MAA products applied by means of absorbent material in a dispenser, such as a pen-like marker, are exempt from this requirement if there is no free liquid in the device and if, under any reasonably foreseeable conditions of use, the methacrylic acid will emerge only through the tip of the device. For more information regarding the child-resistant packaging requirements for MAA, contact the Office of Compliance, CPSC, at 301-504-0608.

Phthalates

Phthalates are a group of chemicals used in a wide variety of products, from toys to carpeting and medical tubing. In nail polishes, they are used primarily at concentrations of less than 10% as plasticizers, to reduce cracking by making them less brittle. Dibutylphthalate (DBP) is used most commonly in nail polishes, but dimethylphthalate (DMP) and diethylphthalate (DEP) are used occasionally.

Toluene In Nail Polishes And Other Products

Toluene is used as a solvent in a variety of nail products, such as nail polish, nail hardeners, and polish removers. Toluene was reviewed by the CIR Expert Panel in 1987, when the Panel determined that it was safe for cosmetic use in nail products when limited to concentrations no greater than 50 percent. The Panel re-evaluated the safety of toluene in 2005 and confirmed its original conclusion.

Reporting Adverse Nail Product Reactions

Consumers, nail technicians, and healthcare providers can report adverse reactions from nail products by contacting MedWatch, FDA's problem-reporting program, on the web (http://www.fda.gov/Safety/MedWatch) or by phone at 800-332-1088.

Chapter 49

Skin Care Concerns For People With Eczema

Bathing And Moisturizing

What is eczema?

Eczema is a chronic recurring skin disorder that results in dry, easily irritated, itchy skin. There is no cure for eczema, but good daily skin care is essential to controlling the disease.

What are the characteristics of dry skin?

When your skin is dry, it is not because it lacks grease or oil, but because it fails to retain water. For this reason, a good daily skin care regimen focuses on the basics of bathing and moisturizing.

What other factors create dry skin?

Wind, low humidity, cold temperature, excessive washing without use of moisturizers, and use of harsh, drying soaps can all cause dry skin and aggravate eczema.

How do I take care of my dry skin?

The most important treatment for dry skin is to put water back in it. The best way to get water into your skin is to briefly soak in a bath or shower and to moisturize immediately afterwards.

About This Chapter: This chapter includes "Bathing and Moisturizing" and "Topical Corticosteroids for Eczema: Myths and Facts," © 2012 National Eczema Association. All rights reserved. Reprinted with permission. For additional information visit www.nationaleczema.org.

Use of an effective moisturizer several times every day improves skin hydration and barrier function. Moisturizer should be applied to the hands every time they are washed or in contact with water.

The goal of bathing and moisturizing is to help heal the skin. To repair the skin, it is necessary to decrease water loss.

Some dermatologists recommend that you perform your bathing and moisturizing regime at night just before going to bed. You are unlikely to further dry out or irritate your skin while sleeping, so the water can be more thoroughly absorbed into your skin.

If you have hand eczema dermatologists recommend that you soak your hands in water, apply prescription medications and moisturizer (preferably an ointment), and put on pure cotton gloves before going to sleep.

If I am on prescription drugs for my eczema, do I still need to moisturize?

Basic skin care can enhance the effect of prescription drugs, and it can prevent or minimize the severity of eczema relapse.

What are the basics of bathing and moisturizing?

Take at least one bath or shower per day. Use warm, not hot, water for at least 10 to 15 minutes. Avoid scrubbing your skin with a washcloth.

Use a gentle cleansing bar or wash, no soap. During a severe flare, you may choose to limit the use of cleansers to avoid possible irritation.

While your skin is still wet (within three minutes of taking a bath or shower), apply any special skin medications prescribed for you and then liberally apply a moisturizer. This will seal in the water and make the skin less dry and itchy.

Be sure to apply any special skin medications to areas affected with eczema before moisturizing. The most common skin medications used to treat skin inflammation are prescription and non-prescription topical steroids or prescription topical immunomodulators (TIMS). Be sure to use these medications as directed. Remember that TIMS can sting if applied to wet skin, so apply a thin coat to affected areas only.

Be sure to apply moisturizer on all areas of your skin whether it has or has not been treated with medication. Specific occlusives or moisturizers may be individually recommended for you.

Moisturizers are available in many forms. Creams and ointments are more beneficial than lotions. Petroleum jelly is a good occlusive preparation to seal in the water; however, since it contains no water it works best after a soaking bath.

How does water help my skin?

- Water hydrates the stratum corneum (the top layer of skin).
- Water softens skin so the topical medications and moisturizers can be absorbed.
- Water removes allergens and irritants.
- Water cleanses, debrides, and removes crusted tissue.
- Water is relaxing and reduces stress.

Is water an irritant or a treatment?

Water *irritates* skin if…

- Skin is frequently wet without the immediate application of an effective moisturizer.
- Moisture evaporates, causing the skin barrier to become dry and irritated.

Water *hydrates* skin if…

- After skin is wet, an effective moisturizer is applied within three minutes.
- Hydration is retained, keeping the skin barrier intact and flexible.

What are some cleansing tips?

- Gently cleanse your skin each day.
- Use mild, non-soap cleansers.
- Use fragrance-free, dye-free, low-pH (less than 5.5) cleansing products.
- Moisturize immediately after cleansing while your skin is still wet.
- Avoid scrubbing with a washcloth or towel; pat instead.

What cleansing product should I use?

Our skin surface is much more acidic than soap: the average pH of soap is 9–10.5 while the normal pH of skin is 4–5.5. Some non-soap cleansers are specially formulated with a lower pH to be less irritating. Following are a few suggestions:

- Aquaphor Gentle Wash and Shampoo
- AVEENO Baby Cleansing Therapy Moisturizing Wash
- Basis Sensitive Skin Bar
- Bella Dry Skin Formula Moisturizing Body Bar
- CeraVe Hydrating Cleanser
- Cetaphil Restoraderm Body Wash
- Cetaphil Gentle Skin Cleanser
- Dove Sensitive Skin Unscented Beauty Bar
- Eucerin Calming Body Wash
- Exederm Cleansing Wash
- Kiss of Nature Oh My Baby!! Moisturizing Castile Body Bar
- Mustela Stelatopia Cream Cleanser
- MD Moms Baby Silk Gentle All-Over Clean Hair and Body Wash
- Neosporin Moisture Essentials Daily Body Wash
- Oilatum Cleansing Bar
- Vanicream Cleansing Bar or Free and Clear Liquid Cleanse

What does cleansing remove?

- Sebum (an oily substance produced by certain glands in the skin)
- Apocrine and eccrine secretions (skin gland secretions, discarded cells)
- Environmental dirt
- Bacteria, fungus, yeast, and other germs
- Desquamated keratinocytes (dead skin cells that are the normal product of skin maturation)
- Cosmetics, skin care products, medications

What is preferable, a bath or a shower? For how long?

Either a bath or shower (about 10–15 minutes long) will keep the skin from drying out.

- DO NOT rub your skin.

- DO NOT completely dry your skin after your shower or bath. Instead, pat yourself lightly with a towel if needed.

What type of bath should I take?

A soak in a tub of lukewarm water for 10–15 minutes will help the skin absorb water. You may wish to try one of the following for specific treatment:

- **Bleach Baths:** Bleach baths make the tub into a swimming pool! Soak for about 10 minutes and rinse off. Use two to three times a week. Bleach baths decrease the bacteria on the skin and decrease bacterial skin infections. Use ½ cup household bleach for a full bathtub, ¼ cup for a half bath.

- **Vinegar Baths:** Add one cup to one pint of vinegar to the bath. Can be used as a wet dressing too as it kills bacteria.

- **Bath Oil Baths:** Oils in the bath are a favorite of some providers and patients. Bath oils can leave the tub slippery—be careful. They can also leave a hard-to-clean film. See if they work for you.

- **Salt Baths:** When there is a significant flare the bath water may sting or be uncomfortable. Add one cup of table salt to the bath water to decrease this side effect.

- **Baking Soda Baths:** Baking soda added to a bath or made into a paste can be used to relieve the itching.

- **Oatmeal Baths:** Oatmeal added to a bath or made into a paste can be used to relieve the itching.

What does moisturizing do?

- Moisturizing improves skin hydration and barrier function.

- Moisturizers are more effective when applied to skin that has been soaked in water.

What are the different kinds of moisturizers?

There are three basic classes of moisturizers:

- **Ointments** are semi-solid greases that help to hydrate the skin by preventing water loss. Petroleum jelly has no additional ingredients, whereas other ointments contain a small proportion of water or other ingredients to make the ointment more spreadable. Ointments are very good at helping the skin retain moisture but they are often disliked because of their greasiness.

- **Creams** are thick mixtures of greases in water or another liquid. They contain a lower proportion of grease than ointments, making them less greasy. A warning: creams often contain stabilizers and preservatives to prevent separation of their main ingredients, and these additives can cause skin irritation or even allergic reactions for some people.

- **Lotions** are mixtures of oil and water, with water being the main ingredient. Most lotions do not function well as moisturizers for people with dry skin conditions because the water in the lotion evaporates quickly.

What moisturizer should I use?

The importance of moisturizing cannot be over emphasized as a treatment for eczema and sensitive skin. Moisturizers maintain skin hydration and barrier function. Generic petroleum jelly and mineral oil (without additives) are two of the safest, most effective moisturizing products.

Following are a few suggestions:

- Albolene Moisturizing Cleanser
- Aquaphor Healing Ointment
- AVEENO Eczema Therapy Moisturizing Cream
- CeraVe Moisturizing Lotion or Cream
- Cetaphil Moisturizing Cream
- Cetaphil Restoraderm Moisturizer
- Crisco Regular Shortening
- Curél Itch Defense Skin Balancing Moisture Lotion
- Eucerin Calming Creme or Original Cream
- Exederm Intensive Moisture Cream
- Hydrolatum
- La Roche-Posay Lipikar Balm
- MD Moms Baby Silk Daily Skin Protection Moisturizing Balm
- Moisturel Therapeutic Cream
- Mustela Stelatopia Moisturizing Cream
- Neosporin Eczema Essentials Daily Moisturizing Cream

- Theraplex Emollient or Lotion
- Triple Cream
- Vanicream Moisturizing Skin Cream
- Vaseline Petroleum Jelly

Apply moisturizer to your skin immediately after your bath or shower and throughout the day whenever your skin feels dry or itchy. Some people prefer to use creams and lotions during the day and ointments and creams at night. If you can't find the product you want, ask a pharmacist to order it for you in the largest container available. Buying your moisturizers in large containers like one-pound jars may save you a great deal of money.

What are proper moisturizing techniques?

- Just as it is important to use proper bathing techniques, it is important to properly apply moisturizers to your skin within three minutes of showering or bathing.

- While your skin is still wet, apply prescription medications, and then apply a moisturizer to all your skin.

- A thick bland product is best.

- Dispense the moisturizer from large jars with a clean spoon, butter knife, or pump to avoid contamination.

- Take a dollop of moisturizer from the jar, soften it by rubbing it between your hands, and apply it using the palm of your hand stroking in a downward direction.

- Do NOT rub by stroking up and down or around in circles.

- Leave a tacky film of moisturizer on your skin; it will be absorbed in a few minutes.

Everyone has different preferences concerning how products feel on their skin, so try different products until you find one that feels comfortable. Continue use of the moisturizer(s) even after the affected area heals to prevent recurrence.

How can I reduce skin irritation?

After bathing and moisturizing, the next important step is to attempt to reduce skin irritation.

Don't scratch or rub the skin. These actions can worsen any itch. Instead, apply a moisturizer whenever the skin feels dry or itchy. A cool gel pack can provide some relief from itch.

Wash all new clothes before wearing them. This removes formaldehyde and other potentially irritating chemicals which are used during production and packing.

Add a second rinse cycle to ensure the removal of soap if you are concerned. Use a mild detergent that is dye-free and fragrance-free.

Wear garments that allow air to pass freely to your skin. Open-weave, loose-fitting, cotton-blend clothing may be most comfortable. Avoid wearing wool.

Wet wrap therapy can effectively rehydrate and calm the skin. Soak in a bath, and then apply moisturizer. Medication should also be applied if currently prescribed. The bandages, moistened in warm water until they are slightly damp, are then wrapped around the area. Dry bandages are wrapped over the wet bandages. In place of bandages, athletic socks, or moistened pajamas worn underneath a set of dry pajamas can be used with children and infants.

Work and sleep in comfortable surroundings with a fairly constant temperature and humidity level. Cooler temperatures are preferred but not so cool as to initiate chilling.

Keep fingernails very short and smooth by filing them daily to help prevent damage due to scratching.

Make appropriate use of sedating antihistamines, which may reduce itching to some degree through their tranquilizing and sedative effects.

Use sunscreen on a regular basis and always avoid getting sunburned. Use a sunscreen with an SPF of 15 or higher. Sunscreens made for the face are often less irritating than regular sunscreens. Zinc oxide or titanium dioxide–based products are less irritating.

Go for a swim, which can provide good hydration. Chlorine can also decrease bacteria on the skin that can cause itching or develop into an infection. Of course, residual chlorine or bromine left on the skin after swimming in a pool or hot tub may be irritating, so take a quick shower or bath immediately after swimming, washing with a mild cleanser from head to toe, and then apply an appropriate moisturizer while still wet.

Topical Corticosteroids: Myths And Facts

The word "eczema" is derived from a Greek word meaning "to boil over," which is a good description for the red, inflamed, itchy patches that occur during flare-ups of the disease. Topical steroids are an important part of the treatment plan for most people with eczema. When eczema flares up, applying cream, lotion, or ointment containing a steroid will reduce inflammation, ease soreness and irritation, reduce itching, and relieve the need to scratch, allowing the skin to heal and recover.

Steroids are naturally occurring substances that are produced in our bodies to regulate growth and immune function. There are many different kinds of steroids, including "anabolic steroids," like testosterone, and "female hormones," like estrogen (both produced in the gonads), and corticosteroids such as cortisol, which is produced by the adrenal glands. Corticosteroids are the type of steroid used for eczema. Corticosteroids have many functions in the body, but among other things they are very effective at controlling inflammation. The way corticosteroids reduce inflammation is very complicated, but it involves temporarily altering the function of a number of cells and chemicals in the skin.

Topical corticosteroids have been used extensively for over 50 years to treat various inflammatory skin conditions. Without a doubt, they remain one of the most valuable currently available treatments, and if used properly, can control symptoms and restore patients' quality of life.

The vehicle (type of base in which the medication is contained) and type of corticosteroid influences the strength of the topical medication more than the percentage of medication dissolved in the vehicle. Given the same percentage and type of topical corticosteroid, the following list generally represents the strengths of the medication, from highest to lowest:

- Ointment (highest)

- Creams

- Lotions (lowest)

Ointments are greasy, but have the lowest risk of burning and stinging with application. Solutions, gels, and sprays are newer, often more complex formulations, some stronger and some weaker than lotions or creams containing the same medication.

Topical corticosteroids come in various strengths, ranging from "super potent" (Class I) to weaker, "least potent" (Class 7). Table 49.1 lists some brand-name choices. Many topical steroids have generic versions. While often more expensive, your doctor may prescribe a branded product if they want you to receive the corticosteroid in a particular formulation for a variety of reasons. You should discuss with your doctor if a generic formulation may be available and would be right for you. The list is not comprehensive, and the strength class listing may vary for some products based on the different tests used to define this.

The majority of topical corticosteroid products have been approved by the Federal Drug Administration (FDA) for adults only because studies are always performed in adults first, and performing studies in children is more challenging.

Topical corticosteroids, like many other medications, are often used for indications and ages that have not been specifically studied. This is referred to as "off-label" use.

Table 49.2 lists the topical corticosteroids that have been approved by the FDA for use with children. FDA approval is awarded based on studies with children in a specific range of ages. These medications are commonly used in younger children.

What are the most common risks of using topical corticosteroids?

Most people immediately think of thinning of the skin (skin atrophy). This is a well-recognized possible side effect. It is true that potent and super potent topical corticosteroids can cause skin atrophy if applied too frequently and for a prolonged time without a break. Although early skin thinning can disappear if the topical corticosteroid is discontinued,

Table 49.1. Topical Corticosteroids: Some Brand-Name Choices

Generic Name	Examples Of Branded Products
Class 1—Super Potent	
0.05% clobetasol propionate	Clobex Lotion/Spray/Shampoo, Olux E Foam, Temovate E Emollient/ Cream/Ointment Gel/Scalp
0.05% halobetasol propionate	Ultravate Cream
0.1% fluocinonide	Vanos Cream
Class 2—Potent	
0.05% diflorasone diacetate	ApexiCon E Cream
0.1% mometasone furoate	Elocon Ointment
0.1% halcinonide	Halog Ointment
0.25% desoximetasone	Topicort Cream/Ointment
Class 3—Upper Mid-Strength	
0.05% fluocinonide	Lidex-E Cream
0.05% desoximetasone	Topicort LP Cream
Class 4—Mid-Strength	
0.1% clocortolone pivalate	Cloderm Cream
0.1% mometasone furoate	Elocon Cream
0.1% triamcinolone acetonide	Aristocort A Cream, Kenalog Ointment
0.1% betamethasone valerate	Valisone Ointment
0.025% fluocinolone acetonide	Synalar Ointment

prolonged use can cause permanent stretch marks (striae). Stretch marks usually occur on the upper inner thighs, under the arms, and in the elbow and knee creases. It should be noted that preteens and teenagers who have never used corticosteroids can also get stretch marks. Permanent skin atrophy from topical corticosteroids is now extremely uncommon when the treatment is used properly. In the past, recommendations did not specify the amount, frequency, and duration to apply topical corticosteroids. We now know that these medications are safest when used intermittently, in an appropriate quantity, and for an appropriate length of time.

Many patients with under-treated eczema have the opposite of skin thinning, and actually develop thickening, and sometimes darkening of the skin (changes known as lichenification). This is the skin's response to rubbing and scratching.

Table 49.1. *continued*

Generic Name	Examples Of Branded Products
Class 5—Lower Mid-Strength	
0.05% fluticasone propionate	Cutivate Cream/Cutivate Lotion
0.1% prednicarbate	Dermatop Cream
0.1% hydrocortisone probutate	Pandel Cream
0.1% triamcinolone acetonide	Aristocort A Cream, Kenalog Lotion
0.025% fluocinolone acetonide	Synalar Cream
Class 6—Mild	
0.05% alclometasone dipropionate	Aclovate Cream/Ointment
0.05% desonide	Verdeso Foam, Desonate Gel
0.025% triamcinolone acetonide	Aristocort A Cream, Kenalog Lotion
0.1% hydrocortisone butyrate	Locoid Cream/Ointment
0.01% fluocinolone acetonide	Derma-Smoothe/FS Scalp Oil, Synalar Topical Solution
Class 7—Least Potent	
2%/2.5% hydrocortisone	Nutracort Lotion, Synacort Cream
0.5–1% hydrocortisone	Cortaid Cream/Spray/Ointment and many other over-the-counter products

Table 49.2. Topical Corticosteroids Approved For Use With Children

Generic Name	Age Group
Clobetasol propionate 0.05% foam	>12 years
Fluocinonide 0.1% cream	>12 years
Fluocinolone acetonide 0.01% oil	>2 years
Mometasone 0.1% cream/ointment	>2 years
Fluticasone 0.05% lotion/cream	>1 year
Alclometasone 0.05% cream/ointment	>1 year
Prednicarbate 0.1% cream/ointment	>1 year
Fluticasone 0.05% lotion/cream	>1 year
Desonide 0.05% foam/gel	>3 months
Hydrocortisone butyrate 0.1% cream	>3 months

What are some other risks?

Frequent and prolonged application of a topical corticosteroid to the eyelids can cause glaucoma and even cataracts. Topical corticosteroids can occasionally cause tiny pink bumps and acne, especially when used on the face and around the mouth. On the body, greasy corticosteroid ointments can rarely cause redness around hair follicles, sometimes with a pus bump centered in the follicle (folliculitis). When corticosteroids are applied to large body surface areas, enough may be absorbed to inhibit the body's own production of cortisol, a condition known as adrenal suppression. The risk of adrenal suppression is highest with high potency (Class 1–2) corticosteroids. Infants and young children have a higher ratio of body surface area compared to their weight, so they are more susceptible to corticosteroid absorption. If a child is given corticosteroids by mouth, in large doses or over a long term, prolonged adrenal suppression can be associated with growth suppression and weakened immune responses. Adrenal suppression does not have a significant effect on a child's brain development.

Myths And Facts

MYTH: Topical corticosteroids should not be used on cracked, broken or weepy skin.

Topical corticosteroids are effective in helping to heal cracked and broken eczematous skin. While these creams and ointments are more easily absorbed through eczematous skin, they are safe as long as they are used according to the advice of your physician and their use is tapered or discontinued when the skin is healed. If your skin is tender and swollen it may be infected; this should be evaluated by your doctor.

MYTH: Topical corticosteroids cause stunted growth and development.

Corticosteroid creams and ointments should not be confused with anabolic steroids infamously used by some athletes. But, babies and very young children are at risk of absorbing topically applied corticosteroids into the bloodstream, especially when these medications are very potent, applied in large quantities too frequently, or used inappropriately under a diaper or other covered (occluded) area. As such there may be a risk of slowing growth (height). Corticosteroids taken by mouth or used for prolonged periods of time are absorbed into the bloodstream. These can reduce the body's production of natural corticosteroids, weaken immune responses, and affect growth, but do not affect brain development. Topically applied corticosteroids used in the appropriate quantity and for the appropriate duration are unlikely to affect growth or the body's ability to fight infections.

It is important to follow the advice of your doctor when using topical corticosteroids in babies and young infants.

When making a decision about the need for topical corticosteroid therapy, it is critical to weigh the potential risks of the treatment against the risks of the disease. Untreated severe eczema can have an enormously negative impact on overall well-being, restful sleep, ability to concentrate and learn, and family dynamics, which can, in turn, impair a child's normal growth and development. When topical corticosteroids are applied correctly, the risks of the disease are far greater than the risks of treatment.

MYTH: Topical corticosteroids cause lightening or darkening of the skin.

Topical corticosteroids rarely cause skin discoloration, which resolves when the treatment is stopped. Skin discoloration is much more likely to result from the eczema itself, because skin inflammation can increase or decrease the amount of tan pigment in the skin. Skin discoloration from eczema will also resolve over time, but may take several months.

MYTH: Topical corticosteroids promote excessive hair growth.

If topical corticosteroids are used for long periods, they can occasionally cause a temporary, mild increase in fine hair growth in the treated areas, although this is rare. Frequent scratching can also cause a temporary, mild increase in fine hair growth.

MYTH: Topical corticosteroids will prolong the eczema and decrease the chances of improvement with age.

There is no evidence that topical corticosteroids change the underlying natural course of the disease.

MYTH: A lot of moisturizer can eliminate the need for topical corticosteroids.

Proper bathing and moisturizing is essential in managing chronic eczema. Although moisturizers are a first-line treatment, when used alone they will only control the very mildest forms of eczema. Moderate or severe eczema cannot be treated effectively with moisturizers alone. Once the skin becomes red (inflamed), additional anti-inflammatory medication is needed to control the disease. Anti-inflammatory treatments include topical corticosteroids, topical calcineurin inhibitors (TCI's such as Elidel or Protopic), ultraviolet light therapy, or systemic medications.

Tips For Using Topical Corticosteroids

- Use the least potent corticosteroid possible to control the inflammation.
- Only apply the corticosteroid to areas of skin affected by the skin disease.
- It is most effective to apply corticosteroids immediately after bathing.
- Emollients may work better if applied to wet skin. Do not wet the skin without applying an emollient afterwards.
- Only use the corticosteroid as often as prescribed by your doctor—more than twice daily increases the risks but not the benefits of corticosteroids; for many topical corticosteroids, once-a-day application is sufficient.
- Do not use a topical corticosteroid as a moisturizer.
- Wherever possible, avoid using large quantities of corticosteroids for long periods of time.
- Be aware that certain areas of skin—the face, genitals, raw skin, thin skin, and areas of skin that rub together, such as beneath the breasts or between the buttocks or thighs—absorb more corticosteroid than other areas.
- Applying dressings over the area of skin treated with the corticosteroid increases the potency and absorption of corticosteroid into the skin. Only use dressings with topical corticosteroids if advised to do so by a physician.
- Once the inflammation is under control, reduce or stop using the corticosteroid. Remember: a proper bathing and moisturizing practice helps prevent flare-ups.

Special Note For Parents Of Children With Atopic Dermatitis

- Applying medications and supervising your child's skin care is often difficult and time-consuming, especially if the eczema is severe. Many parents are concerned about long-term effects of medications. However, the risk of uncontrolled eczema is far greater. When used appropriately, topical corticosteroids have a very low risk of absorption or thinning of the skin.

Source: "Topical Corticosteroids for Eczema: Myths and Facts," © 2012 National Eczema Association.

MYTH: Topical corticosteroids should always be applied in smaller amounts than prescribed.

It is true that only a thin layer is needed, but it is important to apply enough to cover all the red areas. A useful way of knowing the correct amount to apply is the fingertip rule: Squeeze a ribbon of the topical corticosteroid onto the tip of an adult index finger, between the fingertip and the first finger crease. This amount of corticosteroid represents "one fingertip unit," and should be enough to cover an area of skin the size of two flat adult palms of the hand (including fingers).

Chapter 50

Decoding Food Labels:
A Necessary Skill For People
With Food Allergies

Background

True food allergies are immune-mediated systemic allergic reactions to certain foods. According to the Food and Drug Administration (FDA), true food allergies affect less than 2% of the adult population and 2–8% of children. However, the impact of true allergies can be quite severe. Most childhood food allergies are found in young infants and children under three years old. Food allergies have a genetic component and may be more common among those with asthma.

Reactions to a food allergen can range from uncomfortable skin irritations to gastrointestinal distress to respiratory involvement to life-threatening anaphylaxis—a systemic allergic reaction that generally involves several of these areas as well as the cardiovascular system. The number of people with food allergies appears to be increasing, especially among children. To keep pace with this trend, there is an increasing need for preemptive food selection strategies.

Currently, an individual with a food allergy must learn to read labels carefully and critically. This is because a food allergen may take on an unfamiliar name when used for processing purposes. For example, if eggs, one of the most allergenic foods, are used as a binder to retain water in a food product, the term binder, rather than egg, will appear on the food label. Similarly, soy protein may be used for flavoring and listed on the label as natural flavoring.

About This Chapter: From "Decoding Food Labels: Tools for People with Food Allergies," by Amarat Simonne, PhD, and Elizabeth A. Gollub, PhD, MPH, RD. This document is one of a series of the Department of Family, Youth and Community Sciences, Florida Cooperative Extension Service, Institute of Food and Agriculture Sciences Extension, University of Florida, © 2010. Reprinted with permission. The complete text of this document including references and other resources is available at http://edis.ifas.ufl.edu/fy723.

The Food Allergen Labeling and Consumer Protection Act (FALCPA), which took effect on January 1, 2006, requires food manufacturers to use common names to identify major allergens. However, many consumers continue to have problems understanding complicated labeling information.

The goal of this publication is to provide information to help consumers understand ingredient statements on food packages so they can avoid foods and food products that might contain specific allergens. It also differentiates between allergies and intolerances, and discusses the potential for cross-contamination of foods both in and away from the home.

Food Allergy Vs. Food Intolerances Vs. Histamine Sensitivity

Most people experience an adverse reaction to some food at some point in their life. This does not necessarily mean that the individual is allergic to that food. Food intolerances, including sensitivity to elevated levels of histamine in foods, can produce a response similar to an allergic reaction. Adverse reactions and suspected allergens can be identified through a detailed history and specific allergy testing by a physician or qualified specialist (to exclude other causes).

The difference between food allergies and food intolerance is how the body handles the offending food. In the case of an allergy, the immune system recognizes a chemical in the food (usually a protein) as an allergen, and produces antibodies against it.

A response to an allergen may manifest as:

- Swelling of the lips
- Stomach cramps, vomiting, diarrhea
- Hives, rashes, eczema
- Wheezing or breathing problems
- Severely reduced blood pressure

Most common allergens are found in the following food groups:

1. Cow's milk (especially among children)
2. Wheat (especially among children)
3. Soy (especially among children)
4. Eggs

5. Peanuts

6. Tree nuts

7. Fish

8. Shellfish

9. Food additives (not true allergens, but capable of causing reaction or illness specific to a given person)

In most cases, children will outgrow their allergies to milk, wheat, soy, and eggs, but not to peanuts. Adults do not usually grow out of their allergies.

Food intolerance is more common than a true allergy and does not involve the immune system. Intolerance is a metabolic problem in which the body cannot adequately digest the offending food. This is usually because of a chemical deficiency (for example, an enzyme deficiency).

An individual with food intolerance can generally consume a small amount of the offending food without experiencing symptoms. However, the specific amount may be different for each individual. Intolerances, unlike allergies, seem to intensify with age.

Histamine sensitivity may be considered a type of food intolerance. Because histamine is a primary mediator of an allergic response in the body, consumption of histamine can elicit a similar response. Histamine toxicity is most frequently associated with the consumption of spoiled fish, but has also been associated with aged cheeses and red wines. Elevated levels of histamine occur naturally in these foods.

Decoding Allergens In Foods

Eggs

If you are allergic to egg protein, you should avoid any product with the word egg on the label. You should also avoid products with the following terms on their labels:

- Albumin
- Binder
- Coagulant
- Emulsifier
- Globulin/ovoglobulin
- Lecithin
- Livetin
- Lysozyme
- Ovalbumin
- Ovomucin
- Ovomucoid
- Ovovitellin

- Simplesse (Simplesse is a fat substitute made from egg white and milk protein)
- Vitellin

Types of foods that are likely to contain egg protein include:

- Baked goods and packaged mixes
- Breakfast cereals
- Creamy fillings and sauces
- Custard
- Malted drinks and mixes
- Marshmallows
- Marzipan (marzipan might be made with egg whites)
- Meringue
- Pancakes and waffles
- Pastas/egg noodles
- Processed meat products
- Pudding
- Salad dressings/mayonnaise
- Soups

Milk

Milk and milk proteins are also found in a variety of processed foods. Individuals with milk protein allergies should avoid all types of milk, ice cream, yogurt, and cheese, including vegetarian cheese. Allergic individuals should avoid foods with the terms butter, cream, casein, caseinate, whey, or emulsifier on the labels. Additional labeling terms indicating the presence of milk proteins in a food product include:

- Caramel color or flavoring
- High protein flavor
- Lactalbumin/lactalbumin phosphate
- Lactoglobulin
- Lactose
- Natural flavoring
- Simplesse (Simplesse is a fat substitute made from egg white and milk protein)
- Solids

Types of foods that are likely to contain milk protein include:

- Baked goods and mixes
- Battered foods
- Breakfast cereals
- Chocolate
- Cream sauces, soups and mixes
- Custard, puddings, sherbet
- Ghee (Ghee is clarified butter and is frequently used in Indian cuisine.)
- Gravies and mixes
- Imitation sour cream

- Instant mashed potatoes
- Margarine
- Sausages
- Sweets/candies

Wheat

Individuals who are allergic to wheat proteins should avoid any product that contains the term wheat, bulgur, couscous, bran, gluten, bread crumbs, or hydrolyzed wheat proteins on the label. Wheat has binding properties that are very useful in the food processing industry, and this has extended to use in the pharmaceutical industry. Individuals with wheat allergies should discuss the composition of prescription or over-the-counter medications with a pharmacist prior to use. Rye and barley also contain gluten and must be avoided. The presence of wheat protein in a food product may be indicated by the following label terms:

- Cornstarch
- Farina
- Flour-bleached, unbleached, white, whole wheat, all-purpose, enriched, graham, durum, high gluten, high protein
- Gelatinized starch
- Hydrolyzed vegetable protein
- Kamut*
- Malt
- Miso (fermented soy product with up to 50% wheat)
- Modified food starch
- MSG (monosodium glutamate)
- Semolina
- Spelt*
- Triticale*
- Vegetable starch/gum

*Spelt and kamut are both relatives of wheat; triticale is a wheat/rye hybrid. These grains are gaining popularity as wheat substitutes. Spelt-, kamut-, and triticale-containing products are marketed primarily through health/natural food stores.

Types of foods that are likely to contain wheat proteins include:

- Ale/beer/wine/bourbon/whiskey
- Baked goods and mixes—including barley products
- Battered or breaded foods
- Breakfast cereals
- Candy/chocolate
- Coffee substitutes
- Gravy
- Ice cream and cones
- Malts and flavorings
- Pasta/egg noodles
- Pretzels, chips, crackers

- Processed meats
- Soup and soup mixes
- Soy sauce

Soy

Soy can be consumed as a whole bean, a nut, or a cow-milk alternative. Soy can be processed into foods such as tofu, soy curd, yuba (soy film), and soy flour. Soy can be fermented into products such as tempeh, natto, miso, and soy sauce. Soy has a variety of supportive uses in the food industry as well. It can be a thickener, stabilizer, emulsifier, and a protein extender. Allergic individuals should avoid products with these terms on the label, in addition to products containing the terms soy and soybean.

Soybean oil should be protein-free, but this is not always the case, and some allergic individuals must avoid soybean oil and products made with soybean oil (margarine and products made with margarine, salad dressings, and baby foods). The presence of the following terms on the product label may also indicate the presence of soy protein:

- Artificial and natural flavoring
- Bulking agent
- Carob
- Hydrolyzed vegetable protein (HVP)/hydrolyzed soy protein
- Lecithin
- Vegetable broth/gum/starch
- Miso (Miso is a paste made from fermented soybeans used as a flavoring agent in Japanese cuisine.)
- Monosodium glutamate (MSG)
- Protein
- Starch
- Textured vegetable protein (TVP)

Types of foods that are likely to contain soy protein include:

- Asian foods
- Baked goods
- Bouillon cubes
- Butter substitutes/shortening
- Canned meat/fish in sauces
- Canned tuna
- Canned/packaged soups
- Chocolates/candy
- Crackers
- Gravies/mixes
- Hamburger patties
- Ice cream
- Liquid/powdered meal replacers
- Processed meats
- Seasoned salt
- Seasoning sauces
- Snack bars
- Some breakfast cereals

- Tamari (Tamari is a dark sauce that is similar to but thicker than soy sauce.)
- TV dinners

Peanuts And Tree Nuts

Peanuts are one of the most severely allergenic foods available in the marketplace. Peanuts are frequently used as a flavoring/seasoning agent in a variety of products. Peanuts and peanut oil are commonly used in Asian cooking as well as other types of cooking. As with soy oil, peanut oil (occasionally referred to as arachis oil) may very well contain an amount of peanut protein sufficient to elicit an allergic reaction. The terms peanut, peanut butter, ground-nut, flavoring, extract, and oriental sauce on a product label generally indicate the presence of peanut protein.

Types of foods that may contain peanut protein include:

- African dishes
- Asian dishes (for example, Thai/Indonesian)
- Baked goods/mixes
- Barbecue/Worcestershire sauce
- Battered foods
- Candy/candy bars/sweets (read label)
- Cereal-based products
- Chili
- Chinese dishes/egg rolls
- Energy bars
- Ice cream
- Margarine/vegetable oil/vegetable fat
- Marzipan (Marzipan is a paste made of almond and sugar, used on pastry or molded into candy. Marzipan might be made with egg white as well.)
- Meat substitutes
- Milk formula
- Satay sauce (Satay sauce is made with peanuts or peanut butter and soy sauce. It might also be made with other allergenic ingredients such as shrimp paste or fish sauce.)
- Snack foods
- Some breakfast cereals
- Some grain breads
- Soups
- Sunflower seeds (Sunflower seeds may be processed on equipment shared with peanuts.)

Individuals with a peanut allergy may or may not be allergic to tree nuts (almonds, cashews, pecans, walnuts, etc.) as well. Individuals with tree-nut allergies should be cautious of the foods listed above as well as the following: mixed nuts, artificial nuts, nut oils, nut pastes, nut butters, nut extracts, salad dressings, and amaretto products.

Fish And Seafood

The term "seafood" refers to fish and shellfish. Fish is one of the most common causes of allergic reaction in both adults and children. Some species of fish can cause true allergic reactions as demonstrated by increasing production of immunoglobulin IgE in the affected persons. Current research also reveals cross-reactivity among various species of fish. This means that if one person is allergic to one fish species (such as cod), he/she may be allergic to other fish, such as mackerel and herring. However, certain species of fish contain high levels of histidine (an amino acid), which can be converted into histamine by bacteria following improper temperature management. Reactions to histamine can mimic allergic reactions, but are not indicative of a true allergy.

Types of foods that might contain fish/seafood proteins include:

- Caesar salad dressing
- Caponata (Caponata is an eggplant relish that can contain anchovies.)
- Curry paste
- Fish sauce
- Fish stock
- Hot dogs/bologna/ham
- Marinara sauce
- Pizza toppings
- Surimi (Surimi is a fish protein, most commonly made from pollack, that is marketed as imitation seafood. Surimi may contain artificial flavor, sweeteners, egg white, starch, and small amounts of real shellfish.)
- Vitamin supplements (read label)
- Worcestershire/steak sauce

Shellfish

Shellfish tends to be a more potent allergen among adults. Shellfish include mollusks (for example, squid, octopus, clams, and scallops) and crustaceans (for example, crab, lobster, crawfish, and shrimp). Although shellfish might be incorporated into a variety of foods during processing, the product's label generally states this clearly.

Types of foods that might shellfish proteins include:

- Caesar salad dressing
- Caponata (Caponata is an eggplant relish that can contain anchovies.)
- Chitin or chitosan (Chitin or chitosan is a chemical compound, polysaccharide, derived from crab or shrimp shells. It is widely used in foods and other products as a coating agent, bulking agents, or antimicrobial agent. It is often used in making capsules or other drug delivery systems.)
- Curry paste
- Fermented fish stomach
- Fermented oyster sauce
- Fish sauce
- Fish stock
- Hot dogs/bologna/ham
- Marinara sauce
- Pizza toppings
- Shrimp paste
- Surimi (Surimi is a fish protein, most commonly made from pollack, that is marketed as imitation seafood. Surimi may contain artificial flavor, sweeteners, egg white, starch, and small amounts of real shellfish.
- Vitamin supplements (read label)
- Worcestershire/steak sauce

Food Additives

Food additives are frequently incorporated into food products during processing. They may be used as product preservatives, flavor enhancers or sweeteners, coloring agents, conditioners, or stabilizers. Over the years, adverse reactions to certain food additives, casually referred to as allergies, have been reported. Most notably, these include:

- Sulfite-induced asthma
- Monosodium glutamate-induced asthma, or MSG symptom complex
- Aspartame-induced hives and/or migraines

- FD&C Yellow No. 5 (tartrazine)–induced hives and/or asthma
- Reactions to carmine and cochineal

Reactions to these additives are not immunologically mediated. Rather, reactions to these food additives are considered idiosyncratic (affecting different people in different ways) in that the mechanism of these reactions remains unknown.

Sulfites: Sulfites are used as a preservative to prevent browning reactions. Although sulfite-induced asthma is well documented, its mechanisms are not well understood by experts. Sulfite-sensitive individuals should avoid foods with the following terms listed on their label: sulfur dioxide, potassium metabisulfite, sodium metabisulfite, potassium bisulfite, sodium bisulfite, and sodium sulfite.

Monosodium Glutamate (MSG): Glutamate, an amino acid, occurs naturally in many foods, with particularly high levels in dairy products, meat, fish, and some vegetables. Glutamate has a distinct flavor. Monosodium glutamate (MSG) is added to food as a flavor enhancer. MSG symptom complex includes headaches, nausea, rapid heartbeat, vomiting, and a tingling/numbness/burning sensation along the back, neck, arms, face, and chest pains. These MSG-induced symptoms tend to occur in sensitive individuals within one hour of consuming large amounts (more than three grams) of MSG or consuming MSG in a liquid (for example, soup). Individuals with asthma may be predisposed to this syndrome, as well as to MSG-induced asthma attacks. Food products containing MSG will list it on the label. However, MSG may be used in restaurants, especially in Asian cooking.

Aspartame: Aspartame is an artificial sweetener made from two amino acids: phenylalanine and aspartic acid. Aspartame is marketed as a low-calorie sweetener (NutraSweet and Equal are among its popular names). Associations have been reported between aspartame and a list of adverse symptoms, including headaches or migraines, dizziness, rashes, swelling of the lips and/or eyelids, difficulty breathing, rapid heartbeat, and depression. Individuals with mood disorders may be particularly vulnerable to these reactions. Aspartame is listed on the label of food products, beverages, and in medications, where it may also be used as a sweetening agent.

FD&C Yellow No. 5 (Tartrazine): FD&C Yellow No. 5, or tartrazine, is a dye used as a coloring agent in food processing. Among sensitive individuals, tartrazine appears to be a trigger for asthma, runny nose, and hives. The presence of this dye in a food or drug should be clearly indicated by the terms FD&C Yellow No. 5, tartrazine, or possibly E102 on the food product label or drug package insert. Individuals who are sensitive to aspirin may be sensitive to tartrazine as well.

Cross-Contamination Of Foods In And Away From The Home

If you are allergic or live with an allergic individual, then cross-contamination becomes a daily issue. Cross-contamination refers to the situation through which a "safe" food comes in contact with an allergen—even a small amount. At home, this could occur by cutting a peanut butter sandwich on a cutting board. The board is effectively contaminated with enough peanut allergen to elicit a reaction from the next allergic user. In a bakery, this could occur when an employee removes a sugar cookie for an allergic customer with the same tongs that were used to remove a peanut-butter cookie. In a restaurant, this could occur if the steak you ordered is grilled alongside the fish you are allergic to.

To avoid cross-contamination at home:

- Separate allergenic foods from other foods by storing them in a plastic box or container in the refrigerator or on the pantry shelf.

- Clean all pots, pans, and utensils thoroughly with soap and hot water immediately after contact with an allergen.

- Wash plates and utensils used with allergenic foods separately and with a separate set of washing and drying cloths.

- Do not use wooden bowls or utensils because they absorb contaminants.

- Wash hands after contact with an allergen or wear non-latex food gloves during food preparation.

To avoid cross-contamination in restaurants:

- Avoid buffet-style dining.

- Avoid stores or cafes where food products are stored in bulk bins.

- Avoid sliced deli meats, because slicers are used with a variety of products.

- Avoid seafood restaurants if you are allergic to any type of seafood.

- Avoid Asian restaurants (Thai, Indonesian) if you have a peanut or soy allergy.

- Tell your server about your allergy.

- Ask about possible hidden ingredients, especially in salad dressings and sauces.

- Ask about other foods being prepared in the kitchen simultaneously.

- Order simple dishes with sauces on the side.

- Carry a Chef Card—a personalized card with simple instructions to the chef and others, describing your allergy, related ingredients, and cross-contamination issues.

- Don't be afraid to leave a restaurant if you don't feel safe.

Disclaimer

Not all foods and potential allergens have been included in this chapter. Check with your physician or specialist to make sure you have a complete, individualized list. If you are in doubt regarding food label information or product ingredients, contact the food manufacturer.

Chapter 51

Vaccines And Food Allergies

Millions of routine childhood vaccinations are given every year in the United States; allergic reactions from these vaccines are extremely rare. However, some people with certain food allergies may be at higher risk for allergic reactions as a result of vaccines containing certain food proteins.

Up to 8% of children suffer from food allergies, with egg being one of the most common foods to which children are allergic. Many routine childhood immunizations contain traces of egg protein or other food ingredients. As a result, there is the possibility that a child with food allergies will experience anaphylaxis (a severe allergic reaction) as a result of receiving a vaccination.

The following foods are present in small amounts in routine childhood vaccines; other non-routine vaccines containing food proteins are also listed.

Egg

Children with egg allergy present the biggest concern when receiving childhood vaccines. The following routine childhood immunizations may contain egg or egg-related proteins: influenza (flu) and measles-mumps-rubella (MMR) vaccines. In addition, the following non-routine vaccines contain egg protein: yellow fever and typhoid vaccines.

Influenza vaccine contains limited amounts of egg protein, and this amount may vary from year to year and batch to batch. In general, the influenza vaccine should not be given to people with a true egg allergy (people who have a positive allergy test to egg but can eat eggs without experiencing any symptoms are not egg allergic). However, in certain situations, the benefit of receiving this vaccine may outweigh the risks; this may be the case in people with severe asthma and mild egg allergy. In these cases, an allergist may be able to give the vaccine in small amounts over many hours, while closely monitoring the person for an allergic reaction.

The MMR vaccine is produced in chick fibroblast cell cultures; the vaccine likely does not contain egg proteins to which a person with egg allergy would react. Most people, even those with a severe egg allergy, do not have an allergic reaction to the MMR vaccine. Therefore, the American Academy of Pediatrics recommends that children with egg allergy can be given the MMR vaccine without any special measures being taken. It would be reasonable, however, to monitor an egg-allergic child in the physician's office for a period of time after giving the MMR vaccine.

Yellow fever vaccine, a non-routine vaccine given to people traveling to Central/South America and sub-Saharan Africa, does contain significant amounts of egg proteins and should not be given to people with egg allergy. Yellow fever vaccine, which contains the highest amount of egg protein of all the egg-based vaccines, has also been reported to cause allergic reactions in people with an allergy to chicken meat. Similar to influenza vaccine, the yellow fever vaccine may be able to be given to egg-allergic people in small amounts over many hours, under close monitoring by a physician.

Gelatin

Gelatin, like that found in Jell-O, is added to many vaccines as a heat stabilizer. Routine childhood vaccines containing gelatin include MMR, varicella (chicken-pox), influenza and DTaP (diphtheria, tetanus and acellular pertussis). Non-routine vaccines containing gelatin include yellow fever, rabies, and Japanese encephalitis. Allergic reactions to the MMR vaccine are far more likely due to the gelatin in the vaccine rather than to residual egg proteins in the vaccine.

Essentially, any person who has experienced an allergic reaction after eating gelatin food products (Jell-O) should not be given any of the above vaccines. However, as is the case with egg-containing vaccines in egg-allergic people, gelatin-containing vaccines may be able to be given to gelatin-allergic people under the direct supervision of a physician.

Baker's Yeast

Certain vaccines are synthesized by *Saccharomyces cerevisiae*, which is the common bakers' yeast used for making bread. Routine childhood vaccines containing baker's yeast include hepatitis B, and any combination vaccine that contains hepatitis B.

Any person who has experienced an allergic reaction after eating food products containing baker's yeast should not be given hepatitis B vaccine. However, as is the case with egg-containing vaccines in egg-allergic people, yeast-containing vaccines may be able to be given to yeast-allergic people under the direct supervision of a physician.

Sources

Moylett EH, Hanson IC. Mechanistic Actions of the Risks and Adverse Events Associated with Vaccine Administration. *J Allergy Clin Immunol*. 2004; 114: 1010–20.

Cox JE, Cheng TL. Egg-based Vaccines. *Pediatrics in Review*. 2006;27:118–119.

Centers for Disease Control and Prevention. Accessed December 12, 2007.

Chapter 52

Teens With Food Allergies Need To Be Careful About Kissing

How To Smooch Safely With Food Allergies

For most parents of teens, when the topic turns to kissing, over-protective thoughts abound. "I've got two daughters and I think they should never kiss anyone!" exclaimed Roger Friedman, MD, Clinical Professor of Allergy, Immunology, and Pediatrics at Nationwide Children's Hospital in Columbus, Ohio.

All joking aside, parents of food-allergic children have even more cause to be wary of smooching. Today, three to four million children are affected by food allergies, and allergic reactions can be triggered not just by consuming food firsthand. Kissing—ranging from passionate to a peck on the cheek—can also prompt a reaction.

Educate Others

"You're pretty unlikely to have anything severe happen from a kiss. But it can happen and you need to be smart," Dr. Friedman advised.

Kissing becomes a problem when anyone—from a grandparent to a date—consumes an allergen before smooching a food-allergic child or teen.

"A peck on the cheek from a parent or relative will almost always only result in a local reaction such as a welt or hive; it's very unlikely to cause any severe reaction that you'd be worried about," Dr. Friedman explained.

He recommends teenagers, especially, play it safe.

"If you're in a committed relationship that involves passionate kissing, tell your date 'I'm allergic to nuts, please don't eat any before you kiss my face!'" he suggested.

Todd D. Green, MD, Assistant Professor of Pediatric Allergy and Immunology at Children's Hospital of Pittsburgh, agreed.

"If a date cares enough about you to kiss you, hopefully they'll care enough to refrain from eating the food you're allergic to that day," he said.

Avoid Allergens

Kissing (and even sharing utensils, straws, and cups) causes exposure to food allergens through saliva, which can contain enough allergen to cause local and systemic allergic reactions.

In a study published in the *Journal of Allergy and Clinical Immunology*, participants ingested two tablespoons of peanut butter to establish how long the peanut allergen stays in saliva. Researchers collected the saliva of the participants at different times, and also evaluated mouth-cleansing techniques (brushing teeth, rinsing, and chewing gum.

According to the study, "the most effective way to avoid causing an allergic reaction, if you're going to eat the food to which your partner is allergic, is to eat the food several hours before a kiss and have a meal free of the allergen before you kiss—although not eating the food at all would always be the safest approach," said Dr. Green.

Though the risk of having a severe allergic reaction from a kiss is small, there is always a slight possibility, said Dr. Green. "Unfortunately you can't predict the amount of protein that will be transferred during kissing, and it is difficult to predict the reaction," he said. That said, it is better to err on the safe side.

Dr. Friedman reminds parents that a kiss is unlikely to be "the kiss of death."

"Worry about the right things," he advised. "Overall, the risks of developing a severe reaction from a kiss are rare and unusual."

Smooch Safely

Food allergic children and teens should follow these pointers before they pucker up:

- Remind your kissing partner about your allergies.

- Suggest your partner avoid eating serious allergens, if possible.

- Ask your partner to minimize allergen exposure, such as by washing hands and face, or brushing teeth thoroughly, before kissing.

- Carry appropriate medication and know how to use an injectable epinephrine kit.

- Wear emergency medical identification (such as a Medic Alert® bracelet).

Reference

Maloney J., Chapman M., Sicherer S. (2006). Peanut allergen exposure through saliva: Assessment and interventions to reduce exposure. *Journal of Allergy and Clinical Immunology*. 719-24.

Chapter 53

Basic Ingredient Substitutions To Accommodate Food Allergies

Basic Ingredient Substitutions For Food Allergies

Many common allergens are also common ingredients in your favorite recipes. There are some ingredients for which you can easily and successfully use non-allergenic substitutes, and there are others for which satisfactory substitutes do not exist.

Whether or not a "safe" version of a recipe can be successfully made often depends on two important factors. First: What is the role of the allergen in the recipe? For example, you really cannot make an "egg dish," such as fried eggs or omelets, without eggs (although some cookbooks present "egg" recipes based on tofu, the end result does not look, taste, or feel like "eggs"). Second: How many of the recipe's ingredients require substitutions? If the recipe only has five ingredients and you need to swap out four of them, the end result might bear little resemblance to the original dish. The bottom line: sometimes you can create a "safe" version of a recipe, and sometimes you are better off finding a different recipe altogether.

The following is a general guide to using ingredient substitutions for egg allergy. Please verify the ingredients and safety of any products named to ensure that it is safe for your child's unique allergy issues.

If you need additional assistance in finding product suggestions or where to find ingredients for substituting, post a message in the Kids With Food Allergies (KFA) Food and Cooking forum (online at http://kidswithfoodallergies.org/eve/forums/a/frm/f/8160079562 for KFA Family Members) to obtain suggestions from other parents of food allergic children who are also managing the same food allergies.

Cooking And Baking Without Egg Ingredients

Egg Substitutes For Baked Goods

In a typical recipe for baked goods, eggs generally play one of two roles: binder (to hold the recipe together) or leavening agent (to help it rise). Sometimes eggs play both roles at once. Determining which purpose the eggs primarily hold in the recipe you are considering will help you determine what options for replacement you might have.

As a rule of thumb, if a recipe for baked goods calls for three or more eggs per batch (with a typical batch consisting of 36 cookies, one pan of brownies, one loaf of bread, or one cake), egg substitutes generally do not work. The consistency of the finished product comes out poorly. Pound cakes, sponge cakes, angel food cakes, and other popular desserts with relatively high egg content do not turn out well in egg-free cooking. In these situations, it is usually best to make something else.

There are commercial egg replacement products on the market. Be sure that you are considering an egg replacement, not an egg substitute. Egg substitutes are generally marketed in the dairy portion of the grocery store, and are designed for cholesterol-conscious people, rather than for egg-allergic people. They contain egg, and are unsafe for those with egg allergies. Commercial egg replacement products (such as Ener-G brand Egg Replacer, a popular powdered product that is available in natural foods stores across the U.S.) generally will work for either binding or leavening purposes. As with any other product, be sure to read the ingredient statement to ensure that the product is indeed safe for your child.

Eggs As A Binder

For recipes which use eggs primarily as a binder (such as drop cookies), possible substitutions for one egg include:

- ½ of a medium banana, mashed

- ¼ cup of applesauce (or other pureed fruit)

- 3½ tablespoons gelatin blend (mix 1 cup boiling water and 2 teaspoons unflavored gelatin, and then use 3½ tablespoons of that mixture per egg)

- 1 tablespoon ground flax seed mixed with 3 tablespoons warm water; let stand 1 minute before using

- Commercial egg replacement products (see above)

Keep in mind that the addition of pureed fruit may impact both the taste and the density of the finished product.

Xanthan Gum: Xanthan gum can be added to egg-free cakes and cookies, as well as milk-free ice cream, to bind and add texture. Use about one teaspoon per recipe. Xanthan gum is a white powder derived from the exoskeleton of a bacterium. It is cultivated on corn sugar.

Eggs As A Leavening Agent

For recipes which use eggs primarily as a leavening agent you can try a commercial egg replacement product (see above) or the following mixture:

- 1½ tablespoons vegetable oil mixed with 1½ tablespoons water and 1 teaspoon baking powder per egg.

Note: This mixture calls for baking powder, not baking soda. The two products are not interchangeable.

Egg White Glaze

Occasionally recipes will use egg whites as a glaze, with the beaten egg whites brushed onto the top of the item before it is cooked. One good option here is to use melted margarine instead of the beaten egg whites.

Substituting Milk And Dairy Ingredients

The following is a general guide to using ingredient substitutions for milk allergy. Please verify the ingredients and safety of any products named to ensure that it is safe for your child's unique allergy issues.

Substitutes For Dairy Ingredients

Be aware that some brands and varieties of soy-based products (especially soy cheeses) contain dairy or are made in production facilities with equipment shared with dairy and should therefore be avoided by those with a milk allergy.

As with everything that you feed to your child, be sure to carefully read the ingredient statement and look for a Kosher dairy symbol on the products. Although Kosher labeling in general cannot be used as a guide to determining whether a product does or does not contain milk, many parents find they can save time in the supermarket by simply assuming that foods marked as "Kosher dairy" are not safe for a dairy-allergic child.

Substituting For Butter

One of the easiest substitutions to make is for butter: simply use a dairy-free margarine instead. However, you may need to do some searching and taste-testing to find the best dairy-free margarine available in your area, as a good margarine can make a big difference in many recipes. For baked goods, try to find a dairy-free margarine with a low water content and high fat content (for example, if you melt a stick of margarine, it should not be mostly water). Margarines with high water content produce inferior baked goods.

Substituting For Yogurt, Sour Cream, And Cream Cheese

Soy-based "yogurt," "sour cream," and "cream cheese" products are available at natural products grocers. These generally work very well in recipes, although as "stand-alone" products they do not necessarily taste "just like" their dairy-based counterparts.

Substituting For Cheese

Dairy-free cheeses are a bit of a challenge. Soy cheeses do not taste or melt like traditional dairy cheeses. If a child is old enough to remember "real" cheese, you may want to wait a while before introducing the soy version. Younger children will usually adapt more easily. In most cases, soy cheese will not appear melted, but will in fact be melted inside.

Soy cheese does not work well in recipes for cheese sauces. If you would like to make a dairy-free "cheese sauce," check the KFA Safe Eats recipe database for "cheese sauce" recipes based on nutritional yeast or soy (http://www.kidswithfoodallergies.org/recipes/introduction.php).

Substituting For Milk

There are currently a number of commercially produced liquid soy, rice, potato and oat milks, most of which are available in a few different flavors (such as "regular," "vanilla," "chocolate," and "mocha"). All of these milks can be substituted 1-for-1 in recipes.

Although almond milk is also available, careful consideration should be given to the wisdom of introducing tree nuts to an already food-allergic child. Coconut milk is also available, but recently the U.S. Food and Drug Administration (FDA) reclassified coconut as a tree nut. Check with your child's doctor about the suitability of using almond milk or coconut milk before using either for a child with a tree nut allergy.

Alisa Fleming has done extensive taste-testing to determine which types of milks work best in which types of recipes. Her book, *Dairy Free Made Easy* is available at www.godairyfree.org.

Substituting For Evaporated Milk

You can make your own substitute by making a "safe" evaporated milk and adding sugar. Evaporated milk is milk that has water content reduced by 60%. Simmer any quantity of soy or rice milk in a pan until it reduces by 60%. Approximately 3 cups of rice or soy milk will leave 1 cup of evaporated milk left at the end. Be careful not to scald it. Next, mix one cup of evaporated milk with 1¼ cups of sugar. Heat until the sugar is completely dissolved. Cool. It will yield 1½ cups of evaporated milk substitute. It will keep in the refrigerator for several days.

Another alternative for evaporated milk is to substitute coconut milk 1:1 in the recipe. This will impart a coconut flavor to the recipe, so it works in some recipes but not all.

Substituting For Buttermilk

You can make your own buttermilk substitute by mixing one tablespoon vinegar plus 1 cup milk alternative such as rice milk or soy milk.

Substituting For Light Cream, Sweet Cream, Or Heavy Cream

You can use Silk or Mocha Mix brand soy creamers or light coconut milk as substitutes for light cream.

Full fat coconut milk can be substituted for heavy cream. A coconut milk substitute will impart a coconut flavor to a recipe, so it will work for some recipes, but not all.

You can use Kineret brand whipped topping as a substitute for sweet cream if used straight out of the carton and not whipped.

Basic Recipe Substitutions For Wheat Allergy

The following is a general guide to using ingredient substitutions for wheat allergy. Please verify the ingredients and safety of any products named to ensure that it is safe for your child's unique allergy issues.

Wheat Substitutes For Baked Goods

There are a variety of formulas for substituting other flours for wheat flour in baked goods recipes. You may want to experiment to see what works best for you, given all of your child's allergies. You should be forewarned, though, that alternative flours generally do not produce the same texture and consistency as wheat flour. Keep in mind also that these suggestions are for wheat allergy; if you are avoiding gluten, you will need to avoid barley, rye, and other gluten-containing grains. Oats can be contaminated with wheat due to cultivation practices. There are wheat-free oats available as an alternative.

Single-Ingredient Substitutes For Wheat Flour

Generally speaking, you will achieve better results by using multi-ingredient wheat substitutes rather than one-ingredient wheat substitutes. These one-ingredient substitutes are provided for your convenience:

Possible single-ingredient substitutes for 1 cup of wheat flour include:

- ⅞ cup rice flour

- ⅞cup garbanzo bean (chick pea) flour

- ¾ cup potato starch

- 1⅓ cups ground rolled oats

- 1 cup tapioca flour

Multi-Ingredient Substitutes For Wheat Flour

Some cooks feel they get better results when they mix together a few different flours. Some multi-ingredient wheat flour substitution formulas are:

- 4 cups oat flour + 2 cups barley flour + 1 cup rice flour

- 1 cup rye flour + 1 cup potato flour

- 1 cup cornstarch + 2 cups rice flour + 2 cups soy flour + 3 cups potato starch flour

- 2 cups sweet rice flour + ⅔ cup potato flour + ⅓ cup tapioca flour (this combination often works very well)

Rice Flours

There are different types of rice flours available, and there are different suitable uses for each. Rice flour, also known as rice powder or rice starch, may be used interchangeably in recipes although brown rice flour has a nuttier flavor. The texture of rice flour can vary and will affect the consistency of the finished product, ranging from very light and soft to somewhat gritty in texture. You may need to make a few test recipes to determine what will give you the best results.

White Rice Flour: White rice flour is made from rice kernels with the hull and bran layers removed. It is a refined flour with a mild flavor that works well in most recipes. White rice flour can be used as a thickening agent for sauces and puddings as well as for making Asian noodles. It can be used in some baked goods, such as cakes, cookies, and dumplings, although it can be gritty in large quantities, so it's best used in combination with other flours.

Brown Rice Flour: Brown rice flour is made from whole grain rice. It has a slightly more robust flavor than white rice flour, and when used in baked goods, such as cakes and cookies, brown rice flour provides a grainy texture with a fine, dry crumb. Brown rice flour works well in bread recipes.

Sweet Rice Flour: Sweet glutinous rice flour, also known as Mochiko flour or mochi flour, is milled from mochi rice, a short-grained, glutinous rice common in Asia. Although called "glutinous flour" it does not contain gluten. It is often used to thicken sauces and food mixes, providing a strong bonding that can withstand refrigerator and freezer temperatures without separating. It is often used for breading foods prior to frying and for making traditional foods that require flour, such as desserts and baked goods, or rice dumplings referred to as Japanese mochi. Sweet rice flour can also be used as a 1:1 replacement for cake flour.

General Tips For Wheat-Free Cooking

- One of the down sides of wheat-free baking is that the recipes don't rise as much. Wheat-free flours often work best if the recipe is cooked for a longer period of time at a lower temperature than usual. Reduce your oven temperature by about 25 degrees, and you will find the finished product will be a little less flat. If you are not avoiding eggs, adding an extra egg to a gluten-free recipe will help the product rise a little more.

- If you are looking for a protein boost for your recipe, use equal portions of brown rice flour and chickpea flour to make a complete protein.

- Refrigerating dough for half an hour before baking may help improve the texture and flavor.

- Since many wheat-free foods will crumble, you may want to experiment with making foods with smaller surface areas, such as cupcakes instead of cakes.

Basic Recipe Substitutions For Corn Allergy

The following is a general guide to using ingredient substitutions for corn allergy. Please verify the ingredients and safety of any products named to ensure that it is safe for your child's unique allergy issues.

Substitutions For Corn Ingredients

Substituting for corn ingredients is generally fairly simple.

- **Corn Oil:** Substitute corn-free oil, such as soy oil, canola oil, sunflower oil, etc.

- **Baking Powder:** Substitute corn-free baking powder or 1 teaspoon baking soda + ½ teaspoon cream of tartar for each teaspoon of baking powder

- **Corn Starch:** See "Substitutes For Thickeners" [at the end of this chapter].

- **Corn Syrup:** Substitute 1 cup granulated sugar + ¼ cup water for 1 cup corn syrup

- **Powdered Sugar:** Grind 1 cup granulated sugar + 1 Tablespoon potato starch in a coffee grinder, blender, or food processor. Note: This does not turn out as fine as the "real thing," and grinding sugar in this way can burn out the motor of your appliance if it is run too long for this purpose.

- **Vanilla Extract:** Substitute corn-free vanilla extract (can be difficult to find) or make your own: Drop two vanilla beans into a small bottle of potato vodka; let sit for one to two months and then remove the beans.

Soy Substitutes For Cooking And Baking

The following is a general guide to using ingredient substitutions for soy allergy. Please verify the ingredients and safety of any products named to ensure that it is safe for your child's unique allergy issues.

Substitutes For Soy Oil

Soy oil can be substituted with another oil safe for the allergies you are managing. Canola oil has a mild flavor and is a good substitute for baked goods or desserts, while oils with a distinct flavor such as corn oil or olive oil can be substituted in savory dishes.

Substituting For Soy Margarines

Soy-free margarines can be substituted with real butter if you are not managing a milk allergy. For those needing a milk- and soy-free margarine (that is also free of soy oil and soy lecithin), the only options are Earth Balance Soy Free Natural Buttery Spread and Kosher for Passover margarines that are available in the early months of each year when makers of Kosher margarines reformulate their products to be free of legumes. At other times of year, the Kosher margarines will have soy in them, so read packaging carefully. Kosher for Passover margarines freeze well. If you purchase in bulk and double wrap, you can buy a supply that will last from one year to the next. Some Kosher web sites, such as www.kosher.com, may have Passover margarine available throughout the year. Be sure to verify the ingredients to make sure it is the Kosher for Passover version.

Substituting For Soy Sauce

Soy sauce in recipes generally serves the purpose of adding a salty flavor, so any substitute used should have a salty flavor to impart the same quality to a recipe. There is a chick pea-based miso available from South River Miso that works well.

Other options to try that will impart a unique flavor with a salty component are olive brine, umeboshi vinegar (also called ume plum vinegar) or balsamic vinegar plus a fair amount of salt.

Substituting For Teriyaki Sauce

Teriyaki sauce is another sauce for which there is no true replacement; however, two other options to try are a sweet and sour sauce if you can find one with ingredients safe for the allergies you are managing, or a combination of balsamic vinegar, orange juice, white or brown sugar, water, olive oil, and pepper.

Substituting For Soybean Paste (Miso)

For recipes calling for soybean paste, non-soy-based miso pastes are available that are made of chick peas and rice or azuki beans and rice from South River Miso.

Basic Recipe Substitutions For Thickeners

The following is a general guide to using ingredient substitutions for thickeners. Please verify the ingredients and safety of any products named to ensure that it is safe for your child's unique allergy issues.

Substitutes For Thickeners

To replace 1 Tablespoon wheat flour that is used as a thickener for sauces, gravies, and puddings, try one of the following:

- 1½ teaspoon arrowroot starch
- 1 Tablespoon cornstarch
- 1½ teaspoon tapioca starch

- 1½ teaspoon potato starch

- 2 teaspoons quick-cooking tapioca

- 1 teaspoon xanthan gum

Advantages and disadvantages of some of these thickeners are:

Arrowroot

- **Advantages:** Works well with cold acid fruits. Does not need to boil to thicken. Does not need to be cooked to remove the "raw" taste.

- **Disadvantages:** When used in a sauce that is served hot, it does not keep long and does not reheat well.

Cornstarch

- **Advantages:** Used for translucency. Recommended in high-acid fruit environments

- **Disadvantages:** Once they have gelatinized, over-beating or overcooking cornstarch-based sauces will cause them to thin. If the sugar level is too high, cornstarch will not thicken the mixture. Can have a raw taste if insufficiently cooked. Lumps can form if the cornstarch is not properly dissolved in cold liquid before it is mixed with the hot liquid.

Potato Starch

- **Advantages:** Requires less simmering than flour-based sauces. Has some translucency. Makes a more delicate sauce than flour.

- **Disadvantages:** Starts to lose thickening power at high temperatures. Hot sauces will not stand long, as it does not have much holding power.

Tapioca Starch

- **Advantages:** Works well in fillings that are to be frozen, as it does not break down like flour-based sauces do.

- **Disadvantages:** Will get "stringy" if boiled.

Part Six
If You Need More Information

Chapter 54

Resources For Allergy Information

Academy of Nutrition and Dietetics

120 South Riverside Plaza, Suite 2000
Chicago, IL 60606-6995
Toll-Free: 800-877-1600
Phone: 312-899-0040
Website: www.eatright.org
E-mail: amacmunn@eatright.org

AllergicChild.com

6660 Delmonico Drive, Suite D249
Colorado Springs, CO 80919
Website: www.allergicchild.com

Allergic Living Magazine

2100 Bloor Street West, Suite 6-168
Toronto, ON M6S 5A5
Canada
Toll-Free: 888-771-7747
Phone: 416-604-0110
Website: www.allergicliving.com
E-mail: info@allergicliving.com

Allergy and Asthma Information Association

295 The West Mall, Suite 118
Toronto, ON M9C 4Z4
Canada
Toll-Free: 800-611-7011 (Canada Only)
Phone: 416-621-4571
Fax: 416-621-5034
Website: www.aaia.ca
E-mail: admin@aaia.ca

Allergy and Asthma Network Mothers of Asthmatics

8201 Greenboro Drive, Suite 300
McLean, VA 22102
Toll-Free: 800-878-4403
Fax: 703-288-5271
Website: www.aanma.org

About This Chapter: Resources in this chapter were compiled from multiple sources deemed reliable. Inclusion does not constitute endorsement, and there is no implication associated with omission. All contact information was verified and updated in September 2012.

Allergy UK

Planwell House
LEFA Business Park
Edgington Way
Sidcup, Kent DA14 5BH
United Kingdom
Helpline: +13 22 619898
Fax: +13 22 470330
Website: www.allergyuk.org
E-mail: info@allergyuk.org

American Academy of Allergy, Asthma and Immunology

555 East Wells Street, Suite 1100
Milwaukee, WI 53202-3823
Phone: 414-272-6071
Website: www.aaaai.org
E-mail: info@aaaai.org

American Academy of Dermatology

P.O. Box 4014
Schaumburg, IL 60168
Toll-Free: 866-503-SKIN (866-503-7546)
Phone: 847-240-1280
Fax: 847-240-1859
Website: www.aad.org
E-mail: MRC@aad.org

American Academy of Otolaryngology-Head and Neck Surgery

1650 Diagonal Road
Alexandria, VA 22314-2857
Phone: 703-836-4444
Website: www.entnet.org

American Board of Allergy and Immunology

111 South Independence Mall East
Suite 701
Philadelphia, PA 19106
Toll-Free: 866-264-5568
Phone: 215-592-9466
Fax: 215-592-9411
Website: www.abai.org
E-mail: abai@abai.org

American Celiac Disease Alliance

2504 Duxbury Place
Alexandria, VA 22308
Phone: 703-622-3331
Website: www.americanceliac.org
E-mail: info@americanceliac.org

American College of Allergy, Asthma and Immunology

85 West Algonquin Road, Suite 550
Arlington Heights, IL 60005
Phone: 847-427-1200
Fax: 847-427-1294
Website: www.acaai.org
E-mail: mail@acaai.org

American Latex Allergy Association

P.O. Box 198
Slinger, WI 53086
Toll-Free: 888-972-5378
Phone: 262-677-9707
Website:
www.latexallergyresources.org
E-mail: alert@latexallergyresources.org

American Lung Association

1301 Pennsylvania Avenue NW
Suite 800
Washington, DC 20004
Toll-Free: 800-LUNGUSA
(800-586-4872)
Phone: 202-785-3355
Fax: 202-452-1805
Website: www.lungusa.org

American Osteopathic College of Allergy and Immunology

16128 East Kingstree Boulevard
Fountain Hills, AZ 85268
Phone: 480-585-1580
Fax: 480-585-1581

American Osteopathic College of Dermatology

1501 East Illinois Street
P.O. Box 7525
Kirksville, MO 63501
Toll-Free: 800-449-2623
Phone: 660-665-2184
Fax: 660-627-2623
Website: www.aocd.org
E-mail: info@AOCD.org

American Partnership for Eosinophilic Disorders

P.O. Box 29545
Atlanta, GA 30359
Phone: 713-493-7749
Website: www.apfed.org
E-mail: mail@apfed.org

American Rhinologic Society

P.O. Box 495
Warwick, NY 10990-0495
Phone: 845-988-1631
Fax: 845-986-1527
Website: www.american-rhinologic.org
E-mail: arsinfo@american-rhinologic.org

Anaphylaxis Canada

2005 Sheppard Avenue East, Suite 800
Toronto, ON M2J 5B4
Canada
Toll-Free: 866-785-5660
Phone: 416-785-5666
Toll-Free Fax: 888-872-6014
Fax: 416-785-0458
Website: http://www.anaphylaxis.org
E-mail: info@anaphylaxis.ca

Asthma and Allergy Foundation of America

8201 Corporate Drive
Suite 1000
Landover, MD 20785
Toll-Free: 800-7-ASTHMA
(800-727-8462)
Website: www.aafa.org
E-mail: info@aafa.org

Australasian Society of Clinical Immunology and Allergy

P.O. Box 450
Balgowlah NSW 2093
Australia
Website: http://www.allergy.org.au
E-mail: education@allergy.org.au

Canadian Lung Association

1750 Courtwood Crescent
Suite 300
Ottawa, ON K2C 2B5
Canada
Toll-Free: 888-566-5864 (Canada Only)
Phone: 613-569-6411
Fax: 613-569-8860
Website: http://www.lung.ca
E-mail: info@lung.ca

Celiac Disease Foundation

20350 Ventura Boulevard, Suite 240
Woodland Hills, CA 91364
Phone: 818-716-1513
Fax: 818-267-5577
Website: www.celiac.org
E-mail: cdf@celiac.org

Center for Food Safety and Applied Nutrition

Food and Drug Administration
5100 Paint Branch Parkway
College Park, MD 20740-3835
Toll-Free: 888-SAFEFOOD
(888-723-3366)
Website: http://www.fda.gov/food
E-mail: consumer@fda.gov

Environmental Protection Agency (EPA)

Ariel Rios Building
1200 Pennsylvania Avenue NW
Washington, DC 20460
Phone: 202-272-0167
TTY: 202-272-0165
Website: www.epa.gov

Food Allergy and Anaphylaxis Network

11781 Lee Jackson Highway, Suite 160
Fairfax, VA 22033-3309
Toll-Free: 800-929-4040
Phone: 703-691-3179
Fax: 703-691-2713
Websites: www.foodallergy.org;
www.fankids.org; www.faanteen.org
E-mail: kids@foodallergy.org

Food Allergy Initiative

515 Madison Avenue, Suite 1912
New York, NY 10022-5403
Toll-Free: 855-FAI-9604 (855-324-9604)
Fax: 917-338-5130
Website: www.faiusa.org
E-mail: info@faiusa.org

Food Allergy Research and Resource Program

Food Science and Technology
143 Food Industry Complex
University of Nebraska-Lincoln
Lincoln, NE 68583-0919
Phone: 402-472-2839
Fax: 402-472-5307
Website: www.farrp.org
E-mail: farrp@unl.edu

International Food Information Council

1100 Connecticut Avenue NW, Suite 430
Washington, DC 20036
Phone: 202-296-6540
Website: www.foodinsight.org
E-mail: info@foodinsight.org

Kids with Food Allergies

73 Old Dublin Pike, Suite 10, #163
Doylestown, PA 18901
Phone: 215-230-5394
Fax: 215-340-7674
Website: www.kidswithfoodallergies.org

National Center for Complementary and Alternative Medicine

P.O. 7923
Gaithersburg, MD 20898-7923
Toll-Free: 888-644-6226
Toll-Free TTY: 866-464-3615
Toll-Free Fax: 866-464-3616
Website: nccam.nih.gov
E-mail: info@nccam.nih.gov

National Center for Environmental Health

Centers for Disease Control and
Prevention
1600 Clifton Road NE, MS E-17
Atlanta, GA 30333
Toll-Free: 888-232-6789
Toll-Free: 800-CDC-INFO
(800-232-4636)
Toll-Free TTY: 888-232-6348
Phone: 404-639-2520
Fax: 404-693-2560
Website: http://www.cdc.gov/nceh
E-mail: cdcinfo@cdc.gov

National Coalition for Food-Safe Schools

Website: www.foodsafeschools.org
E-mail: info@foodsafeschools.org

National Digestive Diseases Information Clearinghouse

2 Information Way
Bethesda, MD 20892-3570
Toll-Free: 800-891-5389
Toll-Free TTY: 866–569–1162
Fax: 703-738-4929
Website: digestive.niddk.nih.gov
E-mail: nddic@info.niddk.nih.gov

National Eczema Association

4460 Redwood Highway
Suite 16D
San Rafael, CA 94903-1953
Toll-Free: 800-818-7546
Phone: 415-499-3474
Website: www.nationaleczema.org
E-mail: info@nationaleczema.org

National Heart, Lung, and Blood Institute

P.O. Box 30105
Bethesda, MD 20824-0105
Phone: 301-592-8573
TTY: 240-629-3255
Fax: 301-629-3246
Website: www.nhlbi.nih.gov
E-mail: nhlbiinfo@nhlbi.nih.gov

National Institute of Allergy and Infectious Diseases

6610 Rockledge Drive, MSC 6612
Bethesda, MD 20892-6612
Toll-Free: 866-284-4107
Toll-Free TDD: 800-877-8339
Phone: 301-496-5717
Fax: 301-402-3573
Website: www.niaid.nih.gov
E-mail: ocpostoffice@niaid.nih.gov

National Institute of Arthritis and Musculoskeletal and Skin Diseases

Information Clearinghouse
1 AMS Circle
Bethesda, MD 20892-3675
Toll-Free: 877-22-NIAMS
(877-226-4267)
Phone: 301-495-4484
TTY: 301–565–2966
Fax: 301-718-6366
Website: www.niams.nih.gov
E-mail: NIAMSinfo@mail.nih.gov

National Institute of Environmental Health Sciences

P.O. Box 12233, MD K3-16
Research Triangle Park, NC 27709-2233
Phone: 919-541-3345
Fax: 919-541-4395
Website: www.niehs.nih.gov
E-mail: webcenter@niehs.nih.gov

National Jewish Medical and Research Center

1400 Jackson Street
Denver, CO 80206
Toll-Free: 877-CALL-NJH
(877-225-5654)
Phone: 303-388-4461
Website: www.njc.org

Nemours Foundation/ KidsHealth

1600 Rockland Road
Wilmington, DE 19803
Phone: 302-651-4000
Website: www.kidshealth.org
E-mail: info@kidshealth.org

New Zealand Dermatological Society

P.O. Box 4431
Palmerston North
New Zealand
Phone: 06 357-1466
Fax: 06 357-1426
Website: www.dermnetnz.org

Pan American Allergy Society

1317 Wooded Knoll
San Antonio, TX 78258
Phone: 210-495-9853
Fax: 210-495-9852
Website: http://www.paas.org
E-mail: panamallergy@sbcglobal.net

PeanutAllergy.com

Website: www.peanutallergy.com
E-mail: info@peanutallergy.com

Pollen.com

c/o IMS Health Incorporated
1 IMS Drive
Plymouth Meeting, PA 19462
Phone: 610-834-0800
Website: www.pollen.com

U.S. Department of Agriculture (USDA)

1400 Independence Avenue SW
Washington, DC 20250
Phone: 202-720-2791
Website: www.usda.gov

U.S. Food and Drug Administration (FDA)

10903 New Hampshire Avenue
Silver Spring, MD 20993
Toll-Free: 888-INFO-FDA
(888-463-6332)
Website: www.fda.gov

Vickerstaff Health Services

2016 High Canada Place
Kamloops, BC V2E 2E3
Canada
Phone: 250-377-0945
Fax: 250-377-3248
Website: www.allergynutrition.com
E-mail: vickerstaffhs@allergynutrition.com

World Allergy Organization

555 East Wells Street, Suite 1100
Milwaukee, WI 53202-3823
Phone: 414-276-1791
Fax: 414-276-3349
Website: www.worldallergy.org
E-mail: info@worldallergy.org

Chapter 55

Finding Recipes If You Have Food Allergies

Online Recipe Resources For People With Food Allergies

BBC Gluten-Free Recipes
http://www.bbc.co.uk/food/diets/gluten_free

BBC Nut-Free Recipes
http://www.bbc.co.uk/food/diets/nut_free

Cook IT Allergy Free
http://www.cookitallergyfree.com

Eating with Food Allergies
http://www.eatingwithfoodallergies.com/allergyfreerecipes.html

Food Allergy and Anaphylaxis Network
http://www.foodallergy.org/recipes

Food Allergy Kitchen
http://www.foodallergykitchen.com

Kids with Food Allergies
http://www.kidswithfoodallergies.com

Living Without
http://www.livingwithout.com/topics/recipes.html

PeanutFree Recipes
http://www.peanutallergy.com/nut-free-recipes

About This Chapter: Resources in this chapter were compiled from multiple sources deemed reliable. This list is intended as a starting point only, and it is not comprehensive. Inclusion does not constitute endorsement and there is no implication associated with omission. All website information was verified and updated in September 2012.

Cookbooks For People With Food Allergies

Allergen-Free Baker's Handbook, by Cybele Pascal. Celestial Arts: 2009.

Allergy Cooking with Ease: The No Wheat, Milk, Eggs, Corn, and Soy Cookbook, Revised Edition, by Nicolette M. Dumke. Allergy Adapt: 2006.

Allergy Proof Recipes for Kids, by Leslie Hammond and Lynne Marie Rominger. Fair Winds Press, 2003.

Allergy Self-Help Cookbook, Revised Edition, by Marjorie Hurt Jones. Rodale Press: 2001.

Allergy-Free Cookbook, by Alice Sherwood. DK Publishing: 2009.

Allergy-Free Desserts, by Elizabeth Gordon. John Wiley and Sons: 2010.

Complete Food Allergy Cookbook: The Foods You've Always Loved Without the Ingredients You Can't Have, by Marilyn Gioannini. Crown Publishing: 1997.

Everything Food Allergy Cookbook, by Linda Larsen. Adams Media: 2008.

Food Allergy Cookbook, by Lucinda Bruce-Gardyne. Reader's Digest Association: 2008.

Food Allergy Mama's Baking Book, by Kelly Rudnicki. Agate Surrey: 2009.

Food Allergy News Cookbook, by Anne Munoz-Furlong. John Wiley and Sons: 1998.

Gluten-Free Cooking for Dummies, by Danna Korn and Connie Sarros. Wiley Publishing, 2008

Go Dairy Free, by Alisa Marie Fleming. Fleming Ink: 2008.

Kid-Friendly Food Allergy Cookbook, by Leslie Hammond and Lynne Marie Rominger. Fair Winds Press: 2004.

Milk-Free Kitchen: Living Well Without Diary Products, by Beth Kidder, Henry Holt and Co.: 1991.

Ultimate Allergy-Free Snack Cookbook, by Judi Zucker and Shari Zucker. Square One Publishers: 2012.

What's to Eat? The Milk-Free, Egg-Free, Nut-Free Food Allergy Cookbook, by Linda Marienhoff Coss. Plumtree Press: 2001.

Wheat-Free, Gluten-Free Cookbook for Kids and Busy Adults, Second Edition, by Connie Sarros, McGraw Hill, 2009.

Whole Foods Allergy Cookbook, Second Edition, by Cybele Pascal. Square One Publishers: 2005.

You Won't Believe It's Gluten-Free! 500 Delicious, Foolproof Recipes for Healthy Living, by Roben Ryberg. De Capo Press, 2008.

Index

Index

Page numbers that appear in *Italics* refer to tables or illustrations. Page numbers that have a small 'n' after the page number refer to information shown as Notes at the beginning of each chapter. Page numbers that appear in **Bold** refer to information contained in boxes on that page (except Notes information at the beginning of each chapter).

A

X, Z